Mental Illness and Learning Disability Since 1850

In the past three decades the history of mental illness and mental disability has provided scholars with a rich source of discussion and debate. Many of the asylums and residential homes established in the Victorian and Edwardian decades have been closed as policy-makers and practitioners have developed alternatives to institutional care. The abandonment of these institutions and the limits of provisions which have been made in 'the community' contributed to a public concern with the consequences of the policies pursued for those with a wide range of mental disorders. In particular, the historical responsibility of families, neighbourhoods and wider society for the care of their members has become a major theme in historical as well as contemporary enquiries.

This collection of essays provides an assessment of the policies and the practices devised to accommodate and manage a wide range of people with disabilities as well as mental illness. In contrast to some recent accounts, the authors emphasize the complexity of institutional systems, illustrating the influence of medical and legal personnel as well as family members in the care offered to those identified as needing protection and control. Class relationships, gender and regional variations emerge from these essays as significant factors which influenced the kind of provision made for those seen as suffering from a variety of disabling conditions and psychiatric illnesses.

A fresh, stimulating step forward in the history of institutional care, *Mental Illness and Learning Disability Since 1850* is undoubtedly an important resource for students and scholars of the history of medicine.

Pamela Dale is a Wellcome Fellow based in the Centre for Medical History at the University of Exeter. Her postgraduate work examined the implementation of the 1913 Mental Deficiency Act and she is currently working on a project exploring the relationship between health visitors and Medical Officers of Health. **Joseph Melling** is Reader in the History of Industrial Health and Welfare and Assistant Director of the Centre for Medical History at the University of Exeter. He has published widely on the history of asylums and psychiatry and is also researching occupational health and labour relations in British industry. *The Politics of Madness*, based on the Exminster project and co-authored with Bill Forsythe, will be published in 2006.

Routledge studies in the social history of medicine
Edited by Joseph Melling
University of Exeter
and
Anne Borsay
University of Wales, Swansea, UK.

The Society for the Social History of Medicine was founded in 1969, and exists to promote research into all aspects of the field, without regard to limitations of either time or place. In addition to this book series, the Society also organizes a regular programme of conferences, and publishes an internationally recognized journal, *Social History of Medicine*. The Society offers a range of benefits, including reduced-price admission to conferences and discounts on SSHM books, to its members. Individuals wishing to learn more about the Society are invited to contact the series editors through the publisher.

The Society took the decision to launch 'Studies in the Social History of Medicine', in association with Routledge, in 1989, in order to provide an outlet for some of the latest research in the field. Since that time, the series has expanded significantly under a number of series editors, and now includes both edited collections and monographs. Individuals wishing to submit proposals are invited to contact the series editors in the first instance.

1 **Nutrition in Britain**
  Science, scientists and politics in the twentieth century
  Edited by David F. Smith

2 **Migrants, Minorities and Health**
  Historical and contemporary studies
  Edited by Lara Marks and Michael Worboys

3 **From Idiocy to Mental Deficiency**
  Historical perspectives on people with learning disabilities
  Edited by David Wright and Anne Digby

4 **Midwives, Society and Childbirth**
  Debates and controversies in the modern period
  Edited by Hilary Marland and Anne Marie Rafferty

Mental Illness and Learning Disability Since 1850

Finding a place for mental disorder in the United Kingdom

Edited by
Pamela Dale and Joseph Melling

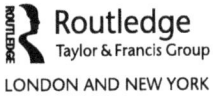

Routledge
Taylor & Francis Group

LONDON AND NEW YORK

First published 2006
by Routledge
2 Park Square, Milton Park, Abingdon, Oxon OX14 4RN

Simultaneously published in the USA and Canada
by Routledge
270 Madison Ave, New York, NY 10016

Routledge is an imprint of the Taylor & Francis Group, an informa business

© 2006 Pamela Dale and Joseph Melling

British Library Cataloguing in Publication Data
A catalogue record for this book is available from the British Library

Library of Congress Cataloging in Publication Data
A catalog record for this book has been requested

ISBN10: 0-415-36491-4 (hbk)
ISBN10: 0-203-01594-0 (ebk)

ISBN13: 978-0-415-36491-1 (hbk)
ISBN13: 978-0-203-01594-0 (ebk)

Contents

Illustrations

Contributors

Frank Crompton taught History at University College Worcester for approaching twenty-two years. He is the Historical Adviser to the George Marshall Medical Museum. His publications include *Workhouse Children* (Sutton, Stroud, 1997), and *An Audioguide to the George Marshall Medical Museum* (Acoustiguide, 2004).

Pamela Dale is a Wellcome Fellow based in the Centre for Medical History at the University of Exeter and is currently working on a project exploring the relationship between health visitors and Medical Officers of Health. Her chapter draws on postgraduate research, supported by the Exeter University Foundation and the AHRB, that examined the implementation of the Mental Deficiency Acts.

Matt Egan conducted his PhD on mental deficiency in late nineteenth and early twentieth century Scotland at the Centre for Medical History, University of Glasgow with funding from the ESRC. He currently works at the Medical Research Council Social and Public Health Sciences Unit, University of Glasgow where he is part of a programme evaluating the impacts of social policy on public health and health inequalities.

Vicky Long is a Research Assistant in the Centre for the History of Medicine at the University of Warwick. She is currently working on a Wellcome-funded project, the Politics and Practices of Health in Work in Britain, 1915–74. Her PhD thesis explored public representations of mental illness in nineteenth- and twentieth-century Britain and was funded by the AHRB.

Joseph Melling is Reader in the History of Industrial Health and Welfare and Assistant Director of the Centre for Medical History at the University of Exeter. He has published widely on the history of asylums and psychiatry and is also researching occupational health and labour relations in British industry. *The Politics of Madness*, based on the Exminster project and co-authored with Bill Forsythe, will be published in 2005–06.

Elaine Murphy is an academic psychiatrist and health services manager by background and an Honorary Senior Research Fellow at the Wellcome Centre for the History of Medicine at University College London. She is also an active crossbench life peer.

David Pearce is a practising psychiatrist working in Devon. He completed his MPhil on the operation of the 1930 Mental Treatment Act in local psychiatric hospitals at the University of Exeter in 2002 and is currently researching health services in Devon during the Second World War.

John Welshman was educated at the Universities of York and Oxford, and is Senior Lecturer in Public Health in the Institute for Health Research at Lancaster University. He has published widely on the history of public health and social policy in twentieth-century Britain, and is currently working on a history of care in the community.

Louise Westwood completed her Doctoral thesis 'Avoiding the Asylum: Pioneering Work in Mental Health Care' in 1999 and is now a lecturer in the History Department of the University of Sussex. She continues to work on the clinical practice of women psychiatrists in the first half of the twentieth century. This research has been supported by grants from the Wellcome Trust.

Acknowledgements

The origins of the present volume lie in a series of seminars organized by the Medical History Regional Research Network arranged between the Universities of Exeter and Southampton. They were sponsored by the Wellcome Trust and jointly organized by Joseph Melling and Bernard Harris. John Malin, Tony Woods and their colleagues at the Wellcome Trust were unfailingly helpful. Some of the present contributors also participated in a Society for the Social History of Medicine postgraduate workshop, organized by Pamela Dale and held at the University of Exeter in 2002. We wish to thank all of the contributors and commentators at these seminars and in particular Jonathan Barry, Mark Jackson, Gordon Langley, Catherine Quinn and Charles Webster. Our colleagues at the Centre for Medical History at the University of Exeter, including Mary Carter and Claire Keyte, have been generous in their support and Christi Hetzler worked tirelessly on the final draft of the manuscript. We owe a particular debt to Anne Borsay and Bernard Harris as the editors of the Routledge series who recommended the text to the publishers and to Terry Clague and Katherine Carpenter for their valuable assistance in the production of the volume. Finally, we wish to thank our families for their patience and kindness. In particular Joseph Melling would like to thank his son, Ross Leslie Sproule, for his enthusiasm and intelligent comments on the subject.

1 The politics of mental welfare

Fresh perspectives on the history of institutional care for the mentally ill and disabled

Pamela Dale and Joseph Melling

Introduction

Scholars continue to be troubled by the history of institutional care. The spread of national models of welfare provision and the rhetoric of the 'welfare state' during the middle decades of the twentieth century appeared to have relatively little impact on the provision of services for those considered mentally unwell or disabled. Yet it was these amenities which bore the brunt of the subsequent assault on state-centred medical institutions by intellectuals who criticized the extent to which the large mental hospitals served the interests of the professional elite who managed the patient population and upheld an unequal social order in which the deviant were consigned to the custody of probation officers, social workers and psychiatric nurses.[1] By the 1970s there were a number of serious challenges to the sympathetic account of the growth of psychiatry and the evolution of institutional care from the Hanoverian and Victorian asylum to the modern mental hospital which scholars such as Kathleen Jones had offered.[2] Critical of such benign visions of the progress of institutional care as an exercise in naive optimism, more radical historians also attempted general if not global models of psychiatric advance and institution-building.[3]

More detailed recent research has led to important modifications of the grander narratives of institutional provision, grounded as they often were on distinctive British and North American experience during the nineteenth century. Elegant general models have been found wanting as different actors come into view, striving for particular goals and reaching a specific accommodation in regard to reform settlements. At the same time, the sheer volume of fresh research on different countries has encouraged a stronger international dimension and attempts at comparative analysis of national initiatives in providing services for those seen as mentally unwell or defective. In a recent collection of national case studies, the editors noted the uneven pace of asylum building as modernizing regimes alternated between promoting and abandoning such projects according to political fashion. Elsewhere they appear to favour a greater emphasis on understanding patterns of provision in terms of the demand created by demographic shocks to the family household and the pathological or behavioural characteristics of the host population.[4]

Similar tensions are apparent within much of the most important recent research on the history of institutional care as researchers attempt to assess the influence of different agents and the political structures within which they acted. Scull's early research emphasized the absolute and relative growth in the number of pauper lunatics identified in the English population from little more than 2,000 in 1807 to more than 86,000 in 1890, equivalent to at least a tenfold increase in the numbers of people certified as insane within the general population.[5] Contemporaries were well aware of the Lunacy Commission's claims that much of this expansion in the numbers held in the asylum and related institutions was due to increasing longevity of long-stay patients, though there remained formidable evidence of a disproportionate and unexplained rise in Ireland as well as England, Wales and Scotland which political critics of the Commission were anxious to publicize.[6] A similar if distinct pattern may be detected in the numbers recorded as suffering from mental deficiency in the late nineteenth and early twentieth centuries.[7] Explanations for the rising numbers classified as insane and/or mentally defective have usually discarded the models of social control and 'total institutions' more popular in the third quarter of the twentieth century, in favour of an institutional complex of regulation.[8] Garland's analysis of the 'penal-welfare system' remains an influential approach, interpreting the evolution of the asylum within a network of controls which portrayed the institution in relation to the growth of the workhouse and the prison, fashioning a heterogeneous population of inmates and monitoring distinct forms of deviant behaviour.[9] Arieno's valuable survey of the broader literature on asylum provision draws attention away from regulation in noting the significance of stress created by poverty and deprivation as well as the concern of elites and legislators to ameliorate such conditions while selecting those most capable of sustaining a productive lifestyle.[10]

Interpretations of the origins and social function of the asylum continue to debate questions of class, and more particularly gender, within the broader discussion of the impact of poverty on admissions to such institutions. Recent research continues to cast doubt on earlier feminist interpretations since evidence from a range of national studies suggests that men as well as women were admitted in roughly proportionate terms, though some variations in diagnosis and treatment are also evident.[11] There is less evidence of the care of both women and men within the boundaries of the asylum, research on the twentieth century indicating that in some instances males rather than females may have received more brutal as well as innovative therapies depending on gendered assumptions about resistance and the suitability of subjects for experiment.[12] The experience of mental deficiency institutions suggests those boys capable of being trained, rather than girls, were seen as the fittest subjects for the idiot asylums established during the nineteenth century.[13] Voluntary initiatives to cater for adult female 'defectives' in the twentieth century reflected the greater concern of the British state with males who were seen as having a greater potential for deviant and criminal behaviour.

Fresh directions and debates

Contrasting interpretations of the structure and function of asylum provision since the nineteenth century have drawn attention, therefore, not only to the different social constituencies which sought to shape and utilize the institutions created in this period, but also the changing concepts of governance and expertise which informed the design and administration of these therapeutic communities. Recent research has stressed the uneven influence of ideology and intellectual culture on specific programmes of legislative change.[14] Bartlett argued that the 1845 lunacy laws were the outcome of inconclusive battles between traditionalists and innovators, while Macnicol and Thomson have each suggested that the Mental Deficiency legislation of 1913 was the unintended consequence of similar battles between intellectual and political adversaries.[15] Earlier scholarship which privileged the growth of empire and imperial defence in schemes to promote national efficiency and social discipline by means of welfare reforms is revisited in Porter's claim that the comparative history of asylum building indicates the concern of metropolitan and colonial states to institutionalize racial, ethnic and other minorities.[16] The language of imperial dominance and eugenic selection finds an echo in discussions of 'colonies' for mental defectives during the early years of the twentieth century, though research on African asylums as well as those within the United Kingdom (including Ireland) registers the remarkable diversity and uneven development in both policies and practices between states.[17]

The interplay between ideas, political agency and institutional reform is apparent in the attempts made by medical scientists to discriminate between insanity and mental deficiency in the Victorian and Edwardian years. During the 1870s there was a renewed interest in the accurate classification of institutional populations, including those lodged in different kinds of asylum. Earlier attempts to distinguish between the lunatic as furiously insane compared to the more passive feeble-minded individual were clearly inadequate, since they depended on a shifting conception of dangerousness. Jackson's study of the period noted the significance of legal definition, the continuing importance of lay opinion and a limited evidence of medical imperialism in provisions made for the mentally deficient child.[18] Thomson similarly emphasized the long history of legal controls over idiots from the thirteenth century, while the history of Bethlem completed by Andrews and others stressed both the well-established distinction between idiocy and lunacy and the tendency for institutional practices to obscure this legal boundary.[19] Bethlem experienced a problem in the early modern period which is often associated with 'chronic' patients in a much later era of asylum provision: namely, the difficulties encountered in discharging idiots from care once they had been admitted.

The growing recognition among asylum historians of the importance of legal as well as medical expertise in framing provisions for those considered insane and mentally defective may also be extended to a consideration of the importance of court cases which drew upon medical expertise.[20] As Scull noted, the asylum doctors recognized that their formidable authority lay in the institutional control of a growing inmate population rather than the professional expertise of psychiatry and even within the institution their power was circumscribed by legal regulations and supervision. Threats of legal action were sometimes made against such institutions by people of modest as well as substantial means.[21] In other instances, medical personnel not only came into conflict with legal experts within the judicial system but could clash with disciplinary regimes in other areas of state power. Even within the closed world of British prisons, doctors could assume the role of the inmates' advocate rather than simply associating with the penal goals of the authorities.[22] Prominent asylum superintendents could sustain their vision of institutional leadership only with the tacit support of the governors, a point sometimes overlooked in studies which construct a chronology in terms of medical personnel.[23] Consideration of the neglected role of the fee-paying asylums, as well as the careers of the most eminent of the Victorian alienists, indicates that the mad doctors were able to capitalize on their reputations by providing private care for the wealthy rather than by demonstrating a capacity to cure large numbers of poorer inmates.[24]

An appreciation of the limits of the intellectual and legal authority which could be claimed by asylum psychiatrists during the nineteenth century has contributed to a broader debate in regard to the effective boundaries of these institutions and the capacity of different groups to influence their policies and practices. It is now commonplace for historians to place asylum provision within a larger, mixed economy of care, moderating earlier perspectives of a single dominant institution.[25] A number of historians have sought to frame questions of agency and of gender within a discussion of the key role of family households in the admission and discharge processes. Studies which emphasize the importance of kinship bonds and the life cycle of the nuclear family include Prestwich's account of Parisian asylum admissions and Wright's analysis of Victorian idiot and lunatic asylums.[26] Complementing Bartlett's argument on the central role of Poor Law authorities in the application and administration of English lunacy laws, these accounts offer support for earlier accounts of sympathetic kinship while criticizing the class-based interpretation of asylum provision developed by Scull and others.

The significance of the Poor Law and the role of families in the transmission of people to and from the asylum feature in a number of the chapters which follow. In an earlier assessment, Bartlett suggests alternative interpretations of the introduction of new lunacy legislation in England during 1845, including a concern to appeal to the 'deserving poor' whose members needed support and the demands of other reformers that the asylums should embody an earlier tradition of care. He concludes that it was the capacity of the asylum to appeal to all shades of opinion rather than fulfilling the aims of any particular ideological camp which explained its enduring success.[27] This analysis usefully draws attention to the impact of Poor Law reform on the lunacy debate in the decade after 1834, though it may be argued that the ideological strands described by Bartlett were less distinctive than he implies and the political struggles within the Poor Law unions and with the emerging asylum authorities remained intense in the years following 1845.[28] Many local Guardians and even the Poor Law Board continued to resist the Lunacy Commission's directive that workhouse inmates be released to the care of the county asylums, while boroughs should build their own specialist institutions for the care of the insane and the mentally defective. The responsibilities accorded to the Poor Law authorities under the lunacy legislation can be explained, in part at least, by their strategic role as the established and most important tax-raising body in local government and the only agency with the experience and staffing to support the magistracy in the administration of asylum committals. They also enjoyed considerable autonomy from the London authorities. The relative cost of care remained an important theme in the attitudes of local Poor Law Guardians and ratepayers to usage of specialist asylums, particularly before the important reforms of local government in 1888. The detention of the less hopeful 'chronic' cases in workhouse accommodation was permitted if not encouraged by legislative changes to the lunacy laws in 1862. The unions came under further pressure to improve their services in the 1880s and by 1900 the long-term care of 'idiots' and 'imbeciles' was concentrated in some areas within specialized workhouses.

In the century after 1845, workhouse provision appears to have been in consistent evolution as sites were dedicated to caring for groups such as adult females diagnosed with mental deficiencies, sometimes alongside illegitimate children.[29] Elaine Murphy's study of Poor Law policy and lunacy provision in Victorian London (Chapter 2) draws out the distinctive patterns and continuities of provision in the Metropolis, amidst continuing debates on policy and practice during this period.[30] There is evidence of diverse and distinctive practices among Poor Law authorities dealing with the complex problem of caring for these groups until the early years of the twentieth century, when the passage of the Mental Deficiency Act altered the terms on which 'idiots' and 'imbeciles' could be accommodated. The Poor Law unions in London as well as Devon, for example, became significant clients of the large Starcross Idiot Asylum discussed in

Dale's chapter (Chapter 8), though after 1914 the bulk of admissions were sent by Devon's county and borough authorities.[31] The impression made by changes in the administrative boundaries as well as the scope of local government, including the major reforms of 1888 and 1929, is rarely discussed in the historical literature on institutional care, though such reforms were fundamental to shifts in Poor Law responsibilities.

The continuing influence of the Poor Law was also registered in the responsibility of Guardians for enforcing the legal duties of families, though the capacity of local authorities to police these obligations were considerably extended by the government reforms and legislative changes seen in the years 1888–1914. In his Earlswood study, Wright emphasized the key role of families in calculating the institutional committal of children while considering the needs of siblings and the household.[32] Prestwich similarly regards the later introduction of the category of voluntary patient in asylum admissions as confirming a fresh relationship between doctors and families rather than physicians and individual patients, with compulsory admissions imposed on those households and kin who were reluctant to cooperate in decisions on the care of patients.[33] Illuminating the role of kinship groups in institutional care offers a useful corrective to earlier interpretations which often privileged class and gender as primary factors in asylum admissions. Evidence drawn from Poor Law and other sources points to the need for caution in assuming that families exercised either a benign or consistent influence in decisions on care. In some instances children and adults were rescued from abuse and neglect where relatives were unable or unwilling to cope with them. Relieving Officers of the Poor Law were capable not only of discussing with relatives the terms on which a person might be admitted to the workhouse or sent to an asylum, but also of actively pursuing reluctant families to enforce contributions to the maintenance of a family member when admitted to the asylum.[34] The role of relatives varied according to the legal requirements for the protection of those seen as suffering from different forms of mental disorder or deficiency. The power of families also depended on their economic resources and the means by which an institution was funded. Distinctions in legal provisions governing the entry and exit of patients to asylums financed from Poor Law rates, private fees and charitable trusts remained even after the important Lunacy Act of 1890 brought the committal procedures for private patients closer to those already in place for pauper inmates. The different economic and legal power available to families of fee-paying versus pauper patients in the control over admissions and discharges is traced in Melling's chapter (Chapter 4), while Pearce's analysis of the impact of the Mental Treatment Act of 1930 documents the efforts of more affluent families to influence the treatment offered to the new grades of voluntary and temporary patients in the public mental hospital (Chapter 6).

Another contrast may be drawn in the provision of specialist pauper asylums for adults and the absence of a universal rate-aided institution for 'idiot' children before 1913.[35] Compulsory elementary education was introduced in 1870–75, while the educational training of mentally deficient children was left to voluntary initiatives such as those which resulted in asylums at Earlswood and Starcross. County and borough lunatic asylums displayed great reluctance to accept children and young persons as inmates even when doctors were willing to certify them as lunatics. Substantial numbers found their way into the workhouse, and (in later life) asylums and prisons, as well as specialist facilities. Asylums appear to have been particularly cautious when accepting children without clear kinship ties, given the clear difficulties in planning a route for subsequent discharge, which posed peculiar problems for vulnerable females who might be discharged on to the open highway if the Poor Law authorities refused to accept responsibility for them.[36] The resurgence of political interest in the care of such children arose in the late Victorian and Edwardian years as the British state sought to address a variety of issues affecting the family household, including poverty arising from unemployment, sickness and old age, as well as the risks of children turning to crime and vice.[37] The protection of the family was frequently emphasized by reformers, though central and local authorities appear to have interpreted the role of the family in restricted ways. Dale's chapter on the care of mentally defective children in the interwar period (Chapter 8) shows many people were taken into institutional care on the death or serious illness of the main carer, often with little obvious effort being made to find a substitute among the wider kinship group.[38] The policies pursued by different local authorities in south west England betrayed a suspicion that more distant relatives and employers could not be readily trusted with the care of vulnerable individuals.[39] Egan's chapter on Scotland (Chapter 7) suggests parental concerns were marginalized as doctors and teachers expanded the definition of defectiveness to encompass ever more pupils despite the stigmatizing effect this had on children and families. The increase in numbers, real or statistical, certainly fuelled contemporary concerns about mental deficiency but Egan makes it clear that the counting exercise did not necessarily have an immediate and discernible impact, beneficial or detrimental, on individuals and most 'defectives' continued to live at home as a matter of policy. Elsewhere, the concern of Plymouth City councillors to enforce what they perceived as family responsibilities in regard to people perceived as suffering from mental deficiency again underlines the point that the duties of the family was a normative standard pursued by political advocates as well as the expression of personal sentiment.[40]

Recent studies in the social history of insanity and mental deficiency have attributed substantial agency to the nuclear family in determining the part played by the asylum in the care of close relatives, while the influence of class and gender relationships in shaping the pattern of admissions and discharges have been the subject of reappraisal and revision.[41] Less attention has been devoted to the ages of those admitted to institutional care, their marital status and their changing role within different kinds of household. While children were rarely seen in the lunatic asylums, a substantial majority of admissions were people in their mature adult life who were usually discharged within a few years of arrival.[42] Older people do not appear to have been admitted in disproportionate numbers, though they more often remained in the asylum until their death. The patient population of the Victorian and Edwardian asylum was clearly ageing as a result of an accumulation of longer-stay residents who claimed an increasing proportion of beds even as these institutions expanded to admit fresh cases. There were clear variations not only in the gender composition of these older residents, females surviving the asylum better than males and frequently living to an advanced age within its walls, but also in the marital status of those arriving and remaining.[43] Unmarried women and men were much more likely to be sent to an asylum and mental hospital than their married counterparts, while wives were generally more likely to be discharged alive than either husbands or spinsters. This appears to be as true of older and younger females and to married women with no or few children at home as of women who left behind a growing family. The profile of female educationalists discussed in Melling's chapter (Chapter 4) provides a case study of women who were mostly unmarried on entry to the asylum, though again noticeable differences may be discovered in a comparison of public and fee-paying establishments in regard to the status of the females admitted and their prospects for discharge. In this instance a relationship to a sister or sister-in-law often appeared to be more important to the unmarried woman admitted than connections to parents or brothers, even though far more teachers and governesses in the general population lived in their parents' family home than with their sisters.

The age of patients also seems important for an understanding of the distinct ways in which those classified as mental defectives were identified and treated, since many of those listed as 'idiotic' and 'imbecilic' in adult life were not institutionalized in asylums before 1914 but could be found in prisons, workhouses, family households and even in gainful employment or married.[44] Research into admissions to both lunatic and idiot asylums reveals the extent to which such institutions participated, at different periods, in a process of selection and discrimination as to those considered most eligible to benefit from their services. Transfers of people between institutions were driven not only by the concern of Poor Law unions, local authorities, fee-paying families and others to use their market place resources most efficiently, but also by concerns to attract individuals who met the criteria of the institutions' managers. Following legislative reforms to lunacy legislation in 1862, 1890 and 1930, asylums such as that at Exminster followed the prompting of the Lunacy Commission and Board of Control in seeking to improve their therapeutic capacity by attracting individuals whose mental illness was thought to be recent rather than 'chronic', removing the latter to workhouses in the mid-Victorian years and targeting the most promising cases for the newer treatments developed in the interwar period, as chapters by Murphy and Pearce show (Chapters 2 and 6). Idiot asylums such as Starcross similarly resisted the growing pressures from the Guardians and local authorities to accept growing numbers of intractable, epileptic and older, chronic patients from the late nineteenth century.[45]

Some county councils resorted to the opportunities presented by the abolition of the Poor Law under the 1929 Local Government Act to convert former workhouses into accommodation for more difficult and chronic cases, though the problems posed by the minority of patients considered dangerous was reflected in the court cases recorded in the interwar years.[46] The role of the courts and the legal system more generally deserves much greater attention from historians of mental illness. Jackson's valuable research on mental deficiency has revealed the importance of legal and lay knowledge, as distinct from medical understanding, in defining the rights and responsibilities of the state towards those individuals considered defective in the nineteenth and twentieth centuries.[47] Studies of asylum care in other countries have frequently noted the importance of police surveillance and legal action in prompting the committal of individuals to institutions as family control broke down.[48] The experience of Starcross again suggests that such establishments adapted to the changing market place of institutional care in the mid-twentieth century by promoting itself as an institution capable of addressing the problem of dangerous and criminal behaviour, ultimately developing a forensic unit with expertise in psychopathic disorders.[49] The theme of dangerousness remained an important issue by which institutions sought to discriminate in favour of the patient groups which their directors considered offered the best prospect of effective development for the establishment and its staff, enabling them to serve their clients rather than merely containing them. Nor was dangerousness the only criterion applied as institutions sought to select out those they considered unsuitable. In the early and middle decades of the twentieth century some mental hospitals expressed concern that the lack of foresight displayed by those suffering mental deficiency was not a condition of mental disturbance which could be effectively treated by psychiatrists and such patients should be returned to their previous institution.[50]

Such an emphasis on non-medical opinion and influence also draws attention to the number of social actors who were involved in the committal, care and release of those identified as insane or defective. We have noted the role of established landed elites and borough notables in the movements to establish both the statutory asylums and the voluntary institutions such as Starcross, including leadership of the magistracy, Poor Law unions, county councils and parliamentary representation. The concerns of the magistracy to uphold public order as well as the terms of lunacy legislation were frequently raised when members of the public were outraged at indecent behaviour or alerted by police constables who discovered insane people 'wandering at large', or those who appeared to be not under 'proper care and control'. The decision to certify and commit such persons might bring the responsible authorities into conflict with the wishes of families, rather than respond to the expressed needs of the kinship household.[51] In considering lay versus scientific and professional opinion, it is worth stressing that the 'laity' of civil society included religious figures whose importance in the committal process was recognized in early legislative provision for Anglican clergymen and Poor Law Relieving Officers to complete a committal order for pauper lunatics where a magistrate was unavailable.[52] Evangelical Christians also assumed a leading place in campaigns for lunacy reform and in founding philanthropic establishments while local clergy frequently figured in the evidence provided to doctors certifying insanity as well as negotiating the entry of children to idiot asylums. In assuming a welfare role previously undertaken by clergy and charitable groups, secular personnel such as the voluntary and local authority social workers discussed in chapters by Dale and Long (Chapters 8 and 9), sought to provide moral guidance and protection as well as material assistance to families which they perceived as distressed or failing. The lay experience as well as specialized knowledge claimed by such personnel leads into Dale's discussion of the 'lay professional'.

By the mid-twentieth century a professional identity was forming among a group of social workers who claimed psychiatric expertise, foreshadowing the expansion of services which were associated with ideas of 'community' provision. Welshman's chapter on hostel development (Chapter 10) suggests that provisions beyond the walls of the asylum remained institutional facilities while claiming to serve the needs of individuals and families within the boundaries of a neighbourhood. He persuasively argues that life inside these less traditional facilities needs to be a priority for future work.[53] Studies of earlier asylums indicate that smaller-scale villa and cottage accommodation was well developed in the Victorian decades, providing a transition from secure facilities to release on a trial or probationary period, while Thomson argues that by the early years of the twentieth century the villa system became a basic model of care within asylums designed for mentally defective people.[54] Such evidence cautions against drawing too sharp a contrast between the large institution and alternative models of personal care, still less between the closed regime of the asylum psychiatrist and the domain of the Medical Officer of Health and the general practitioner as well as the family household or the kinship neighbourhood. For another conduit of 'community' information on the predicament of those who appeared to be suffering mental disorder were friends and neighbours who lived in the proximity, including the landladies and employers who witnessed erratic behaviour among the unmarried domestic employees who figured fairly prominently in the ranks of those committed to Victorian and Edwardian institutions.

The influence of work and employment in shaping attitudes towards the mentally disordered and deficient, as well as in the arrangement of institutional therapy, is a theme shared by a number of the chapters which follow. Scull's earlier argument that we should place the rise of the asylum within the context of the capitalist transformation of British society during the eighteenth and nineteenth centuries may require refinement, though the significance of market valuations of individual labouring capacities and the stress which was laid on a person's capacity to maintain a viable household deserve serious consideration. Chapters by Dale, Long and Pearce (Chapters 8, 9 and 6) all suggest the importance of the broader economic climate of the interwar years in colouring the terms in which occupational therapy and the employment capacities of asylum patients were discussed. Useful employment within the institution was a notable feature of the therapeutic regime of the Victorian asylum from its earliest days, while admissions to the idiots asylum were made on the assumption that educational training was possible and such individuals were later placed in employment as agricultural workers, domestic servants and so forth. The rather different expectations placed on those resident in the fee-paying asylum and the concern that females in particular should be re-educated where necessary in the rules of social etiquette and civilized discourse reveals some of the underlying assumptions regarding class and gender. Ideas of privacy and delicacy which led Victorian medical writers to advocate the treatment of the affluent patient in the private house of a physician or small asylum, continued to inform attitudes to therapeutic practices well into the twentieth century, as Pearce's chapter on the treatment of voluntary patients also indicates.[55]

The interest shown in recent work in the role of the Poor Law in the application of mental health legislation from the 1830s until the 1920s occasionally obscures the diverse social character of those entering rate-aided institutions in these decades. Significant numbers of those considered mentally defective were housed in the workhouse before, or after, admission to idiot and lunatic asylums, though a large majority of those certified as insane were far from destitute and came from self-sufficient households with the means to sustain a respectable existence. Not only were skilled artisans, small trades-people, farmers, educationalists and salaried employees represented but the Poor Law authorities pursued many such families for a contribution to their upkeep in the public asylum.[56] Those entering fee-paying asylums were generally of a higher economic and social status than their counterparts in the county and borough institutions, though the different establishments shared occupational groups in the mixed economy of Victorian care. The introduction of voluntary and temporary grades of patient after the 1930 Mental Treatment Act allowed, as Pearce shows, greater numbers of salaried and lower middle class family members to utilize such public institutions. Similar patterns are evident in the social profile of relatives, usually parents, of those who gained places in the facilities designed for the mentally defective, as well as in the distinctive regimes of care and training offered to the inmates of such establishments.

The new research represented in this collection suggests that we should consider the committal of people to institutional care as the outcome of a transaction which involved a number of distinct agents. Recent scholarship has also attempted to reappraise the value of medical science in the identification of insanity and mental deficiency, some scholars calling for more serious attention to be given to the robust diagnostic categories, with the prospect of establishing continuity between historical and modern understanding of the patient's condition.[57] Such arguments draw our attention to the significant number of historical patients whose insanity was attributed to physical illnesses, bodily changes and similar circumstances which the modern psychiatrist may readily associate with the symptoms of mental illness described. It is also evident that many medical personnel involved with these patients did not possess psychiatric training or expertise and that the treatments offered in the nineteenth and much of the twentieth centuries rarely involved intensive supervision by qualified psychiatrists. Historians frequently note the low status and poor remuneration of the physicians employed by the Poor Law unions to certify individuals, though it is remarkable how resilient were the diagnoses and especially the 'facts of insanity' they reported, as these were faithfully entered into the legal and institutional record.[58] It is also noticeable that in a substantial number of cases the causes of insanity were said to be unknown or indefinite while the diagnoses remained generalized where they were not commonplace descriptions.[59]

The Asylum Medical Officers were responsible for the care of those institutionalized, though from the early days the Superintendents of the asylum were absorbed in complex tasks of personnel and estate management, as well as meeting the political concerns of the magistrates, notables and others who formally governed these large establishments. Idiot asylums might be directed by lay personnel as well as being governed by a traditional elite, showing how limited was the 'medicalization' of such services before the 1930s.[60] The political struggles which occurred within such asylums as well as between institutions and local authorities provide a context in which to read the continuing debates over the boundaries and borderlands of mental health and mental deficiency in the late nineteenth and early twentieth centuries. Concerns in regard to family welfare and social class also informed debates about appropriate treatment and the discharge of patients from care, as the asylum authorities sought to monitor the social circumstances in which vulnerable individuals might be placed. The vigorous exchanges which were seen in the Victorian and Edwardian years in discussions of heredity, eugenics and mental weakness shifted towards a concern with the domestic environment by the 1920s and an increasing tendency for commentators to argue that patients with mental defects might also suffer mental illnesses such as depression when confronted by difficult or undemanding home lives. Voluntary social workers appear to have been particularly involved in these efforts to identify the problematic family background, reformulating the familiar Victorian distinction between the respectable and the residuum and anticipating later discourses on the 'problem family'.[61] Such volunteers provided an important bridge between lay understanding and a fresh professional perspective on the dysfunctional family. It was suggested that excessive care for the child in the attentive home could lead to a weakening of their mental resolve while the poorest groups were frequently viewed as inadequate individuals whose low mental capacity and weak social skills were transferred to their children.[62] Such claims may be compared to the conclusions reached by local physicians that petty criminals were suffering from a form of 'moral imbecility' which qualified them as mental defectives for asylum care, while the more threatening individuals were sent to the secure hospital at Rampton.[63]

The continuing influence exercised by a range of medical and lay actors at local level alerts us to the importance of understanding institutional and intellectual change within a wider context of political accountability as well as class and gender preferences. In the early years of the twentieth century psychiatrists as well as social reformers and voluntary activists became more concerned with the lower middle and middle classes as well as the respectable working class families which faced hardship and the stress of managing domestic budgets. The limited asylum provision for those liable to mental strain was apparent in the Victorian years and by the early twentieth century the vulnerability of non-manual employees to what was increasing termed neuroses, figured in debates which culminated in the passage of the Mental Treatment Act of 1930. Westwood's chapter on female psychiatrists (Chapter 5) demonstrates the contribution which professional women made to this reappraisal of earlier models of psychiatric diagnosis, as well as the limitations placed on their own career development in this period. It is possible to interpret the growing medical control over the services for mentally deficient children as the outcome of a strategic alliance between social workers and medical practitioners to undermine the lay expertise which was embodied in the early management of the idiot asylum. Yet the emphasis on training and employment rather than medical treatment persisted and lay patronage and control was not finally broken in some institutions until the 1940s when as Welshman suggests (Chapter 10) new loci of care were presenting different opportunities for lay involvement.

The final theme in the chapters presented here is the importance of understanding the internal life of the asylum, and its successors, and the personal experiences of the patients who entered such places. Recent debates on the growth and development of the asylum have been primarily concerned to explain its historical function in terms of the uses made of these institutions by distinctive social groups who possessed distinct cultural, ethnic and kinship identities. Detailed analysis is now available of admissions and discharges, including the age, marital status, demographic mobility and ethnic origins of those committed and released. Less attention has been devoted to the structure and quality of the institutional regime which guided the lives of the inmates who spent varying amounts of time within its walls. A growing recognition that the asylum became and remained a contested site for political, professional and personal interests does not demonstrate its responsiveness to patients or their relatives but rather points to the need to understand the variety of calculations which contributed to the legal transactions which committed and released individuals from custodial care. The admission documents formed a key stage in the internal procedures of examination, diagnosis and classification which Crompton's study (Chapter 3) of the Worcester Asylum considers in some detail. In common with many similar institutions, the Worcester City and County Pauper Lunatic Asylum at Powick was absorbed in its early years in receiving substantial numbers of 'chronic' individuals, including those termed idiots and imbeciles, who had often languished in workhouses and private dwellings for many years prior to the foundation of these new facilities. Crompton's analysis makes the point raised in a number of chapters that the practical labour of caring for those considered mentally unwell and disabled fell on the shoulders of employees and voluntary workers with little or no medical training. The language of classification and the everyday management of people within such institutions was more often common sense than scientific and the therapeutic regime continued to consist largely in the judicious separation, segregation and rehabilitation of individuals to different spaces within the buildings and grounds of the asylum, progressing towards probationary periods of leave with family or staff members, rather than in the medical interventions which became more common at the beginning of the twentieth century. The pressures of managing large, often crowded, premises which housed hundreds or even thousands of inmates with a tiny medical staff and one attendant for every ten or twelve patients in public asylums, ensured that personal treatment was necessarily limited.

Retrieving the 'patient experience' from the surviving documentation and personal records available to historians has not proved an easy task, though later survivor testimonies have provided an important resource for researchers into twentieth century care. Personal accounts sometimes confirm the impression that the asylum presented a dark alternative to life in a supportive household or local community, offering a bleak space where the most marginal and vulnerable groups were most likely to enter and to suffer abuse when in residence, though researchers have also stressed the beneficial aspects of the asylum as an integrated community where the confused and neglected were offered friendship as well as medical attention.[64] In the longer perspective of asylum building, expansion, contraction and closure which characterized institutional care in the century and a half since the Lunacy Acts of 1845, it can be seen that different narratives of abuse and refuge have contributed to a wider struggle over the scope and limits of state control. The investigations into scandalous neglect or abuse launched by the Lunacy Commissioners and the Boards of Control which regulated the various asylums and workhouse accommodation before 1930 frequently provided a cue for innovations which were contemplated by reformers, while the reconstruction of health care in 1948 had relatively little impact on those served by mental hospitals and psychiatric services. Within a decade the changing priorities of policy-makers and the opportunities presented by pharmacological treatment of mental illnesses was registered in radical responses to evidence of neglect within the institutions which had served as the mainstay of treatment since the early Victorian years. Close reading of case notes provides various insights into the individual experiences of the regimes which prevailed within such institutions, though a careful interpretation of textual evidence within the chain of transactions which bound the institutional fabric together alerts researchers to different voices within the documentary record. Translation of diagnostic terms and case notes into a modern medical idiom may provide a limited guide to such institutional conversations.

Future directions

There remains the question of how the particular accounts which are documented in these chapters can be understood within the larger chronology of political and social change which we have outlined in these introductory comments. These studies indicate the continuing importance of the relationship between local and central agencies of institutional provision within the British state and the distinctive nations of the United Kingdom. One reason for the role accorded to the Poor Law in the administration of lunacy legislation, we have suggested, was the capacity of local Unions to raise revenue, employ medical practitioners and provide the staffing to enforce the directives of local magistrates. The machinery of administration should not obscure the importance of established elites, lay patrons, local clergy and a range of actors within the boundaries of local governance during the nineteenth and early twentieth centuries, before and after the passage of important reforms affecting the control of asylums and the committal of the insane in 1888–90. Lay knowledge and influence was the work of many hands, particularly where the state was slow to provide for the institutional care of defective children, demonstrating the limits as well as the scope for medical empire-building during the later nineteenth century.

Such knowledge almost inevitably involved a moral economy in regard to personal worth, family respectability and community sentiment which was frequently mediated by notable clergymen as well as voluntary workers who contributed to the formation of the social work and family guidance profession during the early decades of the twentieth century. Informed by shifts in ideology, claims to professional expertise, and the promotion of national or trans-national models of 'best practice' within institutional care, regions and localities continued to develop practices which were grounded in the particular experiences of their district. In this respect, the space claimed by the institution reflected not only the legal framework in which it functioned, or the territory from which it drew its clients, but also the cultural assumptions implicit in serving certain communities. As policy-makers and informed opinion became disenchanted with the achievements of institutional care in the years following the Second World War, so the British state sought to renew the idea of community within the terms of alternative arrangements for the care of those seen as in need of mental health care. As these chapters suggest, the shift towards a 'community' model was transacted by a series of initiatives which involved a fresh political understanding with those using these services as well as the personnel who were involved in enacting the new principles of care. The outcome of these reforms has led some campaigners to call for a return to large-scale institutional facilities as a solution to the perceived problem of large numbers of vulnerable individuals placed in prisons, private nursing homes and unregulated rental accommodation.[65] Such debates frequently express a moral appeal to responsible behaviour within the good community, or the supportive family, which suggests the extent to which discussions of institutional care have historically relied on particular ideals of conduct as well as political calculations of costs and benefits.

Notes

1 Most famously in Erving Goffman's presentation of the total institution but also in a wide range of asylum studies. E. Goffman, *Asylums: Essays on the Social Situation of Mental Patients and Other Inmates*, New York: Anchor Books, 1961.
2 K. Jones, *A History of the Mental Health Services*, London: Routledge and Kegan Paul, 1972.
3 Most famously Andrew T. Scull's, *Museums of Madness: The Social Organization of Insanity in Nineteenth-Century England*, London: Allen Lane, 1979.
4 R. Porter, 'Introduction', in R. Porter and D. Wright (eds), *The Confinement of the Insane: International Perspectives, 1800–1965*, Cambridge: Cambridge University Press, 2003, pp. 1–19. In the same volume the essay by Wright *et al.* takes a similar approach while Ablard offers an alternative perspective, *The Confinement of the Insane*, pp. 100–128 and pp. 226–247.
5 Scull, *Museums of Madness*, Table 8, p. 224. Figures from various sources. Scull lists 2,248 people officially classed as insane in 1807, rising to 86,067 in 1890, equivalent to an increase from 2.26 to 29.26 per 10,000 of the population.
6 W. J. Corbet, MP, *Lunacy: The Residing Tide*, Dublin: Sealy, Bryers and Walker, 1890, pp. 9–12 and passim.

7 M. Thomson, *The Problem of Mental Deficiency: Eugenics, Democracy and Social Policy in Britain c.1870–1959*, Oxford: Clarendon Press, 1998, p. 21 and appendix. Estimates of mental deficiency drawn from the decennial census indicate a notable rise between 1891 and 1901, while numbers ascertained under Mental Deficiency legislation rose from more than 61,000 in 1927 to more than twice this figure by 1938 and a slow increase to 1946 when approximately 134,000 were identified under the legislation.

8 J. Andrews and A. Digby, 'Introduction', in J. Andrews and A. Digby (eds), *Sex and Seclusion, Class and Custody: Perspectives on Gender and Class in the History of British and Irish Psychiatry*, Amsterdam: Rodopi, 2004, pp. 7–44. This discussion makes interesting references to the work of Donzelot for example.

9 D. Garland, *Punishment and Welfare: A History of Penal Strategies*, Aldershot: Gower, 1985, pp. 240–243. Garland's claim that the asylum became a destination of last resort is not always supported by evidence of transfers within or between individual mental deficiency institutions.

10 M. A. Arieno, *Victorian Lunatics: A Social Epidemiology of Mental Illness in mid-Nineteenth Century England*, London: Associated University Press, 1989, chapter 1.

11 Andrews and Digby, 'Introduction', in Andrews and Digby (eds), *Sex and Seclusion, Class and Custody*, pp. 7–44 and other essays. Non-European examples suggest that this gives a preponderance of male admissions to state institutions. Porter and Wright (eds), *Confinement of the Insane*, essays by Deacon and Ablard, pp. 20–53 and pp. 226–247.

12 Diana Gittins notes these factors in the gendered treatment given to patients at Severalls, although more prosaically the availability of trained male or female staff limited the application of some therapies. D. Gittins, *Madness in its Place: Narratives of Severalls Hospital, 1913–1997*, London: Routledge, 1998, pp. 196–197.

13 David Wright discusses a number of reasons for the excess of male cases suggesting the condition may actually have been more prevalent in boys while the admission process possibly prioritized concerns about male behaviour in the home and future earning potential. Wright found twice as many idiot boys were admitted as girls and similar findings were reported by David Gladstone for the Western Counties Institution before 1914. The historical allocation of beds probably explains the continuing excess of male admissions to the Royal Western Counties Institution, Starcross (hereafter RWCI) after 1914 although this is less marked than in earlier periods. D. Wright, *Mental Disability in Victorian England: The Earlswood Asylum 1847–1901*, Oxford: Clarendon Press, 2001, p. 90; D. Gladstone, 'The Changing Dynamic of Institutional Care: The Western Counties Idiot Asylum, 1864–1914', in D. Wright and A. Digby (eds), *From Idiocy to Mental Deficiency: Historical Perspectives on People With Learning Disabilities*, London: Routledge, 1996, pp. 134–160; P. Dale, 'Implementing the 1913 Mental Deficiency Act: Competing Priorities and Resource Constraint Evident in the South West of England before 1948', *Social History of Medicine*, 16, 2003, pp. 403–408.

14 For a list of selected legislation in chronological order see page 224.

15 P. Bartlett, 'The Asylum and the Poor Law: The Productive Alliance', in J. Melling and B. Forsythe (eds), *Insanity, Institutions and Society: A Social History of Madness in Comparative Perspective, 1800–1914*, London: Routledge, 1999, pp. 48–67; J. Macnicol, 'Eugenics and the Campaign for Voluntary Sterilization in Britain Between the Wars', *Social History of Medicine*, 2, 1989, pp. 147–169, p. 168; M. Thomson, *The Problem of Mental Deficiency*, introduction, pp. 1–35.

16 Porter, and Wright (eds), *The Confinement of the Insane*. Earlier literature included B. Semmel, *Imperialism and Social Reform: English Social-Imperial Thought 1895–1914*, London: George Allen and Unwin, 1960.
17 R. Porter, 'Introduction', in Porter and Wright (eds), *The Confinement of the Insane*. In the same volume Elizabeth Malcolm, '"Ireland's Crowded Madhouses": The Institutional Confinement of the Insane in Nineteenth and Twentieth Century Ireland', pp. 315–333.
18 M. Jackson, *The Borderland of Imbecility: Medicine, Society and the Fabrication of the Feeble Mind in Late Victorian and Edwardian England*, Manchester: Manchester University Press, 2000, introduction, pp. 1–20.
19 Thomson, *The Problem of Mental Deficiency*, p. 10; J. Andrews, A. Briggs, R. Porter, P. Tucker and K. Waddington, *The History of Bethlem*, London: Routledge, 1997, pp. 95–97, 326–327. Locke's famous distinction of 1690 was frequently cited: namely, that a lunatic was someone who had possessed but lost the capacity to reason while the idiot never possessed such a capacity.
20 R. Smith, *Trial by Medicine: Insanity and Responsibility in Victorian Trials*, Edinburgh: Edinburgh University Press, 1981; J. P. Eigen, *Unconscious Crime: Mental Absence and Criminal Responsibility in Victorian London*, Baltimore and London: The Johns Hopkins University Press, 2003; P. Fennell, *Treatment without Consent: Law, Psychiatry and the Treatment of Mentally Disordered People since 1845*, London: Routledge, 1996; M. Jackson, 'It Begins With the Goose and Ends With the Goose: Medical, Legal and Lay Understandings of Imbecility in Ingram v. Wyatt, 1824–1832', *Social History of Medicine*, 11, 1998, pp. 361–380.
21 It was liability for claims for damages arising from the actions of patients that most concerned the conference of the original five English voluntary idiot asylums. The superintendents shared and discussed the legal advice taken by the Royal Medico-Psychological Association (RMPA) following the Holgate case, which had raised concerns about responsibility for patients on licence from institutions. Turner to Mayer, 7 March 1938, University of Exeter Library, RWCI archive, box 29.
22 S. Watson, ' Applying Foucault: Some Problems Encountered in the Application of Foucault's Methods to the History of Medicine in Prisons', in C. Jones and R. Porter (eds), *Reassessing Foucault: Power, Medicine and the Body*, 1999 (reprint of 1994 edition), pp. 132–151; cf. J. Sim, *Medical Power in Prisons: The Prison Medical Service in England 1774–1989*, Milton Keynes: Open University Press, 1990.
23 Steven Cherry notes the problem but finds structure irresistible. S. Cherry, *Mental Health Care in Modern England: The Norfolk Lunatic Asylum/St Andrew's Hospital c.1810–1998*, Woodbridge: Boydell Press, 2003.
24 A. Scull, C. Mackenzie and N. Hervey, 'The Administration of Lunacy in Victorian England: Samuel Gaskell (1807–1886)', in A. Scull (ed.), *Masters of Bedlam: The Transformation of the Mad-Doctoring Trade*, Princeton: Princeton University Press, 1996, pp. 161–186.
25 P. Bartlett and D. Wright (eds), *Outside the Walls of the Asylum: The History of Care in the Community 1750–2000*, London: Athlone Press, 1999; L. D. Smith, *Cure, Comfort and Safe Custody: Public Lunatic Asylums in Early Nineteenth-Century England*, London: Leicester University Press, 1999.
26 P. E. Prestwich, 'Family Strategies and Medical Power: "Voluntary" Committal in a Parisian Asylum, 1876–1914', in Porter, and Wright, (eds), *The Confinement of the Insane*, pp. 79–99; D. Wright, *Mental Disability in Victorian England*; D. Wright, 'Getting out of the Asylum: Understanding the Confinement of the Insane in the Nineteenth Century', *Social History of Medicine*, 10, 1997, pp. 137–155.

27 In a similar way Mathew Thomson revealed that the apparently paradoxical nature of support for the admittedly draconian Mental Deficiency Act (embracing as it did modernizers and traditionalists, conservatives and radicals, cross-party and cross-gender alliances, lay activists and professional interests), was in fact the explanation for the implementation of measures in the field of mental deficiency that had been rejected in other policy areas. Thomson, *The Problem of Mental Deficiency*, introduction, pp. 1–35.

28 P. Bartlett, *The Poor Law of Lunacy: The Administration of Pauper Lunatics in mid-Nineteenth Century England*, London: Leicester University Press, 1999; B. Forsythe, J. Melling and R. Adair, 'The New Poor Law and the County Lunatic Asylum – the Devon Experience', *Social History of Medicine*, 9, 1996, pp. 335–356.

29 Walmsley *et al.* note that Somerset was one county where workhouses specialized in idiot and imbecile accommodation, a policy that was elaborated in discussions between the County Council and the RWCI (Somerset correspondence file, RWCI archive, box 30) while Dorset similarly provided for adult females (the problematic nature of these arrangements, involving close scrutiny from the Board of Control, are briefly outlined in Hyde to Mayer, 2 January 1934, RWCI archive, box 30). J. Walmsley, D. Atkinson and S. Rolph, 'Community Care and Mental Deficiency 1913 to 1945', in Bartlett and Wright (eds), *Outside the Walls of the Asylum*, pp. 181–203. For wider context see Anne Crowther for the changing relationship to the respectable poor as well as the residuum. M. A. Crowther, *The Workhouse System, 1834–1929: The History of an English Social Institution*, London: Batsford, 1981.

30 For Murphy it is notable that, despite the objections of the Lunacy Commissioners, the workhouse continued to operate as an assessment and receiving point for the insane with only 'suitable' cases being forwarded to the asylum. Imbeciles remained in the workhouses until the Metropolitan Asylums Board created new provision at Leavesden and Caterham after 1867.

31 Gladstone notes ongoing tension between the admission of local cases and the admission of 'trainable cases' within the context of a need to secure financial stability. In the 1860s and 1870s local cases had predominated, then before 1914 the catchment area was a national one with pauper children admitted from across England and Wales. In her chapter (Chapter 8) Dale suggests the Mental Deficiency Act encouraged a renewed concentration on local cases, now more numerous and heterogeneous. D. Gladstone, 'The changing dynamic of institutional care'.

32 Wright, *Mental Disability in Victorian England*.

33 Prestwich, 'Family Strategies and Medical Power'.

34 J. Melling, B. Forsythe and R. Adair, 'Families, Communities and the Legal Regulation of Lunacy in Victorian England: Assessments of Crime, Violence and Welfare in Admissions to the Devon Asylum, 1845–1914', in Bartlett and Wright (eds), *Outside the Walls of the Asylum*, pp. 153–180.

35 Anne Borsay notes a similar neglect of children with physical and/or sensory disabilities with state provision following many decades after charitable and even commercial facilities developed this type of specialist care in residential and other settings. A. Borsay, *Disability and Social Policy in Britain Since 1750: A History of Exclusion*, Basingstoke: Palgrave Macmillan, 2005, chronology of events, pp. 270–282.

36 J. Melling, R. Adair and W. Forsythe, '"A Proper Lunatic for Two Years": Pauper Lunatic Children in Victorian and Edwardian England: Child Admissions to the Devon County Lunatic Asylum, 1845–1914', *Journal of Social History*, 30, 1997, pp. 371–405. Data on idiots and imbeciles from the 1881 census for Devon reveal balanced gender in identification of idiots and imbeciles.

37 Thomson, *The Problem of Mental Deficiency*, pp. 252–257; M. Thomson, 'Constituting Citizenship: Mental Deficiency, Mental Health and Human Rights in Inter-war Britain', in C. Lawrence and A-K. Mayer (eds), *Regenerating England: Science, Medicine and Culture in Inter-War Britain*, Amsterdam: Rodopi, 2000, pp. 231–250.

38 In only one of the 2,503 admissions to the RWCI, Starcross 1914–39 was it explicitly stated that the patient had no living relatives, although relatives often died or lost contact during long institutional stays. If families were perceived to be caring and respectable they were allowed to provide a home for former patients, but neither social workers nor institution staff were surprised when these arrangements broke down, and re-admissions were designed to be particularly straightforward. For example, Lilian received a trial period of licence in 1934 pending transfer to the guardianship of her sister and brother-in-law, who had recently combined households with Lilian's mother, but soon returned to the RWCI where she remained until transferring to another institution in 1948. (Patient 2861, correspondence from Plymouth Voluntary Association, 7 May 1934, RWCI Archive, box 29).

39 While the remarks made by a Plymouth social worker are somewhat ambiguous they do appear to express satisfaction that 'Kate' had been transferred to Rampton and would no longer be viewed as a suitable case for licence to the care of either relatives or an employer. (Correspondence between the Plymouth Voluntary Association and the RWCI, 5 April 1934, RWCI archive, box 29).

40 The case of the S. family revealed significant tension in the management of mental deficiency as a social problem. The alleged delinquency as well as defectiveness of family members encouraged social workers to seek an institutional placement for Wallace S. who had been discharged from a special school. They used the mental health problems of the step-father and the information that an older child was in an approved school and younger siblings had been taken into care as reasons for his urgent removal from home. In committee, local councillors expressed concern that this would encourage the parents to 'get rid of all their children'. (Case presented in correspondence between the Plymouth Voluntary Association and the RWCI, Lee to Mayer, 10 December 1937, RWCI Archive, box 29).

41 Andrews and Digby (eds), *Sex and Seclusion, Class and Custody*.

42 In the mental deficiency sector the situation was slightly different as permanent care remained an aspiration even though it proved impossible to fully deliver. While adult patients were admitted and discharged, at the RWCI it was children and adolescents who were more visible in both admissions and discharges. This was linked to the arrangements for 'education' cases and the review of each case at the age of twenty-one. While large-scale mixed asylums were common there was also significant provision used more exclusively for specific groups of inmates organized by age and/or sex, and grade of mental deficiency. The RWCI noted Board of Control figures for local authority provision for 1931–32. Only four of the fifty-one institutions listed offered a fully comprehensive service. In terms of gender thirteen were for males, eighteen for females and twenty mixed, while sixteen were for adults, two for children and thirty-three had a mix of ages. (RWCI archive, box 36, loose papers marked Board of Control, A. 171/30/11).

43 From a variety of sources Arieno concluded the typical inmate had a mean age of forty, an even chance of being male or female, had 2.2 children and a stated occupation. This is somewhat at odds with the stereotypical picture of such inmates and as Arieno points out does not suggest such people were unwanted or confined to the margins of society. Arieno, *Victorian Lunatics*, chapter 5.

44 As part of the Exminster project an analysis of Devon 1881 census data was undertaken. A subset of 'imbeciles' living in the community included 193 males (173 were single but there were also nine husbands and eleven widowers) and 172 females (145 single, sixteen wives and ten widows and one 'other') of all ages, some of whom had an occupation listed. A further group of 'idiots' in institutions other than the Devon County Asylum included seventy-nine males and sixty-one females. The ages ranged from small children to the very elderly and while most individuals were recorded as single there were some current and former spouses listed. Interestingly eighteen of the males were 'prisoners' in various jails and several of these, and other, inmates had occupations recorded.

45 Gladstone, 'The Changing Dynamic of Institutional Care; Dale, 'Implementing the 1913 Mental Deficiency Act'.

46 In Devon the workhouses at Axminster and Crediton were taken over for mental deficiency work while the St Thomas institution continued its role as a staging post to the asylum, taking cases en route to Exminster and Starcross after 1914. Evidence from the 1881 Census suggests an increasing concentration of lunatics, imbeciles and idiots in particular Devon workhouses although there was no direct correlation between these earlier populations and the institutions later adapted to this work after 1930.

47 Jackson, *The Borderland of Imbecility*.

48 Catherine Coleborne sees the Police as a key part of legal, medical and administrative measures that both identified and defined insanity. C. Coleborne, 'Passage to the Asylum: The Role of the Police in Committals of the Insane in Victoria, Australia, 1848–1900', in Porter and Wright, (eds), *The Confinement of the Insane*, pp. 129–148.

49 The Butler Clinic was developed in the 1970s and marked the culmination of interest in these issues, although the management of difficult and dangerous patients had been a recurring theme since the 1930s with particular concerns expressed about a group of 'unstable' women patients maintained in an annex during the Second World War.

50 Towards the end of the 1930s Exminster and Starcross began to cooperate in the treatment of patients which finally resolved the problem that Starcross had long sought to discharge patients unable or unwilling to respond to the training programme to Exminster whereas the mental hospital had responded to the Mental Treatment Act by requesting the immediate discharge of hopeless cases to Starcross or other similar institutions. Devon County Council completed a survey of transferable cases at Exminster but failed to deliver significant numbers of beds and it is not clear what the fate of these individuals was. It did however become policy to retain mentally deficient patients with symptoms of complicating mental illness at the RWCI, with transfers to Rampton prioritized when behaviour was unmanageable. The Devon County Council investigations were summarized in a report by J. R. Harper presented to the Mental Deficiency Committee, 18 November 1935, Devon Record Office (DRO), 153/5/1/2. See also Dale, 'Implementing the 1913 Mental Deficiency Act'.

51 Correspondence between the Plymouth Voluntary Association and the RWCI reveals how much personal information was available to the social workers. Concerned neighbours as well as family members reported incidents designed to reveal problems with home care or deviant behaviour. These were supplemented by informal contacts with education, health, welfare, criminal justice and child protection services. Where parents acquiesced to, even sought, institutional care the evidence was used to support their application but the same material was also used to coerce the unwilling. Thus while Mrs S. confided that her husband had beaten her son Rowland and used this to argue that

institutionalization would be better for both of them, it could also have become the basis for child protection work and compulsory admission. Lee to Mayer, 20 February 1939, RWCI Archive, box 29.

52 Andrews and Digby, 'Introduction', in Andrews and Digby (eds), *Sex and Seclusion, Class and Custody*, p. 15 for grouping of families, magistrates and clergy together.

53 Although to date the British assessment of hostel type provision has been more optimistic than comparable American work. An important early survey by Lerman expressed concern about the increasing numbers committed to these quasi-institutions, the emphasis being on cost-saving, the quality of care offered and the transference of responsibility for the vulnerable from the state and public authorities to private and charitable initiatives that may be associated with some loss of the citizenship rights achieved between 1935 and 1962, and here he usefully cites references to comments made by Harry Hopkins of the Federal Emergency Relief Federation in 1933. P. Lerman, *Deinstitutionalization and the Welfare State*, New Brunswick, New Jersey: Rutgers University Press, 1982 (1984 paperback edition), pp. 204–224, p. 213.

54 Thomson, *The Problem of Mental Deficiency*, p. 120. New accommodation constructed at the RWCI in the 1930s followed this model although the original asylum and associated annexes continued to house almost half of the patients.

55 William Wood, *Insanity and the Lunacy Law*, London: Churchill, 1879, pp. 20–22, 34–36 for private and pauper patient treatment, for example.

56 The Mental Deficiency Acts required local authorities to secure similar contributions although this presented many problems. Devon Mental Deficiency Committee accounts record that parents were contributing more than £600 to a total budget of £10,000 in the financial year 1916–17, a figure that had risen to £1,200 in a total budget of £14,000 for 1925–26. The parental contributions then became more difficult to collect while overall expenditure increased significantly to the point where parents were contributing just £1,210 to a total budget of £20,000 in 1929–30. Several parents were able to plead poverty to the committee but evidence collected by social workers suggests families were able to conceal income. Minutes of Devon Mental Deficiency Committee DRO 153/5/1/1 and DRO 153/5/1/2 and correspondence regarding patient 2908 from Plymouth Voluntary Association, 12 September 1934, RWCI archive, box 29.

57 M. S. Micale, *Approaching Hysteria: Disease and its Interpretations*, Princeton: Princeton University Press, 1995; P. Michael, *Care and Treatment of the Mentally Ill in North Wales*, 1800–2000, Cardiff: University of Wales Press, 2003.

58 In a similar way the Medical Officer of Health and School Medical Officer's assistants played a significant role in the diagnosis of mental deficiency. The RWCI, and other institutions, accepted their diagnosis in the case of individual patients although Egan's chapter (Chapter 7) suggests a more important role outside of the institutional sector.

59 The RWCI did not record alleged causes after 1914 apart from a brief survey in 1923–24 included in the register of admission. This showed remarkable continuity with Wright's work on the Earlswood cases with events like difficult, delayed or premature birth, illness and/or accident featuring prominently although many causes were recorded as unknown and documents supplied by doctors and social workers put increasing emphasis on both morbid heredity and a poor home environment. RWCI archive, box 20; D. Wright, '"Childlike in his Innocence": Lay Attitudes to "Idiots" and "Imbeciles" in Victorian England', in Wright and Digby (eds), *From Idiocy to Mental Deficiency*, pp. 118–133.

60 The first Resident Medical Officer was appointed to the RWCI in 1938.

61 J. Welshman, 'In Search of the "Problem Family": Public Health and Social

Work in England and Wales 1940–1970', *Social History of Medicine*, 9, 1996, pp. 447–465; J. Welshman, 'The Social History of Social Work: The Issue of the "Problem Family", 1940–1970', *British Journal of Social Work*, 29, 1999, pp. 457–476.

62 Thomson reviews some of the most important work on the role of the family and increasing professional scrutiny of family life. Thomson, *The Problem of Mental Deficiency*, pp. 258–268.

63 The case of John J., a former grammar school boy but persistent delinquent certified as a moral defective at Exeter Prison in 1938, provoked some lengthy discussion about these issues, Devon MOH report to RWCI 11 November 1938 and covering letter, RWCI archive, box 25.

64 G. Reaume, *Remembrance of Patients Past: Patient Life at the Toronto Hospital for the Insane, 1870–1940*, Don Mills, Ontario: Oxford University Press, 2000; Michael, *Care and Treatment of the Mentally Ill in North Wales*; Cherry, *Mental Health Care in Modern England*; D. Atkinson, M. Jackson and J. Walmsley (eds), *Forgotten Lives: Exploring the History of Learning Disability*, Kidderminster: BILD Publications, 1997.

65 An alternative model developed in recent years, with the intention of supporting vulnerable people without putting them in residential accommodation to do so, has been the 'Supporting People' budget although this funding and associated services are under severe pressure. A case study of Stonham Housing Association and its work with the homeless, people fleeing domestic abuse, refugees, ex-offenders, people with mental health problems and people with physical and learning difficulties is outlined by Kate Allen, 'A Cut Above', *Inside Housing*, 4 February 2005, pp. 24–26.

2 Workhouse care of the insane, 1845–90

Elaine Murphy

Introduction

In England and Wales, workhouses and public lunatic asylums both developed within the framework of the Poor Law. For much of the nineteenth century, these apparently disparate institutions stood shoulder to shoulder along a continuum of care options for Poor Law overseers to choose from when it was not possible to support a mentally dependent person at home on 'out-relief'. The spectrum of institutions also included privately run mad-houses, called licensed houses, and a handful of specialist voluntary hospitals. Workhouses and public asylums catered for a range of overlapping species of lunacy but had markedly different costs. When one part of the system was full or considered too pricey, the other providers were brought into play. The aim of this chapter is to explore the realities of workhouse care, consider the shifting legal and policy framework and suggest why metropolitan London moved away from using workhouses by 1890 in advance of most other areas of England and Wales. Much of the illustrative material is taken from east London, the '*locus classicus*', as Rose put it, of nineteenth century poverty studies, where managing the insane was a major challenge for local Guardians.[1]

Bartlett has pointed out that the traditional view of the management of pauper lunatics as a triumph of an embryonic medical profession of mad doctors flourishing within the capitalist expansion of specialist institutions is not borne out by the evidence from official documents about who made the decisions about the disposal of the insane.[2] In his study in the English Midlands, Bartlett judged that the power of the magistracy, who held the purse-strings around admission to asylums, was at the heart of a bargaining process. Local Guardians' officials and doctors had influence and negotiating powers but were tangential to the core business. My own reading in London however suggests that the Guardians, the parish officials and doctors who worked for them and individual families had considerable power to resist the expansionist drive of the Middlesex magistrates and the county asylums, which the Guardians perceived as expensive and not altogether justified.[3] The local poor budget was held by the union clerk and the Guardians themselves made the final decisions, resisting pressure from central inspectorates, the Poor Law Commissioners and Lunacy Commissioners unless it suited them. And what suited them best was to keep paupers in their own institutions where they had control of the costs unless there were powerful reasons for sending them away.

Elements of this institutional system expanded or contracted according to funding incentives, legislation, pressure from the Lunacy Commissioners and availability of building capital but were fundamentally interdependent.[4] This was not the case for example in Ireland, where asylums developed quite separately from the Irish Poor Law, largely escaping the more repressive associations of the workhouse but awkwardly disconnected administratively. Movement between institutions was hampered; asylums became clogged up with the mildly afflicted; massive growth of asylums followed.[5] The English and Welsh system had the merit of flexibility. Throughout the nineteenth century, workhouses absorbed as many as a quarter of those designated as lunatic and furthermore 15 per cent or so of all admissions to workhouses were as a result of mental infirmity.[6] Assessing and treating insanity and idiocy constituted a substantial daily workload of a Poor Law medical officer.

Wapping workhouse was characteristic of many institutions struggling to provide decent care for the insane in the turmoil of the overburdened poor relief system in the mid-nineteenth century East End of London. Looking for a good story after reading a critical magistrate's comment in a newspaper, Charles Dickens visited the Stepney Union insane wards at Wapping workhouse twice, once in early May 1850 and then a decade later in early 1860.[7] Dickens arrived at the workhouse unexpected and unrecognized. He encountered Jane Megson, the energetic, determined and kindly young woman 'Master' of Wapping workhouse, appointed by Stepney Guardians in spite of opposition from the Poor Law Commission.[8]

> A very bright and nimble little Matron with a bunch of keys in her hand responded to my request to see the House. I began to doubt whether the police magistrate was quite right in his facts when I noticed her quick active little figure and her intelligent eyes. The Traveller, the Matron intimated, should see the worst first. He was welcome to see everything.

They went straight to the 'foul wards'. The 'wretched rooms' of the infirmary and foul wing 'were as clean and sweet as it is possible for such rooms to be; they would be a pest house in a single week if they were ill kept'. Dickens 'accompanied the brisk matron up another barbarous staircase into a better kind of loft devoted to the idiotic and imbecilic'. Two old women and other inmates there seemed well cared for. In the refractory wards he notes a lively bantering exchange between the Matron and her noisy young women charges. Dickens understood Mrs Megson's problems;

he could see that given the dilapidated building, the thousands of pounds that would be required to bring it up to standard and the numbers of people in need, the care of these paupers was reasonably good. Mrs Megson conducted a daily battle with the Stepney Guardians about the 'proper place for lunatics'. Sick and destitute old women, syphilitic, worn-out prostitutes and scabby infected derelicts were all squashed into the same old wards as the female lunatics, suitable neither as an infirmary nor as dormitories for the fit, 'a kind of purgatory' Dickens thought.[9] The Board had no money for upgrading the wards and Mrs Megson was still battling to get some improvements when Dickens visited a decade later.

Wapping was no worse than the majority of workhouses, poorly designed, overcrowded and understaffed. For the next fifty years workhouses played a significant part in providing temporary respite or a permanent home for the mentally ill and dependent, a role barely acknowledged in many histories of mental health services in the nineteenth century. Workhouses were recognized as pivotal institutions in the care of the insane.[10] From the point in 1844 when the Metropolitan Commissioners in Lunacy were permitted to extend their remit nationally, they were determined to understand how the committal system worked in practice, extending their national survey of asylums to 'various workhouses and other places'. As a consequence, the Lunacy Acts of 1845 enabled the new national Commissioners in Lunacy to visit and report on workhouses to the Poor Law Commission, although they had no powers to insist on improvements as they could with lunatic asylums. The annual returns reported a total of 9,162 lunatic workhouse inmates; the Commissioners found 3,053 more on their first round of visits to nearly 600 workhouses, giving a grand total of 12,215.[11]

Some workhouses already had specific licenses for lunatic wards, notably the house of industry for the Isle of Wight at Carisbrooke, where both the accommodation and care were rather good, the workhouses at Devonport and at Stoke Damerel near Plymouth, the houses of industry at Morda near Oswestry and at Kingsland near Shrewsbury, this latter decidedly less good, where eighty to ninety patients were chained to the bed at night. There were also numerous workhouses without a license for the reception of insane paupers which nevertheless contained wards exclusively for lunatics, 'dangerous as well as harmless', for example the workhouses at Birmingham, Manchester, Sheffield, Bath, Leicester, Redruth, Norwich and others.[12]

Lunatic workhouse ward inmates were often 'suitable cases for an asylum', the Commissioners thought and criticized the Poor Law Commissioners' view of them as 'in general, incurable harmless idiots'.[13] The term 'idiot' had been extended to mean more than congenital idiots and included many with acquired insanity. The Commissioners declared the returns were 'simply wrong'. In fact, congenital idiots could also be disturbed and 'dangerous'. At this time, the sanctioning of lunatics and idiots of any kind in workhouses was objectionable to the Commissioners on the grounds that patients had no access to medical treatment, keepers and medical staff were inadequately trained, there was little space and often no place to exercise. They were realists however and understood that until there were sufficient asylum places, workhouses would continue to care for lunatics.

By 1852 there were more insane together in wards in some workhouses than in some county asylums. Manchester, Bristol City, Portsea and Southampton Workhouses all had more insane than Derby County Asylum, Hull Borough Asylum or the Welsh Asylum at Abergavenny.[14] Right from the outset, the Commissioners assumed that if the number of asylum places increased sufficiently, the numbers of insane in workhouses would decrease. Over the next twenty-five years this proved to be a mistaken assumption. The Guardians and their officers were ambivalent about asylums. They recognized the powerful arguments of the advantages of asylums over workhouses but did not want to pay the higher costs or admit that their workhouse care was poor.

The impact of the growth of public asylums on the licensed house trade was however real enough. Between 1850 and 1852, as a consequence of the opening of the second Middlesex County Asylum at Colney Hatch in 1851, the metropolitan private licensed houses suffered a reduction in their 'market share' of the Middlesex pauper lunatic business from 37 per cent to little more than 7 per cent, whereas the percentage in workhouses reduced only from 24 per cent to 16 per cent and that for a very temporary period.[15] Cost as always was a potent factor: Colney Hatch was 8s 2d per week; the Middlesex Justices estimated the average cost of a Licensed House was 11s 2d.[16] Workhouses cost a third or less.

There were other influences on the Guardians and their Clerks, who were in daily contact with paupers seeking relief. They knew many of the families over many years; decisions about committals and removals were taken on a case-by-case basis. There may well have been pressure from families or local workhouse staff to retain certain individuals in the workhouse. When the Hackney Union Clerk haggled with Jeffreason, the Colney Hatch Asylum Secretary, over the number of patients the Union would send to the new asylum and when, their battle of wills culminating in a reduction in the numbers and change of allocated date for transferring the workhouse lunatics, the Clerk refused to comply with the suggested new arrangements. The patients were already anxious and distressed about the forthcoming move, he said, and the Guardians did not think it was fair to upset them further by an unnecessary change of date.[17] Colney Hatch was not the solution the Justices and Guardians expected it to be. More or less the same proportion of notified lunatics was maintained in workhouses in 1860 (25 per cent) as in 1842 (28 per cent).[18] The Middlesex Magistrates began to ruminate about a third County Lunatic Asylum.

Workhouses designed primarily as deterrent institutions were poorly adapted to providing care for the insane. In metropolitan London, work-houses were notoriously cheap and grim. The main pressure on the work-house masters was the inexorable growth in the numbers of paupers. Institutions that had housed three to four hundred inmates in the mid-1830s, by 1850 held double or treble that number. To contain the rising demand in the East End, most unions made alterations and expansions or built new larger workhouses under pressure from the Poor Law Board but never kept up with the inward flow.[19] By 1857 many eastern metropolis workhouses contained over 1,000 paupers: Stepney had several huge and expanding workhouses.

D. R. Green has described the deep pit of inefficiency that the east London unions dug for themselves from 1849 through the 1850s and 1860s as their policies on poor relief diverged from other parts of the country.[20] Apart from Poplar, where the Guardians still relied heavily on outdoor relief, indoor relief as a proportion of total expenditure was consistently higher in London than other regions whilst outdoor relief was lower.[21] Their ready willingness to implement the workhouse test tied them irrevo-cably into an expensive and inappropriate system of poor relief for unem-ployed labourers and their families, who grew ever more numerous during the economic recession of the late 1840s. Green traces the adoption of a strict indoor relief policy in the poorer metropolitan districts to the des-peration of the Guardians during the recession of the 1850s, faced with a tide of paupers they could not cope with. Geographical social segregation between rich and poor classes, which characterized the metropolis as a result of inner urban slum clearance, resulted in poorer unions restricting spending in a narrow doctrinaire fashion.

The poorer unions of east London had negligible cash to spend from meagre poor rates. Shoreditch officials, like many others, coped by becom-ing immune to the dire conditions in their workhouse. The wards became infested with bed bugs, the sanitary facilities gravely inadequate. There were no WCs with trap pans, only open earth closets and smelly old latrines. 'The Insane Wards [were] of a prison-like character', 'the yards [were] surrounded by high walls and comfortless airing courts' which several attempts at planting had done little to soften.[22] By 1863 there were over 100 imbeciles and chronic lunatics in the workhouse.

The Lunacy Commission and the Poor Law Board

The Lunacy Commissioners were mindful that workhouses came under a separate government jurisdiction. Their reports to the County Justices about conditions in asylums were longer, more detailed and certainly more critical than their reports to the Poor Law Board about workhouses. The Poor Law Board was there to concern itself above all else with the man-agement of the able-bodied unemployed poor. The sick, infirm and men-tally incompetent were a complication to be dealt with but something of a side issue in the great national scheme to reduce pauperism. The Lunacy Commission on the other hand conducted their task steeped in their chairman Shaftesbury's evangelical ethos of a public duty to care and cure. Lunatics were deserving of the best conditions that could be afforded, for humanity's sake.

Responsible Boards of Guardians tried to steer a difficult course between the parallel tracks of Poor Law policy for the 'deserving' and the 'undeserving'. Relieving officers and workhouse masters reduced the comforts of paupers to comply with their interpretation of 'less eligibility'. At the same time they were expected to be generous 'overseers' of the needy sick, ensuring medical help was available to all, provide comfortable infirmary wards and kindness to the sick and dying. The two groups of able-bodied and non-able-bodied overlapped to such a degree that it was difficult in practice to draw a clear distinction between them even though on paper they appeared quite separate. The fluctuating availability of work in the boom and bust years of the mid-Victorian age had a particularly stark impact on the employability of those less robust intellectually or emotionally. When work was scarce, the most competent, reliable labourers stayed in work, the less gifted became destitute, candidates for the workhouse.

Relations between the Lunacy Commission and the new Poor Law Board established in 1848 began amicably enough.[23] 'The Poor Law Board have always zealously co-operated with us to ensure this object has been effected.'[24] The Commissioners complained repeatedly about the lack of recent cases being sent to the new public asylums and their filling up with incurables, so they were necessarily cautious in recommending too many transfers from workhouses unless there were statutory reasons for doing so. The two inspectorates maintained a united public front but became increasingly frustrated with each other's attitude. As the Poor Law Board assumed more direct responsibility and executive powers over the Boards of Guardians, they became more sensitive to the Guardians' desire to run the pauper management machine as cheaply as the local rate payers wanted. There was nothing special about lunatics as far as the Poor Law Inspectors could see that justified the extra expense that was invested in them as a result of the Lunacy Acts.

None of this was put into plain words until the Select Committee hearings of 1859 and 1860 but there is enough in the correspondence to suggest that there was simmering resentment by the Poor Law authority of the moral superiority assumed by the Lunacy Commissioners for several years before that.[25] The Poor Law Board were getting a taste of the medicine which they had been ladling out for years to the Guardians and naturally found it unpalatable. From 1854 however, when there was a minor skirmish between the two Secretaries about which of their agencies should be responsible for ensuring the Annual Lunatic Returns were properly filled in by the union clerks and medical officers, the tone of letters between them became more strained.[26]

For a while in the early 1850s the Lunacy Commissioners thought that 'the numbers of insane poor detained in workhouses is diminishing in a very marked degree'[27] but rapidly realized they were wrong, the reverse was true. In spite of the numbers of asylums, an increasing number of unions were opening specialist insane wards.[28] The Lunacy Commissioners advocated separate asylums for chronic cases and imbeciles under the control of the magistrates but had few allies. They wanted the

> erection of inexpensive buildings adapted for the idiotic, chronic and harmless patients, in direct connexion with, or at a convenient distance from, the existing institutions. These auxiliary asylums ... would be intermediate between union workhouses and the principal curative asylums.[29]

Shaftesbury had anticipated that these new asylums would fall under the control of the Justices and the provisions of the Lunacy Act. The Poor Law Board however was anxious to exclude the meddlesome Lunacy Commissioners from its territory and certainly keen to block any moves that Commissioners might make to extend their powers further over lunatics and idiots in workhouses. The Inspectors' view came over powerfully in the Select Committee hearings on Lunatics in 1859 when Andrew Doyle, the Inspector from the North-West, challenged directly Shaftesbury's evidence to the Committee. Doyle said it should be possible to detain lunatics formally in workhouses. Poor Law Inspectors were quite as capable as Lunacy Commissioners of supervising their care he thought.[30] Shaftesbury must have regretted the low-key 'softly, softly' approach which the Commission had taken in their early reports about workhouses. It certainly made it difficult for him to back up his opinion that there was much cruelty and thoughtless treatment of chronic lunatics and idiots in workhouses and that their treatment was detrimental to their health and wellbeing. Doyle's raw attack on Lunacy Commission policy to get lunatics out of workhouses and into asylums stung Shaftesbury into a more frank criticism of the quality of Poor Law Board supervision of their institutions. The final report from Sir George Grey's Committee leaned to Shaftesbury's view but that did nothing to foster harmony between the two inspectorates.

From 1860 on, the Poor Law Board began their campaign to bypass the Lunacy Commissioners by establishing asylums under their own control for the class of chronically insane patients that posed such a heavy nursing burden on their workhouses. In London, Gathorne-Hardy's Metropolitan Poor Bill of 1867, which established the Metropolitan Asylums Board, was the triumphal march of the Poor Law Board over the dispirited Lunacy Commissioners. The legal context in which the Guardians operated shifted marginally as a result of the Lunacy Acts Amendment Act of 1862, which gave the Lunacy Commission power to order the compulsory transfer of lunatics from workhouses to an asylum and conversely to grant permission for chronic untreatable cases to be returned from the asylum to the workhouse, subject to approval by the Secretary of State.[31] A year later, in the Amending Act of 1863, the Commissioners were also awarded a veto over the transfer of lunatics to workhouses in the event of the workhouse having unsatisfactory facilities.[32] Transfers could not be arranged solely by the Guardians. The Committee of Asylum Visitors had to make the formal application, a safeguard against the wholesale removal of patients from asylums as a cost-reducing exercise.

The 1862 Act was the first breach of the Lunacy Commission's treasured principle that all insane patients should be removed from the control of the Poor Law authorities to the protection of the Justices and the Lunacy Act. Until then the Commission had assumed it was merely a matter of time and sufficient expenditure by the Justices before all mentally dependent people were transferred out of the control of the Guardians. Neither the Guardians nor the Lunacy Commission were pleased with the 1862 Act because it appeared to encourage workhouses to turn into small lunatic asylums. The Poor Law Board tried to reassure the Guardians that this was not intended but it seemed likely that an even higher proportion of lunatics would remain in workhouses in the future.[33]

Who were workhouse lunatics? How did they live?

Workhouse patients designated as lunatics have often been characterized as harmless imbeciles, chronically but quietly mad or decrepit old dements. 'The great bulk of persons [in workhouses] are feeble or defective ... being in most cases of a congenital or organic and therefore of a permanent nature ... not likely to benefit from treatment.'[34]

Workhouses were portrayed, not least by Dickens, as stultifying 'waiting' rooms filled with a 'heterogeneous mass of physical and mental wrecks' queuing for their removal to a place in the ever-expanding county asylum system or death.[35] After 1863, when workhouses were sanctioned for harmless chronic cases, those on the way in to the Asylum were housed with the displaced burnt-out chronic wrecks on the way out, extruded to make room for the more desirable 'recent cases'. Scull describes these characters that populate the borderlands of the state of lunacy:

> Chronic alcoholics afflicted with delirium tremens or, with permanently pickled brains, reduced to a state of dementia; epileptics; tertiary syphilitics; consumptives in the throes of terminal delirium; cases of organic brain damage ... the malnourished, the simple-minded.[36]

Mentally incapacitated, heavily dependant idiots and imbeciles were a management strain on the masters but not of very great interest to the Lunacy Commission. Instead of an asylum, the Commissioners prescribed work, which they felt would raise the self-esteem and improve the mental condition of these unfortunates. The main benefit an asylum could offer, these early Commissioners felt in the optimistic days of the 1850s, was treatment and if a patient was beyond treatment the only point in transferring them to an asylum was to control violent and difficult behaviour. The doctors were not keen to take on the care of imbeciles and the chronically insane either. The report of the first meeting of the newly named Medico-Psychological Association (the old Association of Medical Officers of Asylums and Hospitals for the Insane) in 1865 makes it very clear that insane persons came in desirable and undesirable forms.

> Whether a few old and imbecile patients may not properly be left in the workhouse is not a matter of very great moment but what is entirely unjustifiable to keep in the workhouse for one hour longer than is absolutely necessary in acute cases of insanity, anyone who knows what are the requirements of treatment in such cases and what workhouses at present are, must feel strongly.[37]

'Treatability' was what interested the doctors. The acutely mad were welcome in the asylum; idiots and old dements languishing in disgraceful workhouses were not their concern.

Bartlett points out that by 1861 the Lunacy Commissioners recognized that in many workhouses with designated lunatic wards, 'The class of patients found in these wards differs little, if at all, from those met in County Asylums'.[38] In 1867, as part of their campaign to promote the Metropolitan Asylums Bill, the Poor Law Board published an entire decade of reports by the Commissioners in Lunacy to the Poor Law Board from 1856 to 1866 and the correspondence between them on the subject of the Metropolitan Workhouses.[39] The overall impression is of gravely inadequate care in defective institutions, although none of the individual reports is especially shocking or noteworthy. Care in workhouses was not uniformly bad. In some parts of the country, the Lunacy Commissioners accepted that expanding the capacity of special wards at a workhouse might be preferable to expansion of an overcrowded over large asylum. In the mid-1860s, the Commissioners encouraged the expansion of special lunatic facilities at Plymouth workhouse for example, rather than countenance the expansion of the declining Devon Asylum at Exminster.[40]

Frances Power Cobbe, in her mid-1860s critique of the New Poor Law commented:

> Workhouses are lunatic asylums for all except violent cases. Many of them contain scores of insane patients. Here a total different order of things comes in view. The Commissioners mercifully intervene in favour of these poor souls, and compel the Guardians to treat them in a manner superior to other inmates in many respects. The appearance

of their wards, decently furnished and often adorned with prints and supplied with objects for their amusement, is at first a surprise to the workhouse visitor.

Cobbe objected to the lack of specific medical treatment for mental disease in workhouses and wanted the more insane moved to asylums for that reason alone, not because their general care was poor.[41]

The City of London Guardians resisted the notion that public asylums were necessarily an improvement on workhouse care or carefully chosen licensed houses. They argued that their policy of placing patients according to individual needs was better able to respond to variations between patients than to build a remote asylum that would offer only one solution.[42] They could see no sense in building a specialist asylum of their own when there were ample rather good private places locally. They had a point. Bethnal Green Asylum was getting better reports in the 1840s and early 1850s than many public asylums and their own workhouse provided excellent care. The City Aldermen were willing to spend what was necessary to secure their own sense of magnanimity; their workhouse or 'Grand Hotel', the Bow Institution, was 'a house of architectural pretensions'.[43] Most other unions had to make do with less ostentatious beneficence.

The City workhouse was an exception. Lunacy Commissioners' reports chronicle the swings in efficiency of union administration, Guardians' responsiveness to criticism and their changing attitudes to caring for long-term mentally dependent patients. Over a five-year period an effective administration could sink into deplorably poor habits; a good workhouse might become filthy and dilapidated within a few months of losing a competent master. Conversely a determined Board could transform the accommodation, care and therefore the lives of the lunatic inmates. Most workhouses were poorly constructed and unsuitable for the majority of the inmates. Few Boards employed paid nurses or trained attendants to care for lunatics and imbeciles, old women paupers living in the house were 'paid' in extra diet or minor privileges to nurse their fellow paupers. In spite of their manifest inadequacies in managing seriously dependent people, Guardians and officials were reluctant to acknowledge defects in the accommodation or regime or keen to remove difficult patients to expensive asylums. The *Lancet* complained in 1869 that Guardians and workhouse staff could not judge the difference between a disorderly able person and one whose difficult or disorderly behaviour was caused by insanity. The consequence was that harsh rules and punishments were extended to all those who were 'in Bastilles for life'.[44]

The rented workhouse of the St Luke's Old Street Union in the City Road was typical of many.[45] There were so many mentally disordered people in the huge institution that 'the workhouse is substantially a lunatic asylum and ought to have the ordinary comforts and conveniences of one'. The wards were crowded, the yards too small, there were insufficient staff, the diet was inferior, seventy-two patients were in crowded lunatic wards 'in want of such treatment as only an asylum can afford'. The medical officer Harris denied it, claiming that the lunatics were all tranquil and manageable. The Guardians resisted criticism; they disagreed that the wards were overcrowded, the yards they declared adequate, the dietary information the Commissioners had been given was wrong. As to the suggestion that there should be more attendants, the Chairman George Whittle wrote that 'the present attendants ... suffer from want of scope for energetic exertion': there was insufficient work for them to do; it would be pointless appointing more. Conditions remained essentially unchanged until 1867, a conspicuous failure for both central inspectorates.

The workhouse infirmary had a key role as a diagnostic 'station stop' for a diverse assortment of cases brought in by the relieving officers and parish doctors for assessment and classification. About 15 per cent of infirmary admissions in east London were suffering primarily from mental disorder, a hefty chunk of the doctor's workload.[46] The admission procedure established in the mid-nineteenth century, to a local institution followed by discharge home or placement in an asylum, established a pattern of clinical assessment that remained broadly the same in London until the closure of the large asylums in the late twentieth century. The relieving officer would bring in the patient, the workhouse medical officer would decide if he or she needed removing to an asylum, then the committal would be completed by the agreement of a local clergyman. Patients could remain in the workhouse for several weeks while a decision was made about their future, unless their behaviour was so unmanageable that an early transfer to an asylum was arranged. Many unions preferred to delay admission to see if the patient would settle, because they often improved sufficiently to go home within a few days.[47]

The day-to-day admission of the despairing and distressed was what unions believed workhouses were there for. There was a dangerously narrow swing bridge in the docks called locally 'Baker's Trap' after the Coroner William Baker, who was also Union Clerk, had drawn attention to it as a common place for suicides.[48] A 'dirty puffy sallow young man' told Dickens that young women 'took a header in', and were fished out by the police or anyone who would do it. Are they restored?, Dickens asked. 'They're carried into the werkiss and put in a 'ot bath and brought round. But I dunno about restored'.[49]

For thirty years, from their founding until well into the 1870s, every year the Lunacy Commissioners pressed hard for individuals to be taken straight before a magistrate and transferred directly to the asylum. They reported lurid tales about the adverse consequences of insane people being detained in workhouses. A typical example was a man named Lewis, who was admitted to Whitechapel workhouse in 1851.[50] On arrival at the workhouse receiving ward, Lewis had been uncontrollably violent. The staff had no idea how to handle him. 'He was restrained for 8 days strapped down in bed with manacles on his legs and arms and a belt across his waist'. After eight days he was a little less disturbed, so 'he was confined less but by April 12th the Medical Officer reported him dangerously ill. Sloughs had formed on his back and limbs. There were none when he was admitted ... He was removed by friends on 6 May, died on the 11 June'. In this instance, attempts had been made to find a place in a lunatic asylum but no vacancy could be found anywhere in London. Lewis had been kept in the receiving ward from his admission to the day his relatives insisted on removing him.

Few unions took notice of the Commissioners' exhortations not to use the workhouse as an assessment and receiving point for the insane. It was geographically convenient for parish officers, required no formal certification procedure and many patients recovered and went home very quickly. With luck the expense of an asylum stay could be avoided. From the Guardians' point of view, it was plain common sense to ensure that those whose confusion was due primarily to physical illness, or suffering from recoverable delirium tremens, or who were emotionally overwrought as a result of a transient life crisis, should be given the opportunity to recover first, to ensure that only the most suitable cases of insanity went to the asylum. This avoided the extra expense but they also knew that physically sick people fared badly in the asylum. The Commissioners were never convinced of the Guardians' arguments but only a handful of unions ever took the slightest notice of the Commission's exhortations. In east London, only Poplar Union tried to implement the recommended policy.

The effectiveness of the Lunacy Commission in workhouses

The Lunacy Commissioners were good at spotting problems on their intermittent visits to workhouses but not sufficiently influential or powerful to insist on major changes. They could not make the Guardians spend money and they could not insist on staffing levels being increased. They worked on the 'drip, drip' principle of continually criticizing the same things, hoping to wear down the Guardians into accepting their suggestions, but the Guardians were masters of procrastination and not very susceptible to exhortation.

The Commission's bland reports did not shock sufficiently to disturb the Guardians' habitual institutional inertia. By the 1860s the Poor Law was being transformed by the addition of specialist medical services and the rising influence of the medical profession on Poor Law policy. The *Lancet* published a series of dramatic reports through 1865–66 by three doctors, Carr, Anstie and Hart, who visited workhouse infirmaries on the journal's behalf to report on conditions. Grandly called the Lancet Sanitary Commission for Investigating the State of the Infirmaries in Workhouses, every fortnight for a year one or more of the metropolitan workhouses was described in minute horrifying detail.[51] It was marvellous sensationalist reporting.

The *Lancet* Report on St Leonard's, Shoreditch was typical.[52] Three-quarters of the 700 inmates were permanent residents, 130 imbecile or lunatic. The workhouse 'combines the principal merits and defects of the system'. The history of its management was 'paved with good intentions' and there was 'much goodwill and openness. The Master [Mr Painter] is an able, business-like and judicious official. The Medical Officer [James Clark] is a man of considerable vigour, long experience and kindly nature' but:

> If we have to show that the infirmary is a terrible failure and the whole state of things in it disgraceful to the parish and to the country, we must ask that a great allowance be made for the superhuman difficulties of the task which would be involved in a fitting administration by this one gentleman of the duties which are properly incidental to the management of so large a hospital as this.

They commented on the extreme cheerlessness and the desolation of the imbeciles

> moping about in herds without any occupation whatever ... congregated in a miserable day-room where they sit and stare at each other or the bare wall ... treated as we would kennel dogs in decent kennels. We denounce the cruelty of keeping these imbeciles in a cheerless town workhouse.

There was just one medical officer for the 700 and one paid nurse. The male pauper nurses 'struck us as a peculiarly rough, ignorant and uncouth set'. There were no night nurses. The imbeciles were better off than the sick, whose sores and sloughs were covered in rags for want of bandages, the wards 'frequently filthy with crusted blood and discharges'. A man with gangrene lay unattended on a hard straw mattress, medicines were dished out in a haphazard fashion from huge pots with little regard to prescription. The *Lancet*'s visitors pondered how good men with fine aspirations could ignore the frightful conditions. They concluded that the Guardians, the Medical Officer and the Master were 'deadened by long routine'.

This dynamite prose was immediately picked up by *The Morning Advertiser* and *The Times*.[53] The Shoreditch Guardians, as inert a body of men as many other Boards in London, were forced to respond publicly and made much of the progress of the new building, defending the care of imbeciles who they said were 'often taken out in vans into the Forest' for their amusement.[54] They could point to the elegant brand new Offices of the Poor as evidence of their commitment. This stinging public humiliation did the Shoreditch Guardians a power of good. They made major investments, smartened up their public image and commissioned a suitably impressive facade and fashionable mansard 'French chateau' style roof for their new workhouse infirmary building. The *Lancet* had achieved with one article what the Poor Law Inspectors and Lunacy Commissioners had failed to in a decade of reports.

The *Lancet* men concluded: 'the conditions of imbeciles in London workhouses is a deeply painful subject' and blamed the London Guardians for the 'monstrous deficiencies'.[55] Both the Lunacy Commissioners and the self-appointed Lancet Commissioners demonized the Guardians, perhaps unfairly given the cash constraints of the rating system and their impoverished populations. The Lunacy Commissioners deplored the 'disposition to withdraw them from the protection of the lunacy laws and place them under the irresponsible care of the Guardians', language that fifteen years earlier would have been unthinkable.[56] The unions were working with a per-capita budget less than half that available to the Magistrates and modest compared to the budget creamed off later from the Metropolitan Common Poor Fund by the Metropolitan Asylums Board.

The dull hand of central directive had curbed the initiative and enthusiasm of even the best Guardians by the late 1860s. In London, energetic men seeking influence and a challenge had been absorbed by the Boards of Works established in 1855 under the central direction of the Metropolitan Board of Works. 'Public Health' had become a matter of sanitary engineering, clean water and fragrant air.[57] Men interested in the relations between poverty, social justice and health care had been sidelined or converted to the religion of sewers and fine buildings, leaving the Guardians to mop up the spillage of human frailty.[58] Union doctors initially imbued with revolutionary fervour like John Tripe in Hackney, Robert Barnes in Shoreditch and John Liddle in Whitechapel, abandoned their parish 'primary care' role to become employed by the local Boards of Works. In London pauper children were shipped out of town to large residential schools in the newer suburbs such as Norwood and Enfield. The Metropolitan Guardians were left with the sick and the mad.

The old Lunacy Commissioners' cry for more, more, more lunatic places was never satisfied.[59] East London Guardians coped with the burgeoning numbers of mentally dependent paupers by expanding their own workhouses, building new separate workhouse infirmaries as decreed by the Poor Law Board in 1863 and by energetic tracking of 'relieved' and 'recovered' patients through the county asylums and licensed houses, to ensure no-one occupied a place a week longer than was necessary. Lacking in imagination and characteristically inert over policy, the Guardians could be fleet of foot over economics.

Gathorne-Hardy, the newly appointed President of the Poor Law Board, noted with some alarm in 1866 that the London workhouses contained 14,000 people who should not be there, including the 'old and infirm' and fifty children and 2,000 adults classed as insane.[60] He regarded these highly dependent paupers with specialized needs as an unfortunate cause of the overcrowding which lay at the root of most workhouse evils. Gathorne-Hardy cleverly presented his plans for the creation of 'auxiliary asylums' as an endorsement of the Lunacy Commission's recommendation. In effect however the new institutions were to be administered not by the Justices but by a new organization, a District Asylums Board, a hybrid creature ingeniously designed to incorporate local representation elected from the Boards of Guardians but with a healthy core of fifteen central Poor Law Board nominees.

The Metropolitan Poor Bill was primarily designed to address the pressing political demands for decent infirmaries for the 21,000 sick paupers in metropolitan workhouses and the recurrent outbreaks of smallpox, cholera and other fevers. The Bill proposed an entirely new system of medical governance for London that effectively imposed central control over planning but appeared to provide safeguards on local government autonomy. Lunatics, children over two, fever and smallpox cases were to be removed altogether, to new institutions under the management of a central body. All other sick paupers would be provided for in separate workhouse infirmaries in the local district, which would be under the direction of asylum district committees accountable to the new central Board.

The new Metropolitan Common Poor Fund was understandably popular in the East End since the burden of poor relief was to be apportioned between parishes and unions on a proportional basis more evenly according to demand. While the cherished link between local rates and local relief was to be severed, this was highly advantageous to impoverished areas. Since the Common Poor Fund would bear centrally the costs of maintaining infectious and insane patients not only in the new asylums but also in county asylums and private licensed houses, significant potential was created for shifting the cost burden. Many who would previously have been carted off to the workhouse 'refractory' wards could be re-labelled with the approval of the Lunacy Commissioners and handed over to become a charge on the common budget. The Common Fund was available to all paupers with a medical certificate declaring that 'the pauper is a chronic and harmless lunatic, idiot or imbecile'. No wonder the rate of 'insanity' rose dramatically in London over the next few years.[61]

Since the imbecile asylums did not fall within the jurisdiction of the Lunacy Acts for the purposes of certification of patients, the expense and inconvenience of hiring a doctor external to the workhouse to give an opinion and then petitioning the magistrate, the required procedure for a county lunatic asylum, was made simpler. In its place, certification for the imbecile asylums required a simple triple declaration by a relieving officer, the workhouse or district medical officer and a Guardian, that the pauper fitted the criteria for admission.[62] It was all too easy. At the same time, the Poor Law Board had acquired a mechanism for coercing the Guardians into acceding to other central demands through the operation of their powers to veto all capital expenditure through the new board.

Gathorne-Hardy's Bill was ingenious and politically astute. It chained the Guardians to central imperatives but at the same time it created the impression of greater Guardian participation in central decision making; a brilliant piece of administrative sleight-of-hand. The proposed arrangements provided for the erection of new cheaper institutions and gave the Guardians the notion that they were retaining some control over policy and costs. The Metropolitan Poor Act of 1867 was a serious blow to the Lunacy Commissioners. The Bill was clearly designed to sidestep the Lunacy Act and stop the Justices widening their influence over matters of lunacy.[63] Two huge cheap imbecile asylums were built by the Asylums Board, one south of the river at Caterham, Surrey and one in the north at Leavesden, Hertfordshire. Designed to take 1,500 paupers each they were rapidly expanded to absorb the free-for-all created by the Common Poor Fund. Within five years they together had nearly 4,000 beds. Architecturally featureless, barrack-like, with symmetrical blocks of identical wards, these warehouses stand as a testament to mean-spirited committee thrift.

The Act of 1867 was followed in London by a series of structural changes to the metropolitan parishes and unions designed to create organizations of sufficient size to make efficient use of existing workhouses and sustain the new district sick infirmaries. The new workhouse infirmaries became general hospitals. The chronic sick and old were left behind in the grimmer old workhouses, together with manageable epileptics, severely disabled accident victims, those with degenerative disease, the quietly mentally infirm who would look misplaced in the old county or new Metropolitan Asylums, even allowing for the widening admission criteria of the latter. Workhouse inmates received a poorer quality of care, had less staff and very few doctors or trained nurses. The development of the 'hospital service' barely touched the old workhouses, which remained dumping grounds for the decrepit long after the advent of the National Health Service in 1948.

Paralysis and legalism 1871 to 1890

The pattern of care in the metropolis was beginning to diverge from the rest of England and Wales. The financial inducement offered by the Common Poor Fund 'has greatly contributed to swell the removals from workhouses to asylums'.[64] There was no equivalent act outside of London and unions made no special provision for the care of imbeciles. Especially in Lancashire and Yorkshire, the increase in inmates of unsound mind in workhouses continued to grow, so much so that Rochdale Guardians fitted up an asylum inside the workhouse.[65] After the Lancet reports however the Poor Law Board strived to improve workhouses as receptacles for the chronically insane and imbeciles. A circular of 1868 specifically recommended an improved dietary for 'imbeciles and suckling women' similar to that permitted for the aged.[66]

In 1871 the Poor Law Board was subsumed under the new Local Government Board but retained many of the old Poor Law inspectors, whose doctrinaire culture cleaved uncomfortably from the sporadic bouts of humanitarianism that characterized the presidents and senior figures of the new Board.[67] While the object of the inspectors was to reduce the increasing outdoor relief bill, the consequent denial of medical relief as an out-patient led to incessant pressure on beds in the new workhouse infirmaries.[68] The central Board sanctioned the building of an unprecedented number of infirmary beds to address the demand. The number of general hospital, that is union infirmary, beds, rose in London at an even faster rate than lunatic asylum places between 1870 and 1900.[69]

An enabling Act of 1886 encouraged unions throughout England and Wales to build special idiot asylums but very few did. In 1889, boarding out regulations assisted unions to maintain imbeciles and chronic lunatics on out-relief at home with their families and in the same Act, medical officers were obliged to sanction that 'persons of unsound mind' retained in the workhouse were suitably placed there. In reality this was no more than recognition that there were at least 5,000 insane still maintained in workhouses in dubious accommodation.[70] The Local Government Act of 1888 transferred the statutory authority for persons of unsound mind from the unions and county justices to the new County Councils. London County Council did not however have any jurisdiction over the Metropolitan Asylum Board facilities and the dual system of institutions continued in London. The ambitious asylum-building programme initiated by the LCC Asylums Committee finally had the effect the Lunacy Commissioners desired. While the proportion of pauper lunatics resident in workhouses outside London remained at about 16 per cent, the percentage in London fell by the end of the century to 2 per cent.[71] Shaftesbury's life-long ambition to get all insane patients out of the clutches of the Guardians had come to fruition at last, at least in London, a decade or so after his death.

The Lunacy Act of 1890 consolidated the various statutes and provisions for all categories of insanity into one detailed whole, tying up loose ends, protecting against improper detention; in Jones' words, a 'triumph of legalism' over the informality and open encouragement to treatment and care advocated by the medical profession and the Lunacy Commission.[72] Another forty years passed before voluntary treatment and informal care were encouraged by government statute.

Conclusions

The Guardians did not explore what exactly was done to pauper insane patients in the workhouse by their doctors. There is scarcely a mention of the technicalities of medical treatment of the insane. Administrators managed the money and were interested in those aspects of care that influenced cost, that is the number and choice of placements. Clinical care was not their business, although they did regard the physical environment and general daily regime as their concern. Parish and union doctors regarded mental illness as part of their core business and some, like Joseph Rogers, who worked in Strand and Westminster Unions, said an encounter with insanity provided 'an agreeable episode in my daily ration of all but thankless routine'.[73]

From 1853 Poor Law medical officers were obliged to visit and report quarterly to the Poor Law Board on pauper lunatics in workhouses.[74] Union doctors' responsibilities were extended in 1870 to the obligatory examination of all pauper lunatics on admission and discharge from the workhouse or workhouse infirmary and to keeping a report book for inspection by the Commissioners in Lunacy. The St Leonard Shoreditch Register for 1870–74 documented the name, age, diagnosis, date of discharge and destination of the 100 to 150 or so cases a year, providing a brief profile of mentally disordered patients in the workhouse infirmary and documenting their comings and goings.[75] Mr Forbes, the medical officer in Shoreditch responsible for keeping up the admissions report book, seems to have used Bucknill and Tuke's classification scheme in their standard popular text, *Psychological Medicine*.[76] By 1870 Bucknill and Tuke's text was the standard work. Neither of the other popular diagnostic schema of the period, Conolly's and Monro's, had distinctive, readily applicable rules which could be used in the kind of hectic environment that workhouse infirmary doctors worked in.[77] Forbes' nomenclature is very similar to Bucknill and Tuke's.

Using Bucknill and Tuke's categories, Forbes' diagnoses of the 260 lunatics admitted to the workhouse infirmary in 1870–71 reveal that a significant proportion of workhouse admissions (39 per cent) was suffering from the kind of insanity that an asylum doctor would recognize as 'a suitable case for treatment'. What inmates received in the way of medicines however is unknown. Few prescription records exist for these inmates. Union doctors brought their own drugs and kept no official records. The insane may with luck have escaped the heroic doses of emetics, aperients, calomel and sedatives which made up the staple of asylum doctors' prescribing.

Throughout the period, diagnostic distinctions between those with acquired insanity, whether 'recent' or 'chronic', and those with developmental mental impairment from early childhood, that is, 'imbecility' were of increasing importance. The care provided to imbeciles was defined as requiring separate but notably less expensive facilities, fewer staff and less doctoring. The hierarchy of classes of insanity placed imbeciles firmly at the bottom, from which they emerged only a century later.

The importance and complexity of the Poor Law in the process of institutionalization in all its forms is now better understood. Bartlett's study in the Midlands suggested that the magistracy, at the pinnacle of the Poor Law administration, were key players in determining how the insane were managed but in London at least the picture was more complex.[78] Centrally the Poor Law lay at the heart of all policy concerned with the sick, mentally dependent and destitute alike and the insane were merely one group of many to be accommodated and dealt with, hence the friction and rivalry between central agencies responsible for implementing policy. At a local level, the workhouse was the fixed centre at the heart of institutional care as it was for all other dependent people, even after the creation and growth of public lunatic asylums. In London, the magistracy had little overall influence on who was admitted to which institution, the parish and union offices chased the most convenient and cheapest vacancy, although magistrates exercised their right to interfere with the committal process on some occasions. There was little love lost between the magistrates and Poor Law officers; they were consulted as little as possible, even though they were ostensibly responsible for running the asylums through their committees.

Until financial incentive structures in the late nineteenth century made it attractive to transfer the care of the insane into specialist institutions, the majority of admission cases and a significant proportion of the continuing care patients were treated wholly in the workhouse, often with kindliness and concern but all too often in huge, featureless, poorly equipped and inadequately staffed wards, ill-designed to promote sanity in even the most robust character. Some doctors and officers took an interest in insanity, but for most, the job was one of containing difficult behaviour, ensuring that the diet was adequate and that the routine of the workhouse was not disturbed.

Notes

1 M. E. Rose (ed.), *The Poor and the City: The English Poor Law in its Urban Context 1834–1914*, Leicester: Leicester University Press, 1985, p. 9.
2 P. Bartlett, *The Poor Law of Lunacy: The Administration of Pauper Lunatics in mid-Nineteenth-Century England*, London: Leicester University Press, 1999. Chapter 4, 'The Pragmatics of Coexistence: Local Officials and Pauper Lunacy', pp. 112–150.
3 E. Murphy, 'The Lunacy Commissioners and the East London Guardians, 1845–1867', *Medical History*, 46, 2002: pp. 495–524; E. Murphy, 'The New Poor Law Guardians and the Administration of Insanity in East London 1834–1844', *Bulletin of the History of Medicine*, 77, 2003, pp. 45–74.
4 P. Bartlett, 'The Asylum, the Workhouse and the Voice of the Insane Poor', *International Journal of Law and Psychiatry*, 21, 1998, pp. 421–432; Murphy, 'The New Poor Law Guardians'.
5 J. Robins, *Fools and Mad: A History of the Insane in Ireland*, Dublin: Institute of Public Administration, 1986, p. 80; O. Walsh, 'Race, Religion and Irish Insanity', in J. Melling and B. Forsythe (eds), *Insanity, Institutions and Society, 1800–1914: A Social History of Madness in Comparative Perspective*, London: Routledge, 1999, pp. 223–242.
6 See for example: Shoreditch Workhouse Admission Books, vols 4 and 5, 1854–70, London Metropolitan Archive, film X20/170.
7 C. Dickens, 'A Walk in the Workhouse', *Household Words* 25 May 1850, pp.

204–207; C. Dickens, 'The Uncommercial Traveller', *All the Year Round* 18 February 1860.

8 E. Murphy, 'The Administration of Insanity in East London 1800–1870' (unpublished PhD thesis, University of London, 2000), pp. 139–140.

9 Dickens, 'The Uncommercial Traveller'.

10 Report of the Metropolitan Commissioners in Lunacy, British Parliamentary Papers [HL], 1844, xxvi, I, p. 4.

11 Further Report of the Commissioners in Lunacy, British Parliamentary Papers, 1847–48, xxxii, 371, pp. 2, 11, 55, 56.

12 Report of the Metropolitan Commissioners in Lunacy, British Parliamentary Papers [HL], 1844, xxvi, pp. 10, 43.

13 Report of the Metropolitan Commissioners in Lunacy, pp. 95–101, 136.

14 Numbers of Insane Persons Confined in Asylums, Hospitals and Licensed Houses on 1st January 1852, Appendix A, Seventh Annual Report of the Commissioners in Lunacy, British Parliamentary Papers, 1852–53, xlix, I, pp. 38–42.

15 2nd Annual Report of the Committee of Visitors of Colney Hatch Asylum, 1854, Appendix 6, General Summary Returns of Pauper Lunatics in Middlesex 1850–52 (1851 figures collected six months after the opening of Middlesex County Lunatic Asylum at Colney Hatch), London Metropolitan Archive, H11/HLL/A/05/014.

16 2nd Annual Report of the Committee of Visitors of Colney Hatch Asylum, 1854, London Metropolitan Archive, H11/HLL/A/05/014, p. 10.

17 Hackney and Stoke Newington Union Minutes of Meetings, Board of Guardians, 1851, London Metropolitan Archive, Ha BG 11, pp. 484ff.

18 E. D. Myers, 'Workhouse or Asylum: The Nineteenth Century Battle for the Care of the Pauper Insane', *Psychiatric Bulletin*, 22, 1998, pp. 575–577. See Table 1, Lunatics Chargeable to Poor Law Unions in England and Wales 1842–1910, p. 576.

19 D. R. Green, *From Artisans to Paupers: Economic Change and Poverty in London 1790–1870*, Aldershot: Scolar Press, 1995, Chapter 8 'The Crisis of Poor Relief', pp. 210–247, 217–223.

20 Green, *Artisans to Paupers*, pp. 212–216.

21 Green, *Artisans to Paupers*, p. 242.

22 Letter from Commissioners in Lunacy to the Poor Law Board 1 February 1862, PRO MH19 Accounts and papers 1860–80 no. 23, vol. LXI, ms 397.

23 Minutes of Meetings of the Commissioners in Lunacy 1845–March 1851, Public Record Office, series MH50/1–4, indexed MH50/40,41; Correspondence between the Poor Law Board and the Lunacy Commissioners, Public Record Office, series MH19/168, 169, 170; Legal Opinions relating to workhouses requested by Lunacy Commissioners, Public Record Office, series MH51/749,760; Miscellaneous Home Office Papers referring to lunatics and the Poor Law Board, Public Record Office series HO45, see particularly 6686, 7269, 7102, 7512, 7520, 7751, 7592.

24 4th Annual Report of the Commissioners in Lunacy, British Parliamentary Papers 1850 [291], xxiii, 363, pp. 13–14.

25 Correspondence between the Poor Law Board and the Lunacy Commissioners, Public Record Office, series MH19/168, 169, 170.

26 Correspondence, Secretary to the Lunacy Commission to Assistant Secretary Poor Law Board, Public Record Office, MH19/168.

27 6th Annual Report of the Commissioners in Lunacy, British Parliamentary Papers, 1851 [668], xxiii, 353, Appendix D, Visits to workhouses pp. 20–21.

28 Return of Unions in which Sane are intermixed with the Insane and where Lunatic Wards have been Established, Numbers of Lunatics in Each Separate Ward together with Number of Lunatics Received into Workhouses from

January 1861 to January 1862, in 16th Annual Report of the Commissioners in Lunacy, British Parliamentary Papers, 1862 [417], xxiii, I, Appendix G, p. 217.

29 Supplementary Report to the 12th Annual Report of the Commissioners in Lunacy, Evidence to the Select Committee on Lunatics, British Parliamentary Papers, 1859, Session 1 (228) IX, p. 1.

30 Andrew Doyle's Evidence to the Select Committee on Lunatics 1859, 2nd Session, British Parliamentary Papers, (156) VII, pp. 501, 156.

31 Lunacy Laws Amendment Act, 1862 (25 & 26 Vic., c. 111, s. 8).

32 R. Hodgkinson, 'Provision for Pauper Lunatics 1834–1871', *Medical History*, 10, 1966, pp. 138–154.

33 G. M. Ayers, *England's First State Hospitals and the Metropolitan Asylums Board 1867–1930*, London: Wellcome Institute for the History of Medicine, 1971, Chapter 4 *'England's First Imbecile Asylums'*, p. 41.

34 3rd Annual Report of the Commissioners in Lunacy, British Parliamentary Papers, 1849 [1028], xxii, p. 381; Supplementary Report on Workhouses, Appendix A, 1847–48, xxxii, p. 371; 6th Annual Report of the Commissioners in Lunacy, British Parliamentary Papers, 1851 [668], xxiii, 353, Appendix D, Visits to Workhouses, p. 20.

35 A. Scull, *The Most Solitary of Afflictions: Madness and Society in Britain 1700–1900*, New Haven: Yale University Press, 1993, p. 372.

36 Scull, *Most Solitary of Afflictions*, pp. 370–373.

37 'The Medico-Psychological Association', *Lancet*, II, 1865, p. 97.

38 P. Bartlett, 'The Asylum, the Workhouse and the Voice of the Insane Poor', pp. 421–432; 15th Annual Report of the Commissioners in Lunacy, British Parliamentary Papers, 1861 [314], xxvii, I, p. 47.

39 Reports of Commissioners in Lunacy to the Poor Law Board on the State of Imbecile Wards in the Metropolitan Workhouses and of the Correspondence Between, Public Record Office, MH19, Accounts and Papers no. 23, vol. LXI 1867, 194–444 (hereafter 'Imbecile Wards in the Metropolitan Workhouses').

40 B. Forsythe, J. Melling and R. Adair, 'Politics of Lunacy: Central State Regulation and the Devon Pauper Lunatic Asylum, 1845–1914', in Melling and Forsythe (eds), *Insanity, Institutions and Society, 1800–1914*, pp. 68–87.

41 F. P. Cobbe, 'The Philosophy of the Poor Law and the Report of the Committee on Poor Relief', *Fraser's Magazine*, 70, 1864, quoted in A. W. Coats (ed.), *Poverty in the Victorian Age: Debates on the Issue from 19th Century Critical Journals*, vol. 2 English Poor Laws 1834–1870, Farnborough: Gregg International, 1973, pp. 373–394.

42 Letters between Shaftesbury, the Secretary of State and City of London Guardians, 6th Annual Report of the Commissioners in Lunacy, British Parliamentary Papers, 1851 [668], xxiii, 353, pp. 9–10; 7th Annual Report of the Commissioners in Lunacy British Parliamentary Papers, 1852–53, xlix, I, p. 10; 8th Annual Report of the Commissioners in Lunacy, British Parliamentary Papers, 1854 [339], xxix, I, p. 27.

43 'Imbecile Wards in the Metropolitan Workhouses' 1867, p. 194; 'Lancet Sanitary Commission for Investigating the State of Infirmaries in Workhouses: I Metropolitan Workhouses', *Lancet*, II, 1865, pp. 14–22.

44 'Editorial', *Lancet*, I, 1869, pp. 130–131.

45 *Lancet*, I, 1869, pp. 224–251.

46 Figure from Shoreditch Workhouse Admission Books, vol. 5, 1862–70, London Metropolitan Archive, film X20/170.

47 'Imbecile Wards in Metropolitan Workhouses, 1867', pp. 356–361.

48 The joke was that Baker, though a popular and impressively fair union administrator, got paid for each coronial case he heard.

49 Dickens, 'The Uncommercial Traveller', p. 393.

50 Stepney Union Board of Guardians' Minutes of Meetings, London Metropolitan Archives, St.BG/L/16, 13 May 1851, p. 9.
51 'Lancet Sanitary Commission', *Lancet*, II, 1865, pp. 1914–1922.
52 'Lancet Sanitary Commission Visit to St Leonard's Shoreditch, Metropolitan Workhouses III', *Lancet*, II, 1865, pp. 131–133.
53 *The Morning Advertiser* 5 August 1865 and *The Times* 12 August 1865.
54 'Report on Complaints in The Times by the Clerk to Shoreditch Guardians', *Lancet*, I 1865, pp. 187–189.
55 *Lancet*, I, 1867, pp. 215–216.
56 21st Annual Report of the Commissioners in Lunacy, British Parliamentary Papers, 1867 [367], xviii, p. 201.
57 C. Hamlin, *Public Health and Social Justice in the Age of Chadwick: Britain, 1800–1854*, Cambridge: Cambridge University Press, 1998, Conclusion, pp. 335–341.
58 Hamlin, *Public Health and Social Justice*, Introduction, pp. 12–15.
59 P. McCandless, 'Build! Build! The Controversy over the Care of the Chronically Insane in England 1855–70', *Bulletin of the History of Medicine* 53, 1979, pp. 553–574.
60 *Hansard*, vol. clxxxv (3rd series), 8 February 1867, cols 161–170.
61 For a detailed description of the operation of Metropolitan Asylums Board (MAB) finances and the Common Fund, see Ayers, *England's First State Hospitals*, Appendix IV, pp. 313–317.
62 Ayers, *England's First State Hospitals*, 'Poor Law Board Regulations 1870', footnote 1, p. 42.
63 22nd Annual Report of the Commissioners in Lunacy, British Parliamentary Papers, 1867–68 [332], xxxi, p. 47.
64 24th Annual Report of the Commissioners in Lunacy, British Parliamentary Papers, 1870 [340], xxxiv, I, p. 47.
65 S. and B. Webb, *English Poor Law Policy*, London: Frank Cass & Co., 1963 (first published by Longman Green, 1910), pp. 125, 222.
66 Circular, 7 December 1868, quoted in 21st Annual Report of the Poor Law Board, British Parliamentary Papers, 1868–69 [4197], xxviii, I, pp. 41–44.
67 Sidney and Beatrice Webb, *English Poor Law Policy*, p. 148.
68 8th Annual Report of the Local Government Board, British Parliamentary Papers, 1878–79 [2681], xxvi, I, p. 91.
69 P. Cowan, 'Some Observations Concerning the Increase in Hospital Provision in London between 1850 and 1960', *Medical History*, 14, 1970, pp. 42–52.
70 Lunacy Acts Amendment Act 1889 (52 & 53 Vic., c. 41, s. 22–25 and s. 40).
71 A. Cochrane, '"Humane, Economical and Medically Wise", the LCC as Administrators of Victorian Lunacy Policy', in W. F. Bynum, R. Porter and M. Shepherd (eds), *The Anatomy of Madness: Essays in the History of Psychiatry*, vol. 3, London: Routledge, 1998, pp. 247–272.
72 K. Jones, *A History of Mental Health Services*, London: Routledge and Kegan Paul, 1972, p. 153.
73 N. Longmate, *The Workhouse*, London: Temple Smith, 1974, p. 214.
74 Lunatic Asylums Act 1853 (16 & 17 Vic., c. 97, s. 6).
75 Medical Officers Report Book of Lunatics in Workhouses, Shoreditch Board of Guardians, London Metropolitan Archive, Sh BG 138, 1870–74.
76 J. C. Bucknill and D. H. Tuke, *A Manual of Psychological Medicine*, London: Churchill, 1858, pp. 72–89.
77 J. Conolly, *The Treatment of the Insane without Mechanical Restraint*, London: Smith Elder, 1856, pp. 45–68; H. Monro, 'On the Classification of Forms of Insanity', *Asylum Journal of Mental Science*, 3, 1857, pp. 193–218.
78 Bartlett, 'The Asylum, the Workhouse and the Voice of the Insane Poor'.

3 Needs and desires in the care of pauper lunatics
Admissions to Worcester Asylum, 1852–72

Frank Crompton

Introduction

Many recent studies of the lunatic asylum in the nineteenth century have addressed the familiar question of the true purpose of these institutions within the societies which arranged their construction.[1] The tensions between the efficient and economical management of such large, frequently expensive, establishments and the therapeutic goals of individual care figure in case studies such as Cherry's recent account of the Norfolk Asylum. In that study the author suggests that the absence of popular campaigns in support of such reforms as the 1845 Lunacy Acts left the question of standards and care to be determined 'by socially dominant minorities'.[2] Such an interpretation may be contrasted with the strong emphasis placed on the influence of family and kinship groups as well as non-asylum provision by scholars such as Bartlett and Wright.[3] Such debates enable scholars to locate the asylum more firmly within the network of elite and kinship relations which bound together contemporary society, though they also shift the locus of debate away from the internal workings of the establishment and the therapeutic community which existed within the walls of the institution. If we are to assess the effectiveness of care provided by the lunatic asylum and the extent to which it functioned as a curative institution for individuals suffering from insanity (construed according to contemporary assumptions about normality), then we need to investigate the terms in which they were understood and treated within its boundaries as well as the external pressures exerted on the institution. The outcome of unequal struggles between the aspirations and interests of different groups inside and outside the institution depended on particular circumstances, though the concerns of families were frequently muted or stifled and often subordinated to more urgent and powerful agents.

Recovering the patient's experience of a Victorian asylum requires a sensitive reading of the voluminous body of records, almost all compiled by legal and medical personalities. In a rarely cited study of an American lunatic asylum, J. L. Moreno's *Who Shall Survive* used 'sociometric' tools to show that many inmates developed meaningful personal relationships, including an approval or disapproval of the behaviour of their peers within the asylum community.[4] The clients of the institution influenced but did not direct its development. Those managing the institution were inevitably required to balance the therapeutic needs of the inmates against a range of other considerations, including public safety and attitudes towards those resident within the asylum. The inmates themselves often needed protection from the dangerous behaviour of other residents. Care and control was not merely exercised on behalf of those managing the establishment or those beyond its frontiers. The basis for the management of those admitted to the asylum can be traced to the diagnoses agreed in the early period of their entry to the institution. Historians of insanity have been sensitive to the generalized and imprecise character of medical description, though the terms in which an individual was depicted was vitally important. For as Lees has recently noted in her examination of the Poor Law, 'treatment by classification' provided the key to the workings of such establishments in the nineteenth century.[5] In this respect we need to understand the classification and treatment of individuals not only in terms of the contemporary diagnoses made by the medical staff but also the likely impact of their behaviour on others within the institution and on wider society should they be released.

Such an approach distinguishes between the management concerns of the medical personnel within the institution, the political interests of the elites who were responsible for the legal governance of the asylum, demands made by families and kinship groups, and the needs and desires of those who were confined within the establishment. One approach adopted in the present study has been to identify the therapeutic needs of those admitted to the asylum in accordance with Maslow's famous hierarchy of needs: the primary concern was to meet physiological needs such as hunger and thirst, followed by the need for security, succeeded by needs for acceptance and for esteem within a community, leading to the fulfilment of cognitive understanding of the environment and finally the self-fulfilment of the person.[6] Preliminary examination of the sources indicated that the application of such a hierarchy of needs required the exclusion of the highest levels of self-fulfilment which were not expected of the inmates prior to a declaration of recovery. It was also apparent that the analysis of patient records should take into account not only the perception of the patient's capacity to engage in the asylum community by gregarious behaviour but also the prevailing model of the human condition adopted by the senior medical staff. The Powick Asylum examined in this chapter embraced the principles of moral treatment developed by the Tukes at York Retreat and other prominent psychiatrists in the late eighteenth and early nineteenth centuries. Within the constraints of a large and expanding county asylum, these ideals were pursued in the early decades at Powick as they were at many other institutions.[7]

The Worcester Asylum

An analysis of patient records at Powick suggests that the process of classification progressed during the residence of the individual and where the
aspirations of patients were viewed as illegitimate or unimportant then
these were translated as 'desires' rather than as 'needs'. The implication
was that the institution was under less, or no, obligation to meet these
demands than the legitimate needs which were perceived and presented as
conducive to the care and recovery of the person concerned. Unreason-
able desires were also portrayed as a threat to the smooth running of the
Asylum in a number of instances. Whereas a number of 'dements' at
Powick were described as enjoying only an 'animal existence', or the even
less alert 'vegetative existence', and others required forcible feeding, they
were a limited minority of the total patient population and these conditions were frequently identified in the late decline of an inmate and were
rarely if ever present on admission. Most of those who entered the
Worcester Asylum were capable of expressing and meeting basic requirements. We may say that there existed some rudimentary exchange
between the conversations of the inmates and the staff responsible for
their classification and treatment.

The research method adopted in the present study was to investigate in
detail approximately 3,000 individuals admitted to the Powick Asylum in
the second half of the nineteenth century. A textual search was applied to
each patient record, sorting the key words used to describe the inmates
and distinguishing those terms applied to each sex as well as common
words and phrases used to characterize both genders. The aim was not to
provide a retrospective diagnosis but rather to summarize the forms of
behaviour which were associated with particular kinds of classification. It
is argued that this process of classifying the individuals was influenced not
only by medical criteria but was also informed by the management considerations of the institution and critically by assumptions and observations
relating to the social status and expectations of the individual. In this sense
the construction of the internal asylum community was the work of those
assessing the characteristics of people admitted, as well as the responses of
the individual to the environment in which they found themselves. The
findings are discussed within the narrative of the institution's development
provided below.

The Worcester City and County Pauper Lunatic Asylum was built to
fulfil the County's obligations under the 1845 Lunatic Asylums Act,
although it did not open until 1852.[8] An attempt to organize a joint asylum
with Herefordshire failed and a partnership between the county and city
was created instead. This led to the location of the county asylum at
Powick, about two miles west of the borough of Worcester, though this
was not a central point in the county or near its most densely populated
areas.[9] The Poor Law Board approved the thirty-acre site, and the later

addition of a 155-acre farm to provide employment for inmates, conforming to contemporary rhetoric which depicted Powick as a curative institution that would restore patients to health and the local community. Census returns indicated that there were about 180 lunatics maintained by the Poor Law or in private mad-houses within the county. Designed to house 200 inmates, Powick Asylum became an early source of tension between a Lunacy Commission which insisted on adequate curative facilities and the Poor Law Board, reinforced by local ratepayers, which insisted on strict economy in its construction.[10]

The architecture of the new premises reflected some of these competing concerns as well as a concern to maintain medical and personal vigilance of the inmates. Long wards were provided for those held there alongside single locked rooms for violent or intransigent individuals, the whole building being bounded by a corridor from which the Medical Superintendent and his staff could survey the inmates within the Asylum. The original structure of Powick shaped the subsequent development of facilities for inmates in Worcester Asylum, two distinct wings of two (later three) storeys housing male and female inmates. Modelled on Pentonville Prison, the Asylum offered pleasant views of the surrounding countryside from windows on its upper floors as well as open vistas from some of its grounds, gardens and airing-courts. Powick's wards were strictly segregated by gender and with distinct accommodation for those diagnosed with a variety of manias, melancholias, 'dementia' and idiots or imbeciles, including some inmates who suffered severe epileptic fits.[11] Staff were allocated to different wards, including those reserved for inmates said to have 'dirty' habits (including incontinence), while the Asylum Hospital was usually reserved for patients who were physically ill or infirm. The wards, excluding the hospital-wards and the dirty-wards, had galleries, together with four single rooms; two of them padded, and an adjacent day-room, which doubled as a dining-room, work-room and recreation-room. There was also a kitchen, scullery and pantry for each ward, and a corridor, used by staff, connected the wards within a wing to each other, offering access to store-rooms. Airing-courts were entered via a lockable door to control access. Mixed social activities were only encouraged for selected patients who could be trusted to behave in an acceptable way whilst not closely supervised.

The planned environment within the Powick Asylum appears to have been designed to structure not only the behaviour of inmates but also the movement of the attendant staff under the supervision of its head. The composure of the medical notes and the prescription of treatment was the responsibility of the Medical Superintendent and his assistants, though the observations of the attendants who staffed the wards also found their way into the notes compiled for individual inmates.[12] The Medical Superintendent was responsible for appointing his subordinates, though the Visiting Committee of magistrates filled such significant posts as that of the Anglican chaplain to the Asylum. Dr Grahamsley, the first Medical Superintendent appointed to Powick, was trained and had experience in the Scottish Lunatic Asylum system. He was well aware of the adaptations necessary to apply 'moral treatment' in a large public lunatic asylum. The records of Powick indicate a strong adherence to these principles throughout the years 1852 to 1872, and even later, though its sparse staffing levels and practice of leaving only one attendant on duty in each ward during the night attracted the criticism of the Lunacy Commissioners. These attendants were poorly paid and were given little or no formal training though their duties were frequently onerous. Turnover of attendants remained a problem though a core remained for considerable periods of time.

When Worcester City and County Pauper Lunatic Asylum opened in August 1852, it began to admit pauper lunatics who had been housed in a variety of institutions or had been identified within the homes of their families or other relatives and friends. After the 1834 Poor Law Amendment Act these individuals were held in the union workhouses and their relatives frequently received outdoor relief for their upkeep, with the most troublesome and violent cases placed in lunatic asylums where care was more expensive.[13] From its early days the staff at Powick sought to differentiate and classify those admitted according to the categories such as sufferers of dementia (including senile dementia), idiocy, imbecility, mania (often refined to descriptions of acute, chronic, monomania and a variety of other manias), as well as melancholia (see Table 3.1a).[14]

Table 3.1a Admission classes of the patients admitted to Worcester Lunatic Asylum between 1852 and 1872

	Males	*%*	*Females*	*%*		*Total*	*%*
Dementia	380	27.2	354	23.9	Males Females	734	51.8 48.2
Idiocy*	87	6.3	69	4.7	Males Females	156	55.8 44.2
Mania**	785	56.4	821	55.3	Males Females	1,606	51.1 48.9
Melancholia	124	8.9	231	15.6	Males Females	355	34.9 65.1
Others	17	1.2	9	0.5	Males Females	26	65.4 34.6
Total all cases	1,393	100.0	1 484	100.0	Total	2,877	

Source: Worcester City and County Pauper Lunatic Asylum, Powick, Patients' Books.

Notes
*   Including Imbeciles.
** Including Monomania.

These assessments were entered in the columns of the admission registers which all asylums were legally obliged to compile and preserve for the
inspection of visiting Lunacy Commissioners, while the detailed patient
case notes were compiled in different volumes held at the institution. The
Powick admission registers indicate that few inmates were reclassified or
given a fresh diagnosis following their entrance to the Asylum. It is interesting that in approximately thirty cases where inmates were discharged as
cured or recovered, and then readmitted, they were usually diagnosed and
classified in very similar terms and directed to the same ward where they
had formerly been held.

The evidence from Powick indicates that inmates were initially assigned
to particular wards based on an evaluation of their form of lunacy and the
problems of care which they were thought to present. Most inmates
remained in these original wards unless a severe deterioration in their condition or behaviour compelled staff to reallocate them. When particular
wards became overcrowded then individuals seem to have been placed, on
a fairly *ad hoc* basis, in ones where beds were available. In extreme cases,
violent or unruly individuals were transferred not only from particular
wards but to other asylums.

Patient experiences

To understand the creation of an asylum 'community' within an institution
such as Powick, we need to recall the considerable and growing pressure
on the Medical Superintendent to provide care to meet the basic needs of
those admitted. Those arriving were often in a very poor physical as well
as mental condition, having been beaten or injured as a result of their agi-
tated and erratic behaviour or from the abusive attacks of others. Some
individuals arrived without appetite for food and were forcibly fed to
provide basic nourishment.[15] Sustenance available to inmates at Powick
was superior to that obtained in the workhouses, particularly since pauper
asylums were exempt from the Poor Law rule concerning strict diet.[16]
Powick offered many inmates an 'enhanced diet', which might include
beer and other alcoholic beverages, not uncommon among lunatic asylums
at this period.[17]

Attitudes towards the inmates as well as their behaviour were
influenced by the terms in which they were diagnosed or classified and
the wards in which they were placed, though subsequent behaviour
prompted removal of those people who were not conforming with
the basic expectations of staff.[18] From the perspective of the Medical
Superintendent, the Asylum's capacity to provide basic care could be
threatened by the behaviour of a minority of highly disturbed inmates,
which helps to explain their isolation in particular wards and single,
padded rooms, as well as the use of cold baths, opiates and other means
of sedating or confining the violent outbreaks of the unruly. The risk of

violence to both the staff and other inmates remained one of the most important considerations affecting the containment of Powick's residents in these years. An analysis of patient records indicates that those individuals classified as 'dements' frequently posed a serious risk to the staff, particularly in the early years when many chronic cases were admitted after languishing for some time in workhouses and other places where they had received little medical attention (see Table 3.1b). In later years it was more likely for those diagnosed as demented to be admitted only after they had offended public decency or made threats of violence in their family household, local community or in workhouses (see Table 3.1c).[19]

A number of people admitted as suffering from dementia had committed serious violence prior to their arrival and continued to pose a danger to staff and fellow inmates, though this threat was not always apparent in the early years. One inmate died after an epileptic seizure after being confined to bed when he had viciously attacked an attendant, some fifteen years after admission.[20] Twenty-four men diagnosed with dementia displayed violence after their entrance to Powick. Other apparently harmless individuals followed the pattern of later violence, as when William H. killed a fellow inmate in an unprovoked attack some six years after admission.[21] Women who were classified as demented exhibited less violence than men, only three females were recorded as particularly aggressive,

Table 3.1b Admission classes of the first 200 patients admitted to Worcester Lunatic Asylum immediately after the institution opened in August 1852

	Males	%	Females	%		Total	%
Dementia	67	70.5	78	74.3	Males Females	145	46.2 53.8
Idiocy*	3	3.2	5	4.8	Males Females	8	37.0 63.0
Mania**	21	22.1	13	12.4	Males Females	34	61.8 38.2
Melancholia	4	4.2	7	6.7	Males Females	11	36.4 63.6
Others	0	0.0	2	1.8	Males Females	2	0.0 100.0
Total all cases	95	100.0	105	100.0	Total	200	

Source: Worcester City and County Pauper Lunatic Asylum, Powick, Patients' Books.

Notes
* Including Imbeciles.
** Including Monomania.

Table 3.1c Admission classes of the patients admitted to Worcester Lunatic Asylum subsequent to the first 200 committals

	Males	%	Females	%		Total	%
Dementia	312	24.1	276	20.0	Males Females	588	53.0 47.0
Idiocy*	84	6.5	64	4.6	Males Females	148	56.8 43.2
Mania**	765	58.9	808	58.5	Males Females	1,573	48.6 51.4
Melancholia	120	9.3	224	16.2	Males Females	344	34.9 65.1
Others	17	1.2	7	0.7	Males Females	24	65.4 34.6
Total all cases	1,298	100.0	1,379	100.0	Total	2,677	

Source: Worcester City and County Pauper Lunatic Asylum, Powick, Patients' Books.

Notes
* Including Imbeciles.
** Including Monomania.

though they were often reported to be destructive and noisy within the Asylum, and there were a few incidents of serious attacks on staff and inmates. After she was admitted in March 1870, Fanny H. attacked the Assistant Medical Officer in an airing-court, flying at him with 'feet, fists and nails, shouting wildly ... now I'll kill you'.[22]

A much smaller group of admissions in the period 1852–72 were described as 'idiots' or 'imbeciles'.[23] Once again, violence against relatives and neighbours figured prominently in the admission registers and patient notes of these individuals, including seventeen-year-old Edward W., who was certified in March 1868 after he had 'attempted to rape a young girl he met in the road near his home'. The Police Superintendent at the police station where he was brought on arrest, 'knew about his mental state' and he was dispatched to the asylum. Edward remained for fourteen years, before his transfer to Rubery Hill Lunatic Asylum, Birmingham.[24] Female idiots and imbeciles were more often thought to be admitted as children or adolescents unless they were in the kind of moral danger faced by Harriet H. who arrived in 1857, aged sixteen, after sexual assault by a family friend.[25] The idiots and imbeciles presented management difficulties for the staff of the asylum, though sexual aggression towards weaker and younger inmates was more readily identified as a problem than simple violence. Imbeciles were noticeably less violent and threatening than idiots, though masturbation was particularly associated with male imbeciles and females were frequently reported to have removed their clothing.[26] With few idiots and imbeciles employed at labouring tasks on the Asylum estate, this group of inmates tended to be confined to the idiots'-wards and the airing-courts. Individuals such as Jane B. collected rubbish as well as decking themselves 'in the most gorgeous colours and ribbons', attacking anyone who sought to interfere with her finery or other inmates who 'she thinks ... receive more attention than her'.[27] There appears to have been little attempt to provide curative treatment for those characterized as idiots and imbeciles, though some of the 'demented' inmates were put to work.

The group of admissions to Powick which included the most threatening of inmates were those diagnosed and classified as suffering from manias. Many of the early entrants to the Worcester Asylum had been placed in private mad-houses before its opening in 1852.[28] Men suffering from mania had frequently injured relatives or members of the public prior to their committal. John C. from Balsall Heath was only twelve years old when certified as suffering mania and epilepsy in 1868, after he had shown such violence to neighbouring children that he had cut one boy's ear and 'knocked another child down and stamped on it'.[29] Eliza P., a seamstress, was diagnosed as suffering mania after she attempted to poison her illegitimate child in 1865. She was to die in Powick many years later.[30]

Those classified as maniacs (including sufferers from 'monomania') were also seen as significantly more amenable to treatment and recovery than idiots and imbeciles. Only a quarter of the violent males and a fifth of the females who had displayed violence continued to display violence after their admission to Powick.[31] Those who did continue to threaten the order of the Asylum and fellow inmates were secluded and treated with blistering. When William G., the son of a Dudley doctor with a record of assaults on women and asylum committals, came to Powick he became involved in an attempt at a mass escape as well as homosexual activities. Seriously injured in another escape attempt, William remained a continuing risk to the security of the institution until his death some twenty-three years after arriving at the Asylum.[32] An examination of the patient notes for this group of admissions reveals phrases which emphasized the potential disruption of Asylum life posed by maniacs as well as commentaries on their return to normal patterns of behaviour prior to their cure.[33] Frightening delusions were documented, males most frequently claiming aggrandizement of their social station and women frequently expressing fear at the threat of poisoning or serious injury. Maniacs, who were out of control, required constant supervision and clearly proved difficult to manage. They were often extremely noisy, used foul language and had objectionable and destructive habits. They destroyed their bedding, their clothes and the fabric of the asylum building and equipment, sometimes by smearing excrement on themselves and on anything within reach. There was, however, a significant distinction in the description and management of those suffering manias and inmates identified as idiotic or imbecilic. Mania was perceived as a transitory state which was capable of treatment and cure and the capacity for rational conversation and affiliation with other inmates were skills which medical staff saw as vital indicators of their improvement or recovery, more than one third of the patient group being discharged as cured.

Individuals who were certified as suffering from melancholy formed a substantial constituency among those coming to the Worcester Asylum. In contrast to claims made by scholars such as Showalter, the majority of these admissions were males rather than females.[34] In contrast to the maniacs, melancholics were identified as posing greater danger to themselves than to others, although some of those certified were reported to have threatened family members. Suicide was a more common cause of death for them than other inmate groups. Violence against others was not unknown. When Fanny R., a twenty-year-old domestic servant, arrived from Malvern, she was found to be so hysterical that she was periodically isolated in a single room, requiring constant attention because of her propensity to destroy her clothes and kick out at anyone within reach.[35] Other melancholic patients experienced disturbing delusions. Ann S. remained in constant fear that her body was injured and believed that she had given birth to an incredible number of children and animals.[36]

The patient case notes of the Worcester Asylum throw some light on the ways in which the desires, as well as the needs, of its inmates were perceived and represented in the mid-Victorian period. Although these sources made only limited direct references to the sexual and sensual desires of the individuals being cared for within the institution, they included various comments on the 'perversions' displayed by some patients. Daniel Hack Tuke, one of the foremost writers on psychiatry and asylum care in the Victorian years, defined a perversion as an alteration for the worse in 'instincts, feelings, habits, appetite and other previous characteristics of the patient', which was a constant accompaniment of insanity but a peculiar feature of 'moral insanity'.[37] Maniacs of both sexes were frequently noted to have undesirable sexual tendencies, usually implying masturbation in men and 'erotic tendencies' in women. Both were regarded as threats to the 'asylum community', although masturbation was viewed more seriously in the early years because of its supposed association with deteriorating mental health. The delusions of females identified as suffering mania included beliefs concerning their body or sexual organs though they were not presented as erotic inclinations. Betsy B., a housewife aged forty-five from Sparkbrook, was committed in August 1858 suffering from a mania which included her belief that there were 'things and animals in her inside'. These included mangles, sewing machines and other 'ridiculous things in her belly' noted by the Assistant Medical Officer.[38] The impression gained from the entries is that the uncontrolled sexual urges and other delusions of these inmates would cause serious disturbance to the 'asylum community'. Deterrents and healthy activities (asylum sports, recreation and entertainments) were prescribed to address these problems. Melancholic patients were more rarely associated with sexual energy or inclinations, though they did complain more frequently of mistreatment by their attendants and nurses at the Asylum.

There remains the question of the availability and efficacy of treatment at Victorian asylums such as the one established in Worcester. The earlier research of Scull and others argued with some force that these institutions soon failed to redeem the promise of moral treatment and rather than providing a cure for large numbers of inmates, the asylums became mere 'warehouses' for the holding of chronically ill people for whom little or no relief was offered.[39] Other scholars have stressed the porosity of the asylum, as well as the capacity of families and friends to place individuals within the asylum and to provide accommodation for them on their discharge.[40] The perspective taken in this chapter differs from these accounts. The Victorian asylum, it is argued here, retained a statutory responsibility for confining and controlling as well as curing the insane. Violence against relatives, neighbours and the wider community was a recurring theme in the certification of the individuals who were admitted to Powick, alongside the threat of harm to themselves and disgraceful public behaviour. While providing humane and rational treatment of those committed to the asylum, both medical staff and unqualified attendants were expected to manage the incomers in ways which preserved the safety not only of the sufferers but of other inmates and employees. Powick was relatively secure and only a handful of patients escaped. The Worcester Asylum also appears to have met a range of basic needs for different classes of inmates and to have provided treatments which were aimed to protect an internal asylum community as well as manage the behaviour of individuals.

The therapeutic success of the Asylum appears to have been reasonably good if we consider the rate of discharge in these two decades, particularly as some of the early admissions were considered as chronic and intractable cases admitted from private mad-houses and workhouses. More than one third of those who departed from the Asylum were discharged as 'recovered', though substantial numbers of inmates did die within the walls of the institution in the first two decades of its life. Other inmates were discharged to the care of friends 'relieved' or 'not improved' (see Table 3.2).[41]

Only a small number of those completely discharged were re-admitted to Powick in this period, again suggesting a reasonable rate of successful recovery, and possibly the capacity of relatives and communities to engage with those who left the Asylum. Others fared less well, including a number released on a month's trial who returned injured, malnourished and dirty, possibly because their home community could not, or did not wish to, cope

Table 3.2 Outcomes of treatment at Worcester Lunatic Asylum of patients admitted between 1852 and 1872 (total N = 2,877)[1]

Male patients

			Died	State in which patient discharged from the asylum		
				Recovered includes 'cured'	Relieved	Not improved
Dementia	380	N	283	40	25	32
		%	74.2	10.5	6.6	8.7
Idiocy*	87	N	62	6	7	12
		%	71.3	6.9	8.0	13.8
Mania**	780	N	400	292	51	37
		%	51.3	37.4	6.5	4.7
Melancholia	124	N	55	64	4	1
		%	44.4	51.6	3.2	0.8

Female patients

			Died	State in which patient discharged from the asylum		
				Recovered includes 'cured'	Relieved	Not improved
Dementia	354	N	247	52	19	36
		%	69.7	14.7	5.4	10.2
Idiocy*	69	N	54	4	5	6
		%	78.3	5.8	7.2	8.7
Mania**	821	N	351	367	63	40
		%	43.1	44.6	7.6	4.7
Melancholia	231	N	84	132	11	4
		%	36.4	57.1	4.8	1.7

Source: Worcester City and County Pauper Lunatic Asylum, Powick, Patients' Books.

Notes
1 The Worcester City and County Pauper Lunatic Asylum, in the period 1852 to 1914, apparently did not use the standard nomenclature used in Discharge Registers used by other pauper lunatic institution.
* Including Imbecility.
** Including Monomania.
Discharges include patients who were transferred to friends and relatives, who were transferred to workhouses, to other institutions and those who escaped.
Twenty-six inmates, seventeen males and nine females, who were suffering from 'other mental afflictions' are not included in this table neither are five male cases of 'mania' whose records are incomplete.

with them. Having been admitted in many instances because of their threatening behaviour, inmates who returned to their families and neighbours found that they could not achieve the transition from institutional to social life.

The Asylum did seek to provide basic forms of care and sustenance to those housed within its walls. Those identified as demented were provided with a solid diet, occasionally being 'forced with food' as they resisted feeding. Limited participation in the communal life of the institution was possible for those capable of working in the Asylum laundry and at other domestic duties, while all inmates were encouraged to attend the Chapel services on Wednesday and Sunday mornings. The condition of most of those classified as demented deteriorated within a period of their entry, only a limited minority playing any active part in ward life. The patient records indicate that those who did so were regarded as tractable, trustworthy, useful and industrious, so they might be employed in various Asylum departments. Men also took part in entertainments and in various sports, such as bowls and cricket, both sexes walking in the asylum grounds and even outside the institution.

Staff at Powick sought to control offending behaviours and did not expect to transform the condition of idiots and imbeciles. Violence towards themselves and others remained a constant risk, as when Hannah M., who suffered from epilepsy as well as mania, died from severe burns when she fell into a ward fireplace.[42] Threatening inmates tended to be shunned by other patients and staff, though sufferers from mania were also seen as curable. Violent and disruptive inmates were contained, though as the memories of these individuals returned they were encouraged to participate in ward or workshop life and to prove themselves useful and industrious, the quality of women's needlework being used as a significant indicator of their progress. Improvements in sleep, appetite and personal cleanliness were recorded alongside encouragements to read and attend entertainments. In Maslow's terms they were directed towards greater 'personal realization' by assuming positions of trust, as when Walter Edward L. was employed at his former occupation of clerking in the Superintendent's office.[43] An analysis of the patient notes of those diagnosed as suffering from monomania suggests that they were seen as less disturbed and less threatening to Powick's staff, with frequent references to the emergence of an active, agreeable personality capable of employing and amusing themselves as well as engaging in conversation, thereby qualifying them for useful work outside the ward.

Melancholics were perceived as more of a danger to themselves than to others, though prospects for recovery were generally perceived to be fair or good. About two-thirds of people who had been certified as suffering from melancholia were discharged as cured, the highest rate of recovery of any patient group at the Worcester Asylum. A textual analysis of patient records indicates the greater mental and social capacities of these indi-

viduals, who progressed from a depressed condition which involved appre-
hension, confusion and disorientation, leaving them fretful, lachrymose or
verbally abusive. In their early days on the wards they were said to neglect
their bodily and personal needs or to engage in perverted habits, ignoring
their fellow inmates and occasionally showing suicidal inclinations. The
descriptions of the recovering melancholic emphasize their progress
towards being more gregarious, actively conversing with those around
them and becoming more civil in their behaviour and personal care as well
as their social manners. In return for tractable behaviour and regular work
they were given greater trust and access to entertainments as they were
encouraged to leave the ward and undertake labour in the grounds, or to
read and attend to their needlework.

One area where tolerance was rarely conceded to those afflicted with
mania or melancholia was in the display of sexual misbehaviour. Hack
Tuke commended the use of bromides not only to promote sleep but as a
depressant which reduced the sexual vigour of the patient, since 'the
sexual act is in part a skin reflex', and diminished the sexual excitement
which played 'so important a part in the genesis of mental afflictions'.[44]
Potassium bromide and 'anodyne draughts' appear to have been used at
Powick Asylum to control aberrant sexual activity as well as as a sleeping
opiate, though difficult sexual behaviour is mentioned in only a limited
minority of case notes.

Conclusions

Recent debates on the place of the Victorian lunatic asylum within the
social history of insanity have called into question Scull's portrayal of
these institutions as mere 'warehouses for the unwanted' and instead
emphasized their curative potential and their accessibility to a range of
external agencies. This chapter has examined 3,000 patient admissions
which were recorded by the Worcester City and County Pauper Lunatic
Asylum at Powick during the two decades after it opened in 1852. The
retreat from a hopeful optimism associated with moral treatment to the
therapeutic pessimism of the 'hereditary' later Victorian period is not
readily apparent in the records which survive from this Asylum. Powick's
staff faced an early influx of 'hopeless cases' from workhouses in the Poor
Law unions of the county and borough and there was an inevitable accumulation of chronic, incurable cases even though the rates of cure (and
death) within the Asylum remained reasonably high in these years. Some
of the 3,000 cases admitted in the mid-Victorian period were to die at
Powick as late as the 1930s. A close textual analysis of the records of those
admitted in the first two decades of the Asylum's existence indicates how
difficult it was to deliver individual care at Powick and suggests that the
institution adapted to a practice which Lees has termed 'treatment by classification', where people identified in a particular way from diagnosis and

behaviour were 'treated', or rather managed, in broadly similar ways. It is possible to understand the functions of the Victorian asylum more broadly than the needs of those held there, as 'institutional', 'communal' and 'individual'. The therapeutic efficacy of the institution and its capacity for meeting the needs of inmates can also be made by drawing on Maslow's outline of basic and developed human requirements, within the classificatory structure of the asylum established in these years.

The first point made in this chapter is that the identification of the inmate had begun prior to their arrival in the terms laid out by the certificate of insanity and committal order, which were usually translated into the admission registers and case books of the institution. Concerns about violence to relatives, neighbours and the wider community as well as to the individual lunatic figured prominently in such accounts and it seems clear that the Asylum assumed, and was expected to undertake, a responsibility for containing as well as seeking to cure the person committed. In construing the needs of their patients the Asylum governors, who were magistrates acting as the Visiting Committee which employed the Medical Superintendent, were not merely expressing the concerns of a social elite responsible for law enforcement but also the interests of those affected by the behaviour of troubled individuals. Among the external groups and interests to which the Victorian asylum remained sensitive were the Poor Law authorities and those concerned, offended or outraged by the plight of an insane person in their midst. Medical and attendant staff at the Asylum arranged accommodation for those admitted according to the level of threat which they presented to those living and working there, as well as to the outside world. The establishment remained deeply aware of the need to maintain order within its precincts as well as protecting public safety by preventing escapes and controlling those capable of violent or outrageous conduct. These concerns are, unsurprisingly, more apparent in the records of those governing the institution than the needs expressed by individuals or their relatives. It seems important to acknowledge, however, that vulnerable inmates benefited from a controlled atmosphere, offering safety from harm whether by themselves or others and giving them basic maintenance.

The concerns of different social groups and staff are embodied in the range of words and phrases found in the texts of the patient notes which survive for these decades. These documents chart not only the ways in which people were given profiles which placed them within the Powick 'community', made up of the wards and the different groups that shaped the institutional life of the Asylum at this time. Patient care was broadly perceived in terms of the differential capacity of inmates for responsible behaviour and communication, though every group was offered basic care in terms of food, drink, clothing, warmth and some degree of safety.

The progress of individuals was usually measured in terms of their ability to take part within the ordered life of the institution, contributing to that community by responsible conduct, rational communication, willingness to labour, and participation in recreational tasks considered appropriate to their ability. While demented people and those diagnosed as idiotic or imbecilic were generally perceived as having poor prospects for recovery, people afflicted by mania or melancholia were considered to be affected by an attack of insanity which was likely to be transient. Medical reports of their behaviour presented their conduct in terms of a continuum which acknowledged differences in personality but made basic assumptions about the minimal personal and social skills required before an inmate could be judged as moving along the road to recovery. Those who failed to curb their violent impulses or subsided into a morose or incommunicative state were generally left to languish in the institution, sometimes for many decades before their death. Others found a niche which enabled them to secure their different needs, and even to make some choices within the confines of this closed institution. Relations between staff and inmates, rarely discussed in recent accounts though arguably critical to an understanding of the therapeutic impact of the Victorian asylum, appear to have been good except where inmates (or presumably staff) engaged in extremes of violence or made disruptive noises. Other forms of unacceptable behaviour were related to what were construed as outrageous displays of perverted sexual desires and 'dirty' habits which were private or public. In such instances the use of sedative draughts as well as isolation and blistering were undertaken even in this era of 'moral management'.

The evidence drawn primarily from patient case notes of the Worcester Asylum indicates that the models of asylum care offered by earlier scholars such as Scull and Showalter are inadequate as a guide to understanding the complex interplay of diagnosis, behaviour and institutionalization in the world of the Victorian lunatic. More recent studies which have emphasized the porosity of these establishments and the influence of external agents on the passage of individuals through their gates have often underestimated the degree to which the asylum constituted a closed world and a controlled institutional community which was guided by internal classification and relationships as well as the imperative to protect wider society from the disorderly conduct of its inmates. The recovery of individuals was assessed according to the sociability which they displayed within the walls of the institution and in many instances they were at least as vulnerable to injury, mistreatment or abuse in contemporary society as the people who surrounded them inside or outside its walls.

Notes

1 For instance: L. D. Smith, *Cure, Comfort and Safe Custody: Public Lunatic Asylums in Early Nineteenth-Century England*, London: Leicester University Press, 1999; P. Bartlett, *The Poor Law of Lunacy: The Administration of Pauper Lunatics in mid-Nineteenth-Century England*, London: Leicester

University Press, 1999. R. Porter and D. Wright, *The Confinement of the Insane: International Perspectives, 1800–1965*, Cambridge: Cambridge University Press, 2003.

2 S. Cherry, *Mental Health Care in Modern England: The Norfolk Lunatic Asylum/St Andrew's Hospital c.1810–1998*, Woodbridge: The Boydell Press, 2003, p. 5.

3 P. Bartlett and D. Wright, 'Community Care and its Antecedents', in P. Bartlett and D. Wright (eds), *Outside the Walls of the Asylum: The History of Care in the Community 1750–2000*, London: Athlone Press, 1999, pp. 1–18.

4 J. L. Moreno, *Who Shall Survive? A New Approach to the Problem of Human Interrelations*, Washington, D.C.: Nervous and Mental Disease Publishing Company, 1934.

5 In L. H. Lees, *The Solidarities of Strangers: The English Poor Laws and the People, 1700–1948*, Cambridge: Cambridge University Press, 1998. Particularly parts 2 and 3.

6 A. H. Maslow, *Motivation and Personality*, New York: Harper Row, 1954.

7 See Chapter 4 by Melling in this volume for an examination of the celebrated Devon County Asylum where J. C. Bucknill established his reputation as a qualified advocate of moral treatment.

8 Lunatic Asylums' Act, 1845 (8 & 9 Vic., c. 101).

9 Specifically Dudley (a detached area within Staffordshire), Kidderminster, King's Norton and Stourbridge Poor Law Unions. All thirteen Worcestershire Poor Law Unions committed lunatics to Powick in the period 1852–72, although urban areas provided a disproportionately high number.

10 See F. G. Crompton, *Workhouse Children*, Stroud, Gloucestershire: Sutton, 1997, Chapter 5, for a further discussion of the class composition of local elites.

11 Idiots were distinguished from imbeciles because their intellectual impairment was from birth (congenital) as opposed to developing from the perinatal period onwards. Some individuals became imbecile as adults.

12 Worcester City and County Pauper Lunatic Asylum, Powick, Patients' Books are held by Worcestershire County Records' Office, County Hall, Worcester – Accession No. 10127. With the exception of the following volumes: 1. Worcester City and County Pauper Lunatic Asylum, Powick, Patients' Books – the first volume and three Continuation Volumes are held at the George Marshall Medical Museum, in the Charles Hastings' Medical Education Centre, Worcestershire Royal Hospital, Worcester and 2. Worcester City and County Pauper Lunatic Asylum, Powick, Admissions and Discharge Registers are held by the Worcestershire County Records' Office, County Hall, Worcester – Accession No. 8343/9–25.

13 4 & 5 Will. IV, c. 76.

14 While some patients' mental afflictions were complicated by chorea, epilepsy and general paralysis, few inmates were committed to Powick solely with these conditions.

15 For instance, Edwin P., a fifty-four-year-old grocer, from Dudley, committed in November 1866, had to be 'fed with a "naso-oesophageal tube" which sustained his life', although he eventually died of abstinence from food and pulmonary congestion after just over a year in the asylum. Patient No. 1862.

16 The Webbs suggested that since that time pauper lunatics were given 'whatever was necessary' to ensure their health, a decision deplored by some utilitarian ideologues. S. Webb and B. Webb, *English Poor Law Policy*, vol. 10 of English Local Government, London: Frank Cass and Company, 1963, p. 88.

17 'Enhanced diets' implied that the official published 'Dietary' of the Powick Asylum was ignored.

18 Whilst the diagnosis of an inmate's mental affliction, that determined their

lunatic asylum class on committal, altered in the period 1852 to 1914, it remained fairly consistent between 1852 and 1872 and patients were unlikely to be moved unless their physical health or behaviour deteriorated significantly.

19 Among the 3,000 Powick admissions were 766 dements of whom sixty had been said to have exhibited violent and destructive behaviour prior to admission.

20 Patient No. 1872.

21 Patient No. 578. The inquest concluded that William S. had 'Died from the effects of injuries inflicted by William H., who was at the time of unsound mind'. This meant that no further action could be taken in the case. The latter was later transferred to Fisherton House Pauper Lunatic Asylum, which dealt with particularly violent lunatics, following an attack on the wife of an attendant.

22 Patient No. 2591. Fanny H. was removed to the acute ward, where her violence continued, which led her to be considered so 'uncertain' that she was maintained in a special ward and given chloral at night to quieten her.

23 There were sixty-two male and forty-two female idiots, and twenty-five male and twenty-seven female imbeciles admitted in this period.

24 Patient No. 2071. He was said to 'eat all sorts of filth and rubbish', which made him doubly incontinent and undernourished. He died within a year at Rubery Hill Asylum.

25 Patient No. 608. Classified as an imbecile and epileptic. Harriet died in Powick Asylum after a fit twelve years later.

26 Incentives to deter such behaviour included punishments and the repeated application of blisters, though with disappointing results. Such punishments were also applied to other inmate groups.

27 Patient No. 1264.

28 These included Rickett's Asylum, at Droitwich, and the Duddeston Asylum, north of Birmingham. After 1834, when the private mad-house care was carried out by the Poor Law, efforts were made to ensure that only violent individuals were sent to such establishments.

29 Patient No. 2073. He died after eighteen years in Powick.

30 Patient No. 1605. She died of phthisis in 1907 after forty-two years in Powick.

31 106 male maniacs and ninety-four female mania sufferers had been certified after displays of violent behaviour.

32 Patient No. 1910. Transferred from Hanwell Asylum, the county lunatic institution for Middlesex, opened in 1831.

33 A textual analysis of the notes of all those diagnosed and classified as suffering from mania revealed over 1,600 different words and phrases, of which about 350 were used in regard to different forms of mania, and for both male and female admissions. The usage of such words and terms indicated a consistent reference to a continuum of behaviour which ranged from the violently disorderly to the normal.

34 E. Showalter, *The Female Malady: Women, Madness and English Culture 1830–1980*, London: Virago Press, 1987. Among 3,000 admissions examined were 733 melancholics, 379 of whom were male.

35 Patient No. 1955. On occasions Fanny attacked people with a broom, or any other object to hand. She died at Powick from phthisis twenty-eight years later.

36 Patient No. 950.

37 D. Hack Tuke, *A Dictionary of Psychological Medicine*, Philadelphia: Blakiston, 1892, pp. 784–786, p. 935. The author cast doubt on the idea of masturbatory madness but suggested the discouragement of the practice by exercise and (social) intercourse with others.

38 Patient No. 747. Betsy later claimed that the beef tea she was fed was 'made from mens' heads and their brains are used for oyster sauce'. She spent thirty

years in Powick before her death. Thirty-seven women admitted as maniacs and monomaniacs were recorded as suffering delusions, most having misapprehensions which could not be readily classified as erotic.

39 A. T. Scull, *Museums of Madness: The Social Organization of Insanity in Nineteenth-Century England*, London: Allen Lane, 1979, restated with more qualifications in A. T. Scull, *The Most Solitary of Afflictions: Madness and Society in Britain, 1700–1900*, New Haven, CT: Yale University Press, 1993, pp. 335–336, pp. 370–374.

40 Bartlett and Wright, 'Community Care and its Antecedents', for example.

41 In the period 1852 to 1872, 2,827 individuals were admitted to Powick Lunatic Asylum, of whom 2,527 (87.8 per cent) were recorded as having 'died' or 'recovered' there. Of the total intake of patients 54.0 per cent died and 33.4 per cent were 'discharged recovered'. Of the 180 patients discharged relieved only a handful of inmates, all males, escaped from the institution and only two of these were never returned to the asylum. One hundred and seventy patients were discharged 'not improved'. Of patients who died at Powick Lunatic Asylum 51.9 per cent were males and 48.1 per cent female. Of those who recovered 41.9 per cent were males and 58.1 per cent females. Of those discharged relieved 50.6 per cent were males and 49.4 per cent females. Of those discharged not improved 49.4 per cent were males and 50.6 per cent females.

42 Patient No. 1728. An inquest returned a verdict of accidental death.

43 Patient No. 2647, had been a clerk prior to his committal to the asylum in June 1871. His condition improved and he was 'employed with the superintendent's clerk or in the office … [where he] … does simple copying'. He also attended the weekly ball, an opportunity generally only available to trusted inmates. However, whilst this man had returned to 'normality' in the sense that he had taken up employment similar to that he had prior to committal, he was never regarded as sufficiently recovered to be discharged 'cured'. He died in 1901, after around thirty years in the asylum.

44 Hack Tuke, *Dictionary of Psychological Medicine*, p. 1130. Modern pharmacology suggests that potassium bromide depressed the nervous system rather than specifically suppressing the sexual drive. I acknowledge the advice of Joanne Palmer, Addenbrookes Hospital, Cambridge, on this point.

4 'Buried alive by her friends'

Asylum narratives and the English governess, 1845–1914

Joseph Melling

Introduction: uncovering the Victorian lunatic

In October 1896 Helena W. wrote to the governors of the Wonford House Asylum near Exeter. Helena had been a patient at this fee-paying establishment since the beginning of 1895 when she was admitted suffering from recurrent mania. Her letter was written to express concern at the apparent disappearance of a domestic servant who had accompanied some of the Wonford ladies on a recent visit to Exmouth. Miss W. recalled the last sighting of the maid servant, vividly framed in the casement of a seaside residence, as she urged the Wonford authorities to take seriously the anxieties of the lady patients that some disaster might have befallen female servants when they failed to make a train connection.

> I certainly saw her looking out of a window of the house with a garden & greenhouse (about the middle of August) next to Plantation House and not since.... She does not seem to have returned by the 'home' train about that time, some only reached it at Starcross. Should she be found at either of these places, we should at least like to hear from her. The thought that she & others may be buried alive under or near the line is intolerable to us.[1]

Helena was herself a former domestic employee though she had served in the more prestigious position of governess. The manner of her literary address to the directors of Wonford House registers this distance between different ranks of employees, as well as something of the distinctive character of the 'private' asylum in Victorian and Edwardian England.

In common with many other fee-paying establishments, Wonford had been originally a charitable institution financed by public subscription and with a sliding scale of fees designed to subsidize the treatment of poorer inmates. After the building of large public asylums funded by Poor Law rates following the lunacy legislation of 1845, these fee-paying establishments generally appealed to more affluent groups who were ineligible or unwilling to use pauper asylums. The terms of admission and the status accorded to those entering the public and private asylum are indicated in a variety of contemporary asylum texts: the certificates of insanity, the committal and registration arrangements, and the patient notes generated in the care of patients. Inscribed within these different sources are the nice social distinctions of contemporary society alongside the 'facts of insanity' and personal details required by law. Concerned to accentuate their social distance from their public counterparts, fee-paying asylums such as Wonford frequently drew on a vocabulary of rank and gentility which emphasized their distinctive appeal within the competitive world of private care. Wonford admitted a number of governesses from the 1850s until 1914 but only a handful of female domestic servants in this period.[2]

Recent research on the Victorian asylum has explored the responsibilities of the Poor Law for the implementation of lunacy legislation, as well as the influence of family and community networks in the passage of individuals to and from the public asylum.[3] Scholars have challenged earlier research which variously characterized the public asylums as warehouses for incurables and as domesticated receptacles for women who were disproportionately represented within them.[4] A complex historical picture of the asylum is emerging in which different kinds of class, gender, kinship, racial and ethnic identities were represented in the evolution of these institutions. In offering a more rounded profile of those who entered the asylum, some researchers have responded to Roy Porter's appeal for greater attention to the patients' experience of insanity and of institutional care.[5] It is easier to agree that the motives and actions of individual patients should be the subject of enquiry than to document their lives. The great majority of patients have not left personal papers, diaries or letters from which to recover their personal testaments, though an examination of institutional, Poor Law and census documents provides some insights into the changing therapeutic relationship between doctors and patients, as well as the social circumstances of those declared insane. The influence of the contemporary social order on medical care is evident in case studies such as Suzuki's account of the personal care of the insane in the eighteenth century. These reveal not only changing perceptions of the medical subject, they also show servants such as the household governess as suffering fits of insanity as well as witnessing the distractions of their superiors.[6] Historians of psychiatry such as Micale have made a rather different appeal to researchers in urging that the reappraisal of female hysteria and other medical conditions should integrate a robust understanding of the scientific milieu in which diagnostic models or techniques were developed, alongside a careful reconstruction of the biographies of individual subjects.[7]

Porter's call for historians to explore the subjective experience of insanity can be read within his larger argument about the growth of psychiatry in the eighteenth and early nineteenth centuries, which was encouraged by the expansion of an 'empire of imagination' as romantic poets and novelists drew out the hectic pleasures of personal experience.[8] Numerous writers have noted the importance of different genres of writing in the formation of both scientific and literary pursuits during the nineteenth century, including the cultural history of female insanity in the Victorian era where the governess novel has often figured as an example of 'hysterical texts' where the restrictions and frustrations of gender subordination were expressed in the depiction of feminine subjects confined within the domestic sphere.[9] Important feminist interpretations of the ideological and cultural roots of gender inequalities have suggested that the mad woman provided a fundamental reference point for representing femininity within bourgeois society, as well as embodying profound tensions between the domestic ideal of maternal responsibility and a practical necessity for unmarried females to find gainful employment.[10] It has been argued elsewhere that the mid-Victorian 'crisis' of the insane governess may be partly understood in terms of contemporary feminist and radical exchanges regarding access to education and professional qualifications, as well as conflicts between aristocratic and middle class groups over patronage and public duty.[11]

As interest in the governess question declined and the governess figure became the province of sensationalist novels serious discussion of her stressful working conditions diminished, though public concern regarding private mad-houses revived during the 'wrongful imprisonment' scandals around Georgina Weldon during the 1880s.[12] A significant but often neglected feature of these debates was the growing recognition even among the most hostile critics of fee-paying establishments that the rate-funded asylums did not provide appropriate accommodation to service the needs of higher social groups.[13] Charlotte Mackenzie's study of Ticehurst provides a vivid portrait of one of the most expensive and exclusive private asylums in the Victorian years, while Jonathan Andrews has described the important role of 'Royal' asylums in Scotland during this period, though we know less about the more modest private establishments in England and Wales at this time.[14] This is an important omission when we consider the remarkable growth of public and personal services during the later nineteenth and early twentieth centuries, including the expansion of female employment in domestic service and education as well as the growing opportunities for men to wear a wide variety of uniforms in the service of the state or private firms. It is also noticeable that those employed as asylum attendants were heavily drawn from the ranks of military personnel and domestic households.

This chapter uses asylum documents to draw a collective or group portrait of governesses admitted to different asylums in Devon from the mid-nineteenth century until the end of the Edwardian period. The methods of textual analysis used by cultural historians may be extended from an examination of institutional sources to the demographic, statistical, scientific and journalistic evidence which is more often used to provide a context in which to read literary works.[15] In acknowledging the difficulties in recasting the patient's role within the legal procedures which secured them within the asylum, this chapter recalls the arguments of historians of psychiatry concerning the capacity of patients to express opinions, manipulate information and influence outcomes within a therapeutic relationship.[16] Relatively few asylum autobiographies survive and the genre of female confessional narratives seems to have been stronger in the United States, where civil rights and religious campaigns possibly provided a larger audience.[17] The celebrated cases of female hysteria and neuroses which early psycho-analysis created are largely absent in asylum records though a number of Victorian psychiatrists (including J. C. Bucknill at the Devon Asylum) burnished their reputations by publishing cameo studies of interesting stereotypes.[18]

The registration documents and case notes which provide the staple source material for mapping the progress of an individual through the asylum followed a prescribed format, embellished by additional details occasionally supplemented by fragmentary letters and diaries. These texts were evidently the work of many hands. They included testimonies and witness statements from relatives, doctors, clergymen, Poor Law officers, policemen, magistrates and asylum staff. They were written with a particular purpose and a specific audience in view. Recordings of the voice of the patient are largely those made by others. This limitation is recognized as an important constituent of the political process which is being investigated: that patients had few opportunities to present a considered account of their journey, even if they possessed the capacity and expressed the wish to do so. Patient case notes often tell us far more about those observing an asylum inmate than the concerns of the individual committed but they offer a window on the asylum world and an oblique view of the patient's own imaginative grasp on that world as well as their apparent capacity to adapt their language and demeanour to the expectations laid upon them. Many of the descriptions which survive in the case notes include, however, the reported speech of the patient, including florid delusions, selected for their salience and dramatic effect. Any interpretation of reported delusions must be speculative. One approach would be to understand the individual's use of expressions, images and claims to titles of rank and status in relation both to their social experience and as a response to the peculiar expectations laid upon them before and after they entered the asylum. Another way to read these materials is as part of an institutional performance in which the patient participated. The dramatic form adopted by commentators as well as the individual patients is echoed in the writings of psychiatrists, including Bucknill, who retained a keen interest in literary figures drawn from Shakespeare and other sources, though more interesting is the awareness displayed by these subjects within the galleries of the asylum itself that they were rehearsing a role which was keenly observed and assessed for its conformity with approved models of conduct.

As Crompton's chapter in this collection makes clear (Chapter 3), the asylum sought to classify and segregate patients for their effective management within the institution, adapting a shifting vocabulary of terms and descriptions to direct the progress of the patient. Words and phrases such as 'improving', 'deluded' or 'dirty and destructive' were used more readily than technical medical language in patient's notes, recording their conversation, behaviour and social skills. Initial descriptions and decisions relied heavily on information which appeared in the certificates of insanity completed prior to the patient's entry and these documents in turn were frequently drawn up after consultation with a range of relatives, friends and figures of authority. The classification and treatment of individuals formed part of a transaction between earlier perceptions of the person and the concerns of the asylum, including the social rules which governed the interior world of the institution. These were generally designed to regulate behaviour and guide the residents towards an acceptable standard of thought and action in preparation for their continued confinement or eventual discharge. The social regime of the public and private asylum indicates the stress laid on moral as well as social values in assessing mental disorder and also in the patient's capacity to recognize and follow the boundaries of decorum which marked out the road to release. If we assume that a vital qualification for the role of the domestic governess was a judicious and discreet appreciation of the rules of behaviour and etiquette then the insanity of such women and their treatment within the contemporary asylum should provide a deeper understanding of how these social rules were enforced.

Discussion of the asylum governess is arranged in two parts: first, there is a brief outline of the social and personal characteristics of the governesses admitted to three Devon institutions; and second, the ways in which their own opinions and delusions are documented is considered. The composite narratives which may be found in many asylum records include reportage of attitudes, delusions and erratic action in which the observers detected some recurring anxieties, concerns and images. Their reflections provide some insight into the views expressed by these women as well as the constraints and pressures which they faced.

The Victorian governess and the Devon asylums

The portraits of the English governess provided by the Victorian census have the appearance of a fluid and impressionistic work rather than a fixed and consistent classification. The boundaries between the positions of governess, teacher and schoolmistress appear to have shifted in accordance with the titles assumed by and given to these educationalists by a variety of institutions and authorities as well as in response to the growth and contraction in their numbers.[19] An estimated 25,000 females were occupied as governesses in England and Wales in 1851, almost 600 of them living in the prosperous rural county of Devon. More than half of Devon's cohort had been born in south west England, most of the remainder having migrated from the southern and eastern English counties.[20] Their age, marital status and family arrangements may be compared with a smaller group of female 'teachers' and a larger number of 'schoolmistresses' at this time. Teachers were rather younger women, primarily living in their parents' homes, while Devon's schoolmistresses were generally older than governesses. Almost one-third of schoolmistresses were married (mostly women older than thirty), the teachers also including a greater proportion of wives, and one in six teachers headed their own household. The schoolmistresses were more likely than teachers or governesses to have their own household.[21] In comparison to other women employed in education in 1851, governesses were more usually unmarried and more likely to be living in the residence of their employer or their parents.

By 1881 the numbers of female teachers in the Devon census had expanded hugely, mostly it seems as a result of the employment in board (government-funded) schools, while the numbers of those identified as schoolmistresses declined.[22] A large majority of teachers were unmarried, mainly younger women, while schoolmistresses were generally rather older and more often wives. Governess numbers had also risen from less than 600 in 1851 to more than 800. Most of these women were aged between fifteen and thirty, though with a significant number in their thirties and forties. Very few were married. The households in which the governesses lived differed from those of both teachers and schoolmistresses. The very youngest usually lived in the parental home, though the most common relationship to the head of household was that of resident governess. A cluster of mainly town governesses headed their own household. A larger number lived with other female householders, including their relatives.[23] The residential governess usually lived in households of farmers, with 'people of some rank' and status or with householders engaged in education. The Devon evidence suggests that these households were generally more prosperous than the family household into which they had been born.[24] It is also apparent that the governess continued to be distinguished by residential position as well as her unmarried status, though family connections to sisters and to householders engaged in education remained important in the later Victorian years.

Those recording admissions to the asylums in Devon during these decades shared with the census enumerators a concern with classification, though the understanding of cultural and social connotations of rank, status and occupation appears to have varied between public and private institutions. The largest asylum established in south west England during this period was the rate-funded Devon County Asylum built at the village of Exminster in 1845. Exeter established its own Borough Asylum at Digby's Field only in 1886, Plymouth following suit a few years later by building an asylum at Moorhaven. Each of these was administered within the framework of the Poor Law, though direct responsibility for Exminster's governance passed from magistrates to the local authorities in 1888. The most substantial private asylum in Devon and Cornwall was originally established at Bowhill House at the end of the eighteenth century and re-founded as Wonford House Asylum on the outskirts of Exeter in 1869. The pattern of governess admissions to Exminster, Digby and Wonford House Asylums reveal a number of interesting points of contrast.

An obvious point to make about female educationalists who were sent to the Devon County Lunatic Asylum at Exminster is that they constituted only a tiny fraction of the 13,000 admissions recorded between 1845 and 1914. Analysis of 4,000 entries yielded details of more than 2,000 females of whom twelve were governesses. There were almost twice as many schoolmistresses but only three teachers. One governess was admitted as a private rather than pauper patient and it was stated of another that her father's loss of money meant that 'she is unable to go to a Private Asylum'.[25] Each governess was examined by a physician in her home or in lodgings rather than at a workhouse infirmary and they were, with one exception, unmarried. Most were Anglicans aged between twenty-three and sixty-four, half being older than forty. Their nearest relative was most commonly a sister or sister-in-law.[26] There was some fluidity in the use of the title of governess, though a broad comparison with the Exminster schoolmistresses indicates half of the latter were married, which is higher than the average of wives recorded more generally at the Asylum in this period.[27]

These females were certified as 'of unsound mind' rather than as lunatics or imbeciles, two thirds being diagnosed as suffering from mania, only three from melancholy and one from dementia.[28] There were remarkably few direct references to hysteria throughout this period.[29] In only a few governess cases was the cause of insanity given, though hereditary influences did not figure prominently in the detailed cases.[30] Most governess admissions had displayed symptoms for a matter of weeks, a minority having suffered for months or years, being largely cared for within a family home or in lodgings. Mary J. appears to have been living in lodgings before her admission in October 1861. Ten years earlier she had been resident in the household of a Honiton solicitor, teaching his four children. Family members and local physicians were frequently the key figures in decisions to seek a committal. Elizabeth S. was re-admitted in 1883, having first entered the Asylum almost a decade earlier. She spent the years 1881–83 living in retirement with her sister and brother-in-law at Teignmouth, visited by a local doctor each quarter until her growing excitement and visions led to re-certification.[31] Once admitted to Exminster, prospects for recovery were generally bleak for governesses. Schoolmistresses were much more likely to depart recovered or improved, often after a brief period of residence. Marital status also appears significant in that both governesses and schoolmistresses who were wives or widows were more likely to return home than the spinsters.

Exeter's borough asylum at Digby's Field opened in 1886, and was designed to house a minority of fee-paying patients in addition to those supported by the poor rates, offering competitive fees to families with the means to fund the treatment of relatives. During its first decade Digby Asylum admitted almost 100 women to its private beds and three times this number to pauper places.[32] Only two governesses arrived at this time, both registered as paupers on arrival from asylums in the greater London area, though one was immediately transferred to the private list, only being transferred back to pauper status nine years later, presumably on the exhaustion of her private means.[33] Digby also admitted two young female teachers of music and an elderly French teacher, while two schoolmistresses were both recorded as private patients.[34] While very little can be said about Exeter's borough asylum, the records of the largest fee-paying institution in Devon are more abundant. The legal provision for committal to a fee-paying establishment differed significantly from pauper admissions before 1890. Relatives or close friends were able to petition for entry providing two qualified physicians had independently certified an individual. There was also provision for voluntary boarding, with the agreement of the patient, in private asylums. After the Lunacy Act of that year, reception orders for one year with provision for annual renewals approved by the asylum's Committee of Governors, were also required for private patients.[35]

Relocated to an impressive new building in the village of Wonford in 1869, Bowhill House and Wonford admitted almost 900 females and about 800 males in the six decades after 1855.[36] The small scale of the institution is revealed by the 1881 census which lists fifty female and forty male patients in its handsome premises, under the Superintendent, Sutherland Philipps, and surgeon Dr Shapley. There were twelve Attendants of each sex and a large domestic staff, resulting in an attendant–patient ratio more than twice as high as that found in the County Asylum.[37] These amenities did not reach the standards of luxury found in the prestigious private asylum at Ticehurst, where few governesses or schoolteachers appeared among those admitted. Even the modest scale of charges required at Wonford could burden respectable families in polite society.[38] The mother of Mary C., a teacher, wrote to Dr Drake in 1909, anxious to learn the 'lowest figure' that the Superintendent could accept, since the family was entirely dependent on the pension of her husband, 'a retired civil servant (English)' of the India Office.[39]

A greater emphasis on the privacy allowed to the Wonford clients is evident not only in its design but its apparent reluctance to disclose their personal details to census enumerators in 1881. The future prospects of men and women whose employment depended on their reputation may have figured in the discretion displayed by private establishments.[40] Another remarkable feature of the Wonford admission registers is the identification of almost a third of all females as 'gentlewomen', which remained the most common status for women until its abrupt disappearance from the registers in 1907.[41] This status was given to a tiny fraction of the Devon population in the Victorian census and in other respects the occupational titles of those admitted to both pauper and private asylums appear to have displayed reasonable consistency with census returns.[42] In this particular regard Wonford appears to have opted for a genteel, even archaic manner of depicting its female educationalists. While governesses were more prominent than other female educationalists, there is little evidence that significant numbers of women who were otherwise known as 'teachers' were translated by admission registers into a more genteel status.[43]

Governesses dominated the Wonford educationalists. More than thirty were admitted between 1855 and 1912. They were almost all unmarried females older than thirty, including a few elderly ladies, primarily living in Devon and south west England.[44] Their health ranged from good to feeble, almost two thirds certified as suffering from mania, while dementia and delusional insanity also claimed more entries than melancholy.[45] The most frequent causes of insanity given were: overwork (or over study); female bodily cycles or bad health, including menopause and childbirth; anxiety, mental strain or worries; and disappointments or grief.[46] Overwork was seldom mentioned as a cause among other female admissions, while heredity, previous attacks, religion and old age figured less prominently in the governesses.[47] Table 4.1 indicates the relative weight given to different causes of insanity among Wonford females.

There were also clear differences between the sexes which may be detected in the way patients were certified and the causes attributed.[48] In common with almost half of all females entering Wonford, the most common diagnosis of the governess was that of mania.[49] The recurrence of 'overwork' as a cause of insanity among Wonford governesses suggests the strains which could arise from the delicate contractual position of the governess as an employee and her dependence on the resources of relatives, as well as the household of her employer. Close family and household relationships can be identified in most cases as well as some evidence of the contractual dependence of the governess on domestic employers. Governesses were rarely certified when at an employer's household, returning to lodgings or a relative's home some time before committal. Strains of overwork and the vulnerability of an unmarried, often impecunious woman illustrate the importance of tolerance if not support from relatives (particularly mothers and sisters), landladies, local clergy and friends.

The Wonford governesses also varied from the mass of the female intake in their marital status, a significant minority of those admitted being wives compared to only a tenth of governesses, possibly affecting rates of recovery and release.[50] One of the few married governesses was Eleanor A., wife of one artisan engraver and mother of another. She left at least one younger child at home when she was admitted in 1884, remaining for

Table 4.1 Wonford admissions 1855–1914, major reported causes of insanity

Cause of insanity selected	Count					
	Males	%		Females	%	
Alcohol, alcoholism	22	4.63	2.78	9	1.60	1.01
Anxiety and overanxiety	19	4.00	2.41	20	3.56	2.24
Childbirth, confinement, puerperal			0.00	40	7.12	4.48
Disappointment			0.00	8	1.42	0.90
Domestic trouble			0.00	8	1.42	0.90
Drink, dipsomania	14	2.95	1.77	2	0.36	0.22
Epilepsy	17	3.58	2.15	4	0.71	0.45
Heredity	55	11.58	6.96	65	11.57	7.29
Hysteria			0.00	4	0.71	0.45
Ill health or injury	18	3.79	2.28	13	2.31	1.46
Influenza	19	4.00	2.41	15	2.67	1.68
Intemperance	20	4.21	2.53	11	1.96	1.23
Mental anxiety, excitement, shock, stress			0.00	15	2.67	1.68
Old age	10	2.11	1.27	14	2.49	1.57
Over study, strain, overexertion,	16	3.37	2.03	13	2.31	1.46
Overwork	40	8.42	5.06	11	1.96	1.23
Pecuniary loss, troubles	10	2.11	1.27	3	0.53	0.34
Previous attack	34	7.16	4.30	53	9.43	5.94
Religion, religious excitement, religious mania	16	3.37	2.03	26	4.63	2.91
Sun stroke	12	2.53	1.52		0.00	0.00
Syphilis	13	2.74	1.65		0.00	0.00
Trouble	6	1.26	0.76	14	2.49	1.57
Unknown	151	31.79	19.11	169	30.07	18.95
Worry	24	5.05	3.04	41	7.30	4.60
Total with above causes	475	100.00	60.13	562	100.00	63.00
Total in Wonford admissions	790	60.13	100.00	892	63.00	100.00

Source: Wonford House Admission Registers.

eighteen months before discharge and returning after a brief period with her family.[51] Married women were almost invariably committed on the authority of their husband, while the entry of the unmarried was usually sanctioned by mothers, sisters, fathers or brothers. Most governesses appear to have been admitted from a family home or lodgings.[52] Mary V. was the daughter of a farmer and sister of another governess while Mary G.'s relatives settled in the well-established textiles centre of Colyton.[53] Eliza I.'s parents were also natives of Colyton, though she was born in Teignmouth. There she lived with an elderly mother and unmarried sister in 1881 before they returned to Colyton and admitted Eliza to Wonford a decade later. Others made a longer journey, including Charlotte Anne C. who arrived in 1882 from Helston, where her family seem to have been substantial drapers. Ellen L. also came to Wonford from Cornwall in 1884.[54]

The domestic arrangements of those who came to Wonford more than once suggest a number of contrasts in the migration patterns of governess families. Susannah R. first entered in 1858 and was re-admitted five times, her final visit in November 1883 ending with her death almost twenty years after. Her early admissions were authorized by her mother, with whom she lived near Exeter, though from 1863 her sisters and a friend approved her committals. In the 1881 census Susannah headed the family household of four 'annuitant housekeepers', living in some hardship.[55] Julia S. also made her first visit in the 1850s, being re-admitted in 1873 on the authority of her mother and returning in 1883, authorized this time by her sister in Exmouth.[56] The connections of the Victorian governess with seaside towns can be detected in admissions to Wonford as well as the regime of rehabilitation designed for its patients. From the fragmentary descriptions and testaments established prior to admission and elaborated within the documentary record of the host institution, it is also possible to gain some insight into patients' responses to the remedial regime in which they were placed. The concern of legal and medical personnel to assess an individual's capacity for rational conversation and orderly behaviour led them to offer detailed and often florid descriptions of patient behaviour and delusions. The next part of this chapter assesses the extent to which we may read such materials as a patient commentary on the social circumstances which had apparently led to insanity and on the treatment offered by the medical authorities who monitored their progress.

'Dirty and destructive': governesses and narratives of patient treatment

It was argued earlier that the Victorian asylum was engaged in imaginative social construction as well as scientific and commonsense methods of classification in their efforts to explain and address the insanity of their patients. The gentility which the admission registers of Wonford House bestowed on their inmates can be usefully compared not only with the census classifications but also the contemporary legal fiction that those who entered the public asylum were pauper lunatics. Very few of those admitted to the public asylums in Devon appear to have arrived from destitute households or from the workhouse itself, though the Poor Law was the key administrative vehicle by which they were transported to the asylum. The transactions involved in the passage of such individuals to and from the asylum were necessarily an expression of status and regard as well as wealth or social power, particularly where the employment prospects of female educationalists depended on respectable connections and personal recommendation as much as formal qualifications. Fundamental to the distinction between the public and private asylum for most of this period was the greater legal authority given to doctors as well as the relatives of fee-paying individuals as compared to those supported by ratepayers.

There were also distinctive institutional concerns, as Crompton and Pearce have noted in their chapters in this collection (Chapters 3 and 6), evident in the admission, classification and management of patients as distinct from the medical criteria involved in the diagnosis and treatment of individuals. The asylum records were composed by integrating the historical information drawn from certificates and committal orders, together with information available when the patient was examined on admission. These entries provided a basis for initial diagnosis and decisions in regard to the accommodation and early treatment of the person within the institution, while case book entries noted their subsequent progress. By the early twentieth century a medical examination could include detailed description of the physical features of the patient.[57] A comparison of case notes which survive for Exminster and Wonford House suggest that more detailed and florid entries were composed for the fee-paying individual, even though most private patients spent significantly less time in the fee-paying establishment than did the average patients admitted to the pauper institution. Another distinguishing feature in the documentation of patient experience in these different kinds of asylum lay in the power of the relatives or friends of private patients to petition for their discharge as well as initial admission. The respective power of petitioners, governors and physicians was altered by the requirements of the 1890 Lunacy Act that fee-paying as well as rate-funded patients should be committed on legal authority, though in the case of private patients a distinction remained in the form of an annual renewal of a committal order up to five years after admission.

From the certificates and case books of Exminster as well as Wonford we gain some perspective on the interior world of the Victorian asylum patient. Violent delusions emerge as a memorable theme in the admission of Exminster governesses, vigorous outbursts having led to certification usually after the intervention of landladies, neighbours and clergymen as well as relatives concerned at the risks posed by their erratic conduct. Frictions with employers were less evident than disruption of lodgings and family households. The peculiarities of the governess were often depicted in terms of their 'exalted' ideas about their status, monetary means or religious authority. There were very few private patients admitted to the Devon Asylum, mostly in the early years when J. C. Bucknill's eminence attracted individuals such as Charlotte T., an unmarried governess who arrived in February 1849 suffering from melancholy rather than mania. One of the two certificates completed by her doctors explained her disturbance at an unexplained noise in the night, while the second described the 'strong mental delusions' of his patient. She entertained, he said:

> The idea of being buried alive by her friends; this idea working on a mind naturally excitable had produced such feelings as to induce her to say it were better to be killed or to kill herself than to undergo such a procedure.[58]

Appearing in good physical health, she died within a few weeks of admission. Other Exminster governesses were more robust in their claims and their capacity to survive the Asylum. Mary J. alarmed her Honiton landlady when her 'mild & retiring disposition' altered a few days before her admission to violent threats against her relatives and a fierce denunciation of the local clergyman as Judas. Resisting all attempts to restrain her, Mary left recovered within weeks.[59] Susan L.'s condition had been of much longer duration when she entered Exminster in 1872, her landlady having reported her screams from the window at night, threatening to burn down the house and cut the throats of everyone in it. Introducing herself as Queen Victoria, Susan expressed indignation at her new surroundings and gazed at them 'as though she was the monarch of all she surveyed'. Within a short period she also showed signs of improvement, was placed in the more liberal regime of North Cottage on the Asylum estate and continued there as 'one of the best-behaved Patients' until her death twenty-five years later.[60] Elizabeth S. similarly assumed royal titles, though only after she was re-admitted for claims that she was in intimate conversation with heavenly visions. Thereafter she devoted herself to sending letters to the Prince of Wales.[61]

Three of the ten Exminster governesses recovered within a year or so of their arrival, while six died at the Asylum, often after many years of residence.[62] Younger women had better prospects of release. Florence J. was admitted in 1888 acutely melancholy and suicidal, her condition attributed to over study. Progressing from close observation to an open ward, she relapsed for a period before being moved to the Cottage in early 1889. After an escape attempt she returned to a closed ward but was discharged within months.[63] Mary P.'s insanity in 1903 was traced to her father's breaking of her engagement, followed by death of her former fiancé. She frequently left the family home to wander alone in the gardens of Buckfast Abbey, believing herself to be at another place. The certifying physician noted that Mary knew 'that she is insane and admits the fact'. After a brief relapse she left on trial in July 1903, being absolutely discharged the next month.[64] Most governesses did not leave the Asylum before their death. Some of these fatalities could be explained by their poor health on arrival, or by the onset of acute illness. Catherine W. was certified as suffering 'epileptic mania' in 1903, prompted by the sight of a person covered in blood and leading to her attempts at suicide. After a few months of intense fits, violent behaviour and sexual delusions she died at the Asylum.[65] Mary H. transferred to Devon from Lancaster Asylum in 1884 after two earlier periods in English asylums and a protracted stay in a Belgian institution. She had long complained of murderous nightly visits but settled down to years of quiet solitary existence only ending in her death.[66]

The Exminster records reveal the importance attached by the Asylum authorities to placing the female patients in different wards, galleries, airing courts and cottage accommodation according to their capacity to associate and converse with others. Similar practices are evident in the terms in which the Wonford governesses were certified and managed during these years. Great attention was paid to the personal characteristics of individual females and psychological language became more evident at the end of this period. Most of the case notes were composed in common-sense language, documenting an unsoundness of mind in refusals to show moral and sexual decorum (in dress as well as behaviour) on the part of the governess patient. Erotic as well as neurotic tendencies were emphasized in accounts of careless actions, though overwork or mental strain might be detailed as the primary cause of insanity. Maud R. initially entered Wonford as a voluntary boarder before her certification in 1900, as her 'eccentric and neurotic' behaviour deteriorated towards the hysterical and suicidal. She complained of nightly voices and that a 'will power over [her] body suddenly seized her in bed and compelled her to come downstairs in dishabille'.[67] Sophie F. was stricken with grief when admitted in the same year, refusing food and exposing her legs 'without any regard for whoever is present'. Edith Y. simply neglected her personal appearance and health, though her re-admission in 1909 was justified after reports that 'she was going about in public not sufficiently dressed'. After complaints against Wonford medical staff she was transferred to Plympton House Asylum.[68]

In common with the Exminster governesses, those coming to Wonford tended to be middle-aged rather than young or elderly females. The prospect of their leaving alive was much better than those who entered the Devon Asylum. Depictions of the Wonford governess often combined a description of her bodily condition as a 'predisposing' cause, while detailing social circumstances or events which had provided the 'exciting' cause for the onset of insanity, most characteristically an attack of mania. Mental disorders were also traced to physical illness and the female life cycle. Charlotte C. was admitted in 1882, claiming to be Queen of England, though she had been under a doctor's care for twelve years, her original insanity being attributed to an attack of 'rheumatic fever'.[69] Emily L. was an older woman previously admitted 'when passing through her critical period', being re-admitted in 1865 and 1866, on fears that intruders entered through the windows of her seaside lodgings. Daughter of a family of modest means, she appeared 'a lady possessing a kind heart with great refinement of character'.[70] Another woman disturbed by voices and delusions in the walls of her bedroom was Catherine L., admitted in 1868 after an addiction to laudanum led her to trouble 'the Police and her neighbours'. Claiming to be the victim of a conspiracy by her sisters, Catherine continued to be plagued by delusions after admission.[71] Constance Eleanor B. insisted that she was never insane on admission in 1891, being discharged shortly afterwards and complaining that her illness had arisen from 'too many doctors, all prescribing different things'.[72]

The effects of overwork and over study along with financial hardships were among the factors most frequently identified as a cause of governess insanity. Helena W.'s transfer to Wonford in 1895 followed her 'very hard situation as governess [where she] was very hard worked & underfed, the poor financial condition of her family preyed on her mind & she developed delusions'. Sophie A. had deep anxieties about her work, though her employers had made no complaints, leading to her return home and suicidal melancholy.[73] Over study was similarly noted when Edith Y. transferred from Plympton House in 1900.[74] A common thread in Susannah R.'s many visits to Wonford was fatigue from teaching and pecuniary anxieties. Susanna was an old Wonford hand by the time she developed a tense abdomen and ovarian tumour at Wonford in the 1890s, dying of 'senile decay' in 1902.[75] As numerous as references to overwork were conditions associated with bodily illness and the female life cycle, as a predisposing or direct cause of distraction, including fevers, fits and surgical interventions. In many instances it was the symptoms rather than the causes of insanity which alarmed family, friends and neighbours, particularly where a governess displayed a shocking disregard for sexual propriety. Julia S. was identified as a governess in 1873 at the second of her three admissions to Wonford, when she was in her forties. The particular form of her mania lay in a lack of any 'power of control' over sexual feelings when in male company, though she claimed that she had recently visited several medical men regarding her inability to restrain 'her sexual passions' and secure a husband. The continuation of her 'flighty, erotic and somewhat idle' behaviour at Wonford was variously attributed during her Asylum stay in the 1870s to her menstrual cycle and the onset of menopause.[76]

The personal visions and delusions of the Wonford governesses were expressed and reported in ways which suggest certain recurring themes in the lives and imagination of these educated women. Bodily functions and personal capacity were connected in some cases to ideas about physical or mechanical power, as when Susannah R.'s worries about lack of money and delusions of regal authority were preceded at an earlier period in her patient career by beliefs 'regarding perpetual motion' and 'a desire to prove her muscular superiority over other people'. The sense of personal isolation in a domestic setting and a deserted landscape of mechanical power figured in various accounts of anxieties about employment, family arrangements and personal safety. Auditory delusions of nightly voices troubled Eversell W., who recognized them as Satanic whispers against her chastity following an imagined legal victory.[77] Ellen L.'s voices were heard in 'telephonic messages when there is no telephone near', contributing to her irritable impatience with pupils.[78] Emily B. complained of acute headaches as well as loud voices which constantly called to her. She confessed to her mother that she longed for death, commenting that Wonford Asylum accommodated 'a lot of drivelling Idiots & one or two nice people but the Heavens defend our House'.[79] As well as expressing her alarm at absent domestic servants, Helena Mabel W. pencilled a note to her sister describing, 'The Little House, Siberia' where she lived. There she watched a man work a big machine in freezing conditions, while another person suffered a fracture, 'perhaps in the Deserted Village'.[80]

Another of Helena's concerns was that the staff at her previous asylum practised 'the "willing out" system on her' by use of hypnosis when she claimed that the house was on fire. Treatment offered to the governesses at Wonford appears to have included hypnotism by the late Victorian years, though only in cases where patients were considered 'susceptible', and where compulsion was not necessary.[81] Suicidal patients were secluded in padded cells, sometimes in strait jackets, while those refusing food, displaying violence or simply requesting sedatives were administered opiates including paraldehyde.[82] These various forms of medical treatment are less obvious even in the patient case notes than descriptions of the behaviour of these women in the galleries and public rooms of the Asylum, where association was governed by clear rules of etiquette including language and demeanour. Serious lapses would lead to their exclusion from shared spaces and to detention in a 'refractory gallery' or even locked wards and rooms where they would be kept under closer observation for misbehaviour.[83] Such activities were usually characterized as 'dirty and destructive', as when Susannah R. marked the walls of the day room and continued for some months 'murmuring defection but much of the Lady in manner and address'. Finally allowed to consort with other ladies in the First Gallery, it was said she was 'scarcely fit to be there', while on a later visit to Wonford many years later her dirty habits were held to exclude her from association with other patients.[84] Violence appears less commonly, though Ellen L. was removed from the First Gallery after slapping faces, which continued when sent on convalescence to Dawlish in her lengthy residence at

Wonford. Mary C. was less troublesome but seized the opportunity of lax supervision to drink a substantial amount of brandy and whisky 'which had been incautiously left about'.[85] Outrageous conduct in the grounds of the Asylum was another source of concern, as when Julia S. was said in the 1880s to have seized a male visitor by his genitals, declaring 'that old gentleman has done plenty of work in his time, you know, though I am not married I have had some of that kind of thing in my time'.[86]

The rehabilitation of the Wonford governesses followed a pattern which was familiar to other female patients at the Asylum: advancement up a ladder of simple tasks and association, with conduct monitored by the reading of letters to relatives as well as the staff and governors. Tea with the Superintendent and Housekeeper appears to have preceded convalescent visits to Dawlish, including a stay at Plantation House mentioned by Helena W. Such excursions served as a prelude to the arrangement of 'leave' outside the Asylum, sometimes under the direct supervision of senior staff, and to formal discharge under the care of relatives.[87] Asylum physicians were clearly reluctant to accede to the request of some relatives that the patient be released. Eversell W. was discharged 'relieved' in 1902, though her doctors warned that her condition warranted only 'a very guarded prognosis'.[88] The governess patients could also influence the terms and timing of their release in a variety of ways. The display of an intelligent understanding of their condition and circumstances was important, though such a talent did not always secure the desired outcome. Julia S. spent two trial periods at Christmas with her mother, returning each time 'saying she was not well enough to live at home' until her discharge after a third attempt, in 1872. Re-admitted the following year, she continued in the Asylum while undertaking periodic trial periods until a release in 1881, only to return in 1883. Always a lively conversationalist, Julia offered a lucid account of her condition during this final residence at Wonford:

> States that she is of a very nervous temperament. That her nervousness comes on at times that she needs some excitement which she gets by having intercourse (sexual) with gentlemen. Her mania seems to be purely of an erotic character, which feature is most decidedly marked.[89]

In such instances the condition of the patient took on the appearance of an intelligent conversation between the physician and his subject which is more often associated in historical accounts with the early days of psychoanalysis.

Conclusions

Recent writing on the history of the English lunatic asylum has located the growth of these institutions within a network of political and social relationships, drawing attention to the importance of demographic change, family connections and sex differences in shaping the way the asylum was utilized in the Victorian and Edwardian decades. Historians of psychiatry have placed greater emphasis on the interplay of scientific evidence and social understanding in the evolution of therapeutic treatment in what is sometimes called a 'golden age of hysteria'. There has remained the elusive promise of recalling the patient experience amidst a massive research effort to delineate the distinctive pattern of admissions and discharges to the asylum. Historians such as Porter have called upon asylum scholars to retrieve the 'patient's voice' from the complex and involved narratives of asylum care, though the methods by which this may be achieved are not always specified. For the individual subject of early psycho-analysis was a peculiar bourgeois construction in which personal and sexual relations between therapist and subject were dramatized in particular cultural terms. It is rare for private asylum personalities to be delineated so carefully, still less for the pauper inmate to claim such biographical detail. The institutionalized governess figured in an institutional narrative which framed her journey within the contractual and personal bonds of contemporary society as well as the social order of the asylum to which she was committed.

This chapter has drawn to a limited extent on methods of textual analysis to consider the ways in which institutional authors represented the female educationalist and her social connections. A comparison of census and asylum records for Devon in these decades suggests that different authorities were engaged in a social representation of the governess in relation to notions of rank and gentility as well as professional status and competence. There were also substantive differences in the rate of admission of women variously described as teachers, schoolmistresses and governesses to the public and private asylum. In terms of domestic employment, age profile and marital status the governess appears to have occupied a distinctive place in contemporary society, as well as in the Victorian asylum. Contrasts can also be drawn between life in the pauper and fee-paying institution, Exminster governesses remaining for considerable periods and usually dying within the institution, while a majority of the Wonford group were resident for limited periods and left alive, even if some were subsequently re-admitted. The personal circumstances of the asylum governess can be discovered only with difficulty, though their mania was most commonly attributed to poor bodily health and overwork, themselves often connected to financial anxieties. Almost all were examined in their lodgings or the home of a relative, authority for certification being given usually by their sister, mother or other family member. More shocking than the spectacle of a governess living a life of quiet despair, behaving oddly in the family home or even drinking laudanum, appeared to be the offence of public decency in expressing religious excitement or, more lethally, by exhibiting sexual enthusiasm. The public and private behaviour of spinsters as well as bachelors and the medical consequences of sexual activity remained a source of serious concern at this time.[90]

An important difference in the certification and committal of the asylum patient remained, even after the important Lunacy Act of 1890, in the provisions for the admission and discharge of the fee-paying versus the rate-aided patient. Exminster's Superintendent largely decided the date and terms of the release of his patients, subject to the direction of the Lunacy Commissioners, while his counterparts at Wonford were more inclined to respond to the petitions of relatives and friends in accepting both the admission and release of a patient even where they retained deep reservations. Social status and the resources associated with the wealthier classes remained a vital element in the unequal power of families in the Victorian and Edwardian decades. Marital status also appears to have figured in patterns of admission and discharge, wives leaving the asylum in greater numbers than spinsters in the educational profession as in other occupations. Social rehabilitation into domestic routine and personal discipline is more apparent than psychiatric intervention in the fee-paying as well as rate-aided institution at this period. The patient case notes do include references to restraints, opiates and hypnotism as well as more elaborate psychiatric terms by the end of the nineteenth century, though the descriptions of governess visions, delusions and behaviour remained literal rather than technical. Disciplined access to the shared and private space of the asylum was embodied in an architecture which included padded cells secluded away from the order of the shared galleries and day rooms through which the improving patient was expected to progress on their way to tea with the Housekeeper and trial periods in estate cottages and seaside villages before their final discharge. Those considered 'dirty and destructive' were liable to be excluded from the polite society of the main galleries, at Exminster as well as Wonford, confined to their rooms and even restrained while they were forcibly fed and injected.

A recurring image from the certificates of insanity completed for the Devon governesses is that of domestic transgressions as they broke glass, screamed from windows and rushed into the street or the sea wearing their night gowns, while even in the imagined landscapes of remote Siberian villages they were menaced by mechanical contraptions as they occupied the 'Little House'. The recorded delusions of these women appeared to express their collective as well as personal narratives of anxiety and strain within the isolated confines of domestic employment. Auditory hallucinations may echo family and public expectations of propriety and domestic obligations. One possible thread connecting Charlotte T.'s dreadful experience of being buried alive with the worries expressed by Helena W. half a century later was a morbid fear of suffocation within the bounds of household service. It was this troubled vision of their world which the tightly ordered regime of the asylum sought to correct. Julia S.'s reflections on her condition suggest that such educated women often retained a clear grasp of the constraints which would confront them beyond the controlled life of the public gallery. Faced with the evidence of their own deviance, some governesses sought to dramatize their predicament by use of droll humour rather than gothic exaggeration. Beatrice N.'s physician noted in 1911:

> She thinks she is at Torquay & on the stage & has tired herself out with trying her part. As the patient close by shouts out 'I am being suffocated', she says 'Never mind dear I am being suffocated too.'[91]

Notes

1 Devon Record Office, Wonford House Asylum, Register and Admissions Certificates and Orders for Reception (hereafter Wonford and admission number of patient), Admission 1271, Helena Mabel W., 5 January 1895. Mainly from DRO 3769 A/H2 series.

2 Wonford House Asylum had been founded in the 1790s. Six women were registered with an occupation given as 'domestic' or 'servant', five of them in 1854–56. Two 'retired servants' arrived in 1891–92.

3 A. Scull, *The Most Solitary of Afflictions: Madness and Society in Britain, 1700–1900*, New Haven: Yale University Press, 1993, pp. 26–29, 32–34, 105–107. Critical assessments of Scull include, P. Bartlett and D. Wright, 'Community Care and its Antecedents', in Bartlett and Wright (eds), *Outside the Walls of the Asylum: The History of Care in the Community 1750–2000*, London: Athlone Press, 1999, pp. 1–18, p. 12.

4 J. Andrews and A. Digby, 'Gender and class in the Historiography of British and Irish Psychiatry', in J. Andrews and A. Digby (eds), *Sex and Seclusion, Class and Custody: Perspectives on Gender and Class in the History of British and Irish Psychiatry*, Amsterdam: Rodopi, 2004, pp. 7–44.

5 R. Porter, 'The Patient's View: Doing Medical History from Below', *Theory and Society* XIV, 1985, pp. 175–198; 'Introduction' to *Patients and Practitioners*, Cambridge: Cambridge University Press, 1985, pp. 1–5 and passim; *Madness*, Oxford: Oxford University Press, 2002; *Mind Forg'd Manacles: A History of Madness in England from the Restoration to the Regency*, Harmondsworth: Penguin, 1990, pp. 36–38 and passim.

6 A. Suzuki, 'Framing Psychiatric Subjectivity' in Melling and Forsythe (eds), *Insanity, Institutions and Society, 1800–1914: A Social History of Madness in Comparative Perspective*, London: Routledge, 1999, pp. 115–116, the sister reporting that the vicious habit had been acquired 'under the evil influence of the worthless maid servant'. Also Suzuki, 'Enclosing and Disclosing' in Bartlett and Wright, *Outside the Walls*, pp. 120–121. In protecting the wealthy and the weak-minded the governess could play a critical role in the proceedings.

7 M. S. Micale, 'Hysteria and its Historiography: The Future Perspective' *History of Psychiatry*, 1, 1990, pp. 33–124, pp. 47–48, 98–99, 110–111 and passim. Edward Shorter, 'Mania, Hysteria and Gender in Lower Austria, 1891–1905', *History of Psychiatry*, 1, 1990, pp. 3–31, pp. 30–31.

8 Porter, 'Love, Sex, and Madness in Eighteenth-Century England', *Social Research*, 53 (2), 1986, pp. 231–232, 241–242; Also *Mind Forg'd Manacles*, p. 282: 'Above all, budding Romanticism gave coherent expression to that new sense of self as something inner, private and potent … [M]adness could be recuperated within the literary and cultural vision.'

9 M. Poovey, *Uneven Developments: the Ideological Work of Gender in mid-Victorian England*, London: Virago, 1989, pp. 136–138, 141–143.

10 M. Poovey, *Making a Social Body: British Cultural Formation, 1830–1864*, Chicago: Chicago University Press, 1995, pp. 99–102, 127, 136–137, 144–156; J. Swindells, *Victorian Writing and Working Women. The Other Side of Silence* Cambridge: Polity Press, 1985, p. 33; Sally Shuttleworth, *Charlotte Bronte and Victorian Psychology*, Cambridge: Cambridge University Press, 1996, pp. 219–244; P. Horn, 'The Victorian Governess', *History of Education*, 18(4), pp. 335–337 and passim; A. Neustatter, *Hyenas in Petticoats: A Look at Twenty Years of Feminism*, Harmondsworth: Penguin, 1990, pp. ix–x, for Walpole's description of Mary Wollstonecraft in 1792; Charlotte Bronte's 'Preface' to *The Professor*, Letchworth: J. M. Dent, 1969, p. xvi, for her complaint that realism should be preferred to the sensational; H. Rogers, *Women and the People: Authority, Authorship and the Radical Tradition in Nineteenth-Century England*, Aldershot: Ashgate, 2000; and E. Gordon and G. Nair, *Public Lives: Women, Family and Society in Victorian Britain*, New Haven: Yale University Press, 2003, for recent critical perspectives on 'separate spheres'.

11 J. Melling, 'Sex and Sensibility in Cultural History: The English Governess and the Lunatic Asylum, 1845–1914', in J. Andrews and A. Digby, *Sex and Seclusion, Class and Custody*, Amsterdam: Rodopi, 2004, pp. 177–222. For an excellent discussion of female employment in education see H. Bradley, *Men's Work, Women's Work: A Sociological History of the Sexual Division of Labour in Employment*, Cambridge: Polity Press, 1989, pp. 205–209, 339, including a nine-fold increase in female elementary teachers between 1875 and 1914.

12 W. L. Parry-Jones, *The Trade in Lunacy. A Study of Private Madhouses in England in the Eighteenth and Nineteenth Centuries*, London: Routledge & Kegan Paul, 1972, pp. 231–232; R. Porter, 'Georgiana Weldon and Louisa Lowe', in R. Porter, H. Nicolson and B. Bennett (eds), *Women, Madness and Spiritualism*, London: Routledge, 2003. For contemporary controversies involving the imprisonment of men see Gilbert Scott's letter to *The Times* 12 May 1884, 14b, for the celebrated architect who went into French exile to escape the English lunacy laws. *The Times*, 'A Lunatic's Freak', 18 July 1883, 20 September 1883, 27 September 1883, for male and female escapes from Brookwood Asylum.

13 J. L. Hammond and B. Hammond, *Lord Shaftesbury*, London: Constable, 1923, pp. 203–210.

14 C. Mackenzie, *Psychiatry for the Rich*, London: Routledge, 1992; J. Andrews, *'They're in the Trade of Lunacy ... They "Cannot Interfere" – They Say': The Scottish Lunacy Commissioners and Lunacy Reform in Nineteenth-Century Scotland*, London: Wellcome Institute for the History of Medicine, Occasional Publication No. 8, 1998.

15 J. Melling, 'The Body in Question: British Cultural Formation, 1830–1864', *Journal of Victorian Culture*, 4(1), 1999, pp. 164–173.

16 Micale, 'Hysteria', pp. 70–77, including a discussion of the 'secret clinical romance' of therapist and patient.

17 J. L. Geller and M. Harris (eds), 'Introduction' to *Women of the Asylum. Voices from Behind the Walls, 1840–1945*, New York: Doubleday, c.1975, pp. 7–11.

18 J. C. Bucknill and D. Hack Tuke, *A Manual of Psychological Medicine*, Philadelphia: Blanchard and Lea, 1858.

19 Devon Record Office, Exminster Asylum, Register and Admissions Certificates and Orders for Reception (hereafter Exminster and admission number of patient), 6233, Elizabeth S., for example.

20 The 1851 census identifies 572 governesses, 332 being natives of the county.

21 There were 288 female 'teachers' of all kinds identified in the 1851 census, including music and dancing teachers. This compares with about 1,400 schoolmistresses. More than a third (36 per cent) of the latter were heads of household, while daughters of the householder constituted more than a quarter (27 per cent) and wives less than a quarter (23 per cent). About one in six schoolmistresses were widowed heads of households. A similar proportion were unmarried heads of households.

22 More than 1,300 (1,357) teachers of various descriptions were found in the 1881 census compared to less than 1,000 (930) schoolmistresses. By 1891 the number of female teachers in Devon rose to 3,835.

23 More than 270 females (271–278) were given as a 'governess' in the household, while in less than 100 they were given the status of 'servant' (93), a similar number identified as boarders or lodgers (94). Fewer governesses (220) were daughters of the householder, only about fifty having their own household, many in Exeter, Plymouth and substantial towns.

24 Almost all the employers' households employed residential servants, averaging four per household. A substantial majority of the 122 farmers employing a resident governess farmed more than 100 acres. Governesses also lived in at least 176 female-led households, notably with sisters employed in education.

25 Six of the eleven governesses charged to a Devon union were from Newton Abbot, including the Torbay coastal area. Exminster 10173, Hannah Fallows W., had her certificate 'pauper in receipt of relief' crossed out. Exminster 10034, Mary Winifred P.'s father had lost money.

26 Ten of the twelve cases showed kin relatives, five being sisters or sisters-in-law, two or three mothers and two fathers.

27 Of the three female teachers among more than 2,000 female admissions, only Jessie M. was clearly identified as a teacher at school, another being a music teacher and a third a teacher of French. There were seventeen schoolmistresses, one National Schoolmistress and two 'former' schoolmistresses, plus one wife of a school teacher who *may* have assisted in the classroom.

28 In 1880–82 a total of 538 admissions were recorded at Exminster, 276 being female. Among those females identified as pauper admissions, 181 were certified as of unsound mind compared to fifty-six lunatics. Among the 'non-paupers' there were twenty-five cases of unsound mind and only three lunatics.

29 The sample of just over 2,000 females at Exminster in 1845–1914 indicated that more than two fifths (42 per cent) suffered from mania, over a quarter (27 per cent) melancholy, and one in six (16 per cent) dementia. Analysis of the 276 female admissions for 1880–82 revealed a similar proportion of mania cases (41 per cent), with slightly more melancholy sufferers (32 per cent) and the same proportion of dementia sufferers (16 per cent). Hysteria was almost always referred to after a diagnosis of female mania, for example in four clear references in the female admissions (two in 1870 and two in 1893–94), where the principal diagnosis was mania. Among the females admitted in 1880–82, there was one diagnosis of 'hysterical mania' among 114 recorded cases of mania.

30 In seven governess cases the cause of insanity was said to be unknown and in another the admission certificate is missing. Among the 1880–82 intake 62 per cent of females and 58 per cent of males were admitted with the causes of their insanity not stated.

31 The 1851 census shows that Mary J.'s hosts were the Townsend family. John Honeywood Townsend lived with his wife and four children, along with three other servants and a gardener. Exminster 6233, Elizabeth S., had previously entered in 1874, Exminster 4642, described as a 'retired schoolmistress' in the 1881 census.

32 Amongst the 312 Digby pauper list females, more than seventy were given no occupation, almost as many described as servants, together with a dozen in laundering and fifty occupied in some form of dressmaking or needlework. More than half of the private list females were given no occupation, another quarter described as wives or widows. There were two governesses, two music teachers, one former ladies companion, two clerks, three nurses and one farmer on the female pauper list.

33 Devon Record Office, Digby Hospital Register and Admissions Certificates and Orders for Reception (hereafter Digby pauper or Digby private with admission number and name) pauper case 404, Isabel H., admitted in 1890 and discharged 'not improved' in 1895. Digby pauper case 596, Alice J. admitted 4 February 1893 and transferred to the private list.

34 Digby private, 182, Marianne Albure C., was aged fifty-eight when admitted as a private patient in 1895 and was finally transferred to the pauper list in 1919, a year before her probable death. Private cases 42, Rosabella J. aged thirty-two, and 126, Frances Emma L. aged twenty-eight. Both were unmarried schoolmistresses suffering 'mental strain'.

35 Wonford 1424, Maud Isobel R., a governess who was a voluntary boarder before certification 13 August 1900. Wonford 1565, Grace F., was admitted from St Andrews Hospital, Northampton in 1905 but discharged in February 1906 when the Reception Order was not 'properly continued'.

36 The present chapter uses 'Wonford House' for all admissions after 1855. In the comparative period 1845–1914, Exminster admitted 7,000 females and 6,000 males.

37 In addition to a Housekeeper and ten house maids (one also a Nurse), five women were employed in the laundry.

38 Mackenzie, *Psychiatry for the Rich*, pp. 170–171, Table 6.1.

39 Wonford House files, 3992F/H32/11, Letter to Dr Drake of Wonford House from Lilias C., 27 March 1909, concerning Mary Wilhelmine C., a Digby patient 1901–03. She added that 'Dr. Jackson of Plymouth would also interest himself on our behalf if he has returned from Egypt'.

40 One Plympton House Asylum resident in 1881, Charlotte C., may have been a governess. Four governesses boarded at St Raphael's Home in Tormoham.

41 'Gentlewoman' accounted for 272 of 892 female admissions, disappearing in 1907.

42 Comparison of a sample of Exminster admissions and census returns in 1881 suggests that half of the cases (fifteen of thirty) matched exactly or very closely, a small number of entries fairly closely (four), in some (six or seven) there was an entry in one of the records. Wonford examples where variance was found include Mary V., described as a governess on admission in 1855, having appeared as a 'Domestic Teacher' in 1851. But her relationship to the head of the household was given in the census as 'governess'. The first female school teacher appeared at Wonford in 1894, followed by four others. Six schoolmistresses arrived before 1897 and only one after.

43 One Wonford governess was entered on admission as 'gentlewoman governess', a second as a 'gentleman's daughter' and a third as a governess and 'lady clerk'.

44 Twenty governesses were admitted from Devon, particularly coastal towns. A comparison with 258 'gentlewomen' shows 200 of the latter came from Devon and south west England.

45 There were thirty-four governess admissions, though only twenty-nine women were involved (four being admitted more than once), five in their twenties and only two older than sixty. Twenty-nine of the admissions were unmarried women, four being married. They were equally divided between good and weak health. Twenty suffered from mania, five each from dementia and delu-

sional insanity, four from melancholy. Twenty-five admissions had suffered for six months or less (six for two weeks or less), while seven others had been suffering for up to a year, only seven for longer.

46 Overwork, fatigue and over study figured as the first factor in six instances (though for five individuals), physical illness (including one of opium abuse) and changes in life or childbirth in seven cases, worry, strain, anxiety, fright and trouble in five cases, and grief and disappointment in love in three admissions. In eight cases the cause was unknown.

47 Among 657 Wonford female admissions 'cause of insanity' was unknown in more than a quarter. One tenth was supposedly due to heredity, one in twelve to previous attacks, one in eight to childbirth or menopause, compared to less than 4 per cent due to overwork and over study.

48 Examples of ambiguous diagnoses include Julia Eleanor J., a lady's companion, Wonford 1041, admitted in October 1887, said to suffer 'suicidal but not epileptic' mania.

49 Among Wonford female admissions, 49 per cent were certified as suffering mania, 30 per cent melancholia, 10 per cent dementia and 7 per cent delusional insanity.

50 Almost 500 of the 900 women admitted to Wonford were unmarried, 100 others being widowed.

51 Eleanor A., aged thirty-eight in 1884, had a daughter of seven months as well as an adult son recorded in the 1881 census.

52 Among twenty-six unmarried governess admissions, mothers figured in eight admissions, sisters (or sisters-in-law) in five, fathers and brothers in three each. In other cases the authority was not apparent or no relation.

53 William Hex V. and his wife Margaret farmed at Whimple, where he employed five men and two boys as well as resident house servants in 1851. Mary Elizabeth G.'s family had settled in the textile village of Colyton, with two unmarried daughters recorded as governesses in the 1881 census, living with their parents and a brother at St Andrews Square. Mary had returned from Wonford Asylum in 1877, after only a few weeks in residence, on the authority of her mother, Martha Elizabeth.

54 Charlotte is reported in Wonford records as a governess aged forty-four in 1882, admitted on the authority of her brother, who seems to be the unmarried Thomas N. C., a substantial outfitter in Helston, though in 1881 Charlotte Anne C. is given as an outfitter's daughter aged thirty. Ellen L. arrived in 1884 having lived near Bude.

55 Susannah R.'s first entry in 1858 was as case 286, and her final admission in November 1883 was case 944. She also appears as case 372 and 373, 503, 785 and 855, as well as spending time at Brislington Asylum, near Bristol. Her sisters Jane and Bridget, and William Pine (a friend) approved her admissions from 1863. She died in Wonford aged eighty-four in 1902.

56 The family connections of Julia S. remain obscure. I. E. Tozer is given as her sister in the admission documents for 1883, Julia having lived in 'Burridge's cottage' in Exmouth. Tozer was a substantial builder and inn keeper in Exmouth. Sarah and Frank Burridge lived in Exmouth in 1881, with Sarah's son, Henry Thomas Tozer. An unmarried Eliza Tozer was also a boarder in the Burridge household. Evrell W. admitted in 1901 on the authority of her sister Emma had also lived in Exmouth in 1881.

57 Mary P.'s examination in 1903 noted the insanity of her mother as well as her small head, pointed ears and an appearance which included 'lower part of the face "weak"; upper incisor teeth prominent'.

58 Exminster 619, Charlotte T., Certificates of Henry H. Hele, 17 February 1849 and Thomas Lyle. Handwritten. Charlotte died on 13 April 1849.

59 Exminster 2398, Mary J., Medical certificate of Thomas H. Jerrard 19 October 1861.
60 Exminster 4278, Susan L., Certificate of William H. Rawlings, 4 March 1872. Case notes, 6 March 1872–22 May 1872.
61 Exminster 6233, Elizabeth S., admitted 27 November 1883, previously 1874, possibly 4642. Case notes 27 December 1883, July 15 1884, 7 March 1892, 26 January 1900.
62 Two governesses died within three or four months, another after five years. Three lived on for more than twenty years.
63 Exminster 6939, Florence Miriam J., admitted 15 September 1888. Case notes 23 September 1888, 14–26 October 1888, 2 February–2 March 1889.
64 Exminster 10034, Mary Winifred P., admitted 24 February 1903. Certificate of T. Massey Pearce. Case notes 10 March 1903, 7 July–4 August 1903.
65 Exminster 10033, Catherine Edith W., admitted 23 February 1903. Certificate of R. J. Andrew. Case notes, 22 May 1903, 20 August 1903.
66 Exminster 6336, Mary Elizabeth Ann H., admitted 22 August 1884. Previously fourteen years at M. Julieus Institute, Bruges, Belgium. Case notes 30 August 1884, 6 January 1888.
67 Wonford 1424, Maud Isobel R., certification notes, 13 August 1900.
68 Wonford 1408, Sophie Maud F., admitted 22 February 1900. Case notes 3 March 1900. Wonford 1618 and 1680, Edith Emily Y., admitted 9 September 1907, re-admitted 26 October 1909. Case notes 30 October 1909, 1–11 February 1910.
69 Charlotte Ann C. was said to have been 'Very strong as a child. Always amiable temperate & industrious. No nerves nor disappointment'.
70 Wonford 407, Emily L., admitted 29 June 1865, re-admitted 2 August 1866.
71 Wonford 472, Catherine L., admitted 28 March 1868. Certificate and case notes 5 June–20 August 1868, 16 January–23 April 1869.
72 Wonford 1186, Constance Eleanor B., admitted 22 October 1891.
73 Wonford 1271, Helena Mabel W., Case notes 10 January 1895. Wonford 417, Sophie Jane A., admitted 18 September 1865. Case notes 4 December 1865, 'says her hands are gone and that everything is changed about her'.
74 Wonford 1618 and 1680, Edith Emily Y., admitted 9 September 1907, re-admitted 26 October 1909, 'on an emergency order'. Transferred case notes 5 June–16 September 1907.
75 Wonford 944, Susannah R., admitted 7 November 1883. Case notes 20 August 1895, 2 March 1898, 1 September 1900.
76 Wonford 236, 594 and 945, Julia S., Admitted 11 July 1856, re-admitted after a year's discharge in 15 July 1873, 9 November 1883. Case notes 14 July 1865, 10 February 1867. On 15 May 1867 it was noted, 'Mental condition unaltered, has no control over her feelings, her desires before every Gentleman, is altogether untrustworthy.'
77 Wonford 1463, Eversell W., admitted 26 November 1901. A predisposing cause of menopause. Certificate of John Cook, 27 November 1901, case notes 27 November 1901.
78 Wonford 971, Ellen L., admitted 2 August 1884.
79 Wonford 1510, Rose Emily B., admitted 5 June 1903, discharged 8 January 1905, recovered. Medical certificates of J. Gloster and Russell Coombe, 7 June 1903. Case notes 11–28 June 1903. Undated letter from 'Dear Emily'.
80 Helena Mabel W. Pencilled note 29 December 1896 in case book.
81 Wonford 1408, Sophie Maud F., Case notes 3 March 1900, 18 July 1900, imply she was fed by rectal injections, considered 'a raving maniac' and 'singularly unsusceptible to hypnosis'.
82 Wonford 954, Eleanora A., admitted in July 1884, held in a padded cell for two

months. Wonford 1408, Sophie Maud F. Case notes 3 March 1900, 18 July 1900, noted 'several fits of a hysterical type'. Placed in a padded room and fed through the nose. Wonford 732, Lavinia E., admitted 9 October 1877, hyocyamine to induce conversation. Wonford 1659, Mary Wilhelmine C., teacher, admitted 4 May 1909, letter from Bethlem physician, 17 April 1909.

83 Wonford 472, Catherine L., admitted 28 March 1868, accused Dr Shapley of conspiracy and smashing objects she was removed to a 'Refractory Gallery', sprinkling her urine about. Wonford 1463, Eversell W. Case notes 3–13 December 1901. Smashing glass and placed in seclusion, she tore her clothes and remained naked, 'very dirty in her habits and also very destructive'.

84 Wonford 503 and 855, Susannah R., admitted 31 October 1869 and 22 February 1882. Case notes 26 December 1869, 2 April–28 June 1870, 20 March 1882.

85 Wonford 971, Ellen L. Case notes 4 August–5 September 1884, 3–13 June 1895, 12 May 1893, 20 March 1896. Wonford 1659, Mary W. C. Case notes 5 May 1909.

86 Wonford 945, Julia S. Case notes 25 November–28 December 1883.

87 Wonford 472, Catherine L., admitted 28 March 1868. Case notes 12 July 1869, 9 October–27 December 1869. Wonford 417, Sophie Jane A. Case notes 8 December 1865–68, January 1866, for letters. Also Wonford 971, Ellen L. and Wonford 1510, Rose Emily B. Case notes 5 June 1903, 12 October–November 1903, 17 May 1904, for Dawlish visits. Emma T. also wrote to Dr Shapley from Raleigh Lodge, Exmouth, 23 June 1879.

88 Wonford 1463, Eversell W., discharged 18 February 1902 at request of her sister. Also Wonford 1618, Edith Emily Y., discharged on petition of her brother 5 May 1908 but re-admitted as 1680 on 26 October 1909 and transferred to Plympton House 1 February 1910. On other occasions the governors refused to continue the residence of patients, as when Wonford 472, Catherine L., was discharged relieved on 30 November 1871, after application by her sisters 'to extend the time of her remaining'.

89 Wonford 594, Julia S. Case notes 15 October 1879, her 'mind seems strong enough but morals are very low'. Case notes July 1880–April 1881, for a period with Asylum Housekeeper in Torquay, and 25 November–28 December 1883, 10 June 1884, for final admission. Also Rose B., Wonford 1510. Case notes 23 January–15 February 1904, 17 May 1904.

90 Michael Mason, *The Making of Victorian Sexuality*, Oxford: Oxford University Press, 1994, pp. 183–184, 215–219, for medical discussions on masturbating men.

91 Wonford 1733, Beatrice N., admitted 2 May 1911. Certificate G. P. D. Hawker.

5 Separatism and exclusion
Women in psychiatry, 1900–50

Louise Westwood

Introduction

In the history of psychiatry, women are far more visible as patients than practitioners. Many commentators have argued that women were more likely than men to be certified as insane and institutionalized in asylums.[1] A definite bias towards female admissions was found in the records of the Brighton County Asylum from 1919–35, but recent work suggests that while gender was a key factor in the construction of individual cases, as well as ideas about insanity, the gender imbalance may be less striking than was previously thought.[2] This casts some doubt on the thesis, advanced by Chesler and Showalter, that the male-dominated sphere of mental health care simply oppressed women.[3] Although the debate on admissions has concentrated on the gender composition of patients diagnosed with various forms of mental disorders and confined in private and public institutions there is clearly a need for further analysis of age, profession, economic and marital status. The role of women within the psychiatric profession itself is still relatively neglected, although there is now increasing recognition that women have long been associated with the care of the insane as superintendents of asylums, proprietors of private madhouses and voluntary workers.[4]

This chapter seeks to understand the obstacles that prevented more women from practising in the medical specialities, with particular emphasis on psychiatry, and the restrictions which prevented them from moving out of the prescribed feminine paths of general practice and public/community medicine. While it may be argued that 'overt and covert discrimination has kept out all but a handful of women', it may also be true that the strategies pursued by women who did break into the field precluded them from developing a high profile within the profession.[5] This analysis develops Liz Walker's conclusion that

> women doctors were pioneers in the sense that they crafted the terms of their inclusion into the profession, albeit within constraints imposed by its male members. They were not simply victims of a patriarchal profession, but also actors in the profession.[6]

This chapter also challenges the idea that women psychiatrists were simply operating at the margins of the profession and therefore their contribution can safely be overlooked. Instead it is argued that the competing strategies of integration and separation played to the advantage as well as disadvantage of women doctors as they sought to enter new specialisms and achieve clinical autonomy. These goals were often realized by working in an all-female environment, and with children, but the models of practice developed raised wider questions about the future of psychiatric treatment in institutional and community settings.

Witz concludes that the 1858 Medical (Registration) Act excluded women because 'it failed to provide for the compulsory admission of women to universities, medical schools or qualifying examinations'.[7] It is certainly true that Sophia Jex-Blake and others struggled to obtain admission to the medical school in Edinburgh in the 1870s and this battle for equality continued through to the second decade of the twentieth century.[8] University College London pioneered medical co-education but did not admit women to the medical faculty until 1917.[9] Women were therefore forced to rely on their own London School of Medicine (later renamed The Royal Free), opened in 1874. By 1906 there were 750 qualified women doctors and more than half of these had trained at the Royal Free.[10] Elston states that approximately 1,000 women trained between 1887 and 1914 and refers to these women as second-generation medical women.[11] Towards the end of the nineteenth century medical women were entering the mental health field. In 1888 Dr Jane Waterson became the first woman to be granted the certificate of psychological medicine and in 1893 the Medico-Psychological Association voted to admit women, but it was nearly half a century before the first woman, Dr Helen Boyle, became president.[12] There is virtually no reliable data on the total number of medical women working in mental health at the start of the twentieth century, but figures are available for those qualified for less than four years and working in lunatic asylums; in 1899 there were ten and in 1907 there were eight.[13] However, it should not be assumed that an asylum appointment immediately after qualifying was an indicator for a career in mental health care. Dr Letitia Fairfield (1885–1978) qualified in 1907 and initially spent seven months at the Birmingham City Asylum before moving to positions in general medicine, surgery, paediatrics and finally into public health.[14] For women paid work was clearly desirable in the initial stages of a career wherever it was available. However, the doctors who remained in asylum work or moved to other psychiatric practice had made a positive choice to stay in this medical speciality. But by 1926 there were still only forty three female medical officers (MOs) as opposed to 503 male MOs in mental hospitals in England and Wales.[15]

The gradual increase in the number of women practitioners did raise the question of how women should work with male colleagues and the merits of either a separatist or integrationist approach. Separatists firmly believed that women had a right to be treated by women doctors. Separatism also appeared to ensure a measure of clinical freedom away from the competitive sphere of medicine where women doctors faced unequal pay, patriarchy and poor career opportunities. In Britain many campaigns were fought over these issues by organizations such as the Medical Women's Federation (MWF), the Women's Freedom League (WFL), the Open Door Council (ODC) and the National Union of Societies for Equal Citizenship (NUSEC).[16] The number of organizations campaigning for women's rights in the workplace prior to the Second World War is a measure of the opposition to unequal pay, restricted career opportunities and the notorious marriage bar.[17]

Women doctors were attracted to the separatist approach in medicine, because of their exclusion, or at least marginalization, by the male dominated profession. Louella McCarthy states that in the USA during the nineteenth century separatism for women in medicine 'blossomed' but it had declined by the First World War because of a more 'integrationist' medical system.[18] In Australia separatism remained appealing for women doctors. In Sydney in 1922 the Rachel Forster Hospital was opened and run exclusively by women for women. McCarthy suggests that there was government disapproval at this approach, evidenced by their lack of support. The doctors involved were themselves divided on the need for government involvement, with at least one fearing that it would lead to 'male intervention'.[19] In England Dr Isabel Hutton noted and approved of international trends towards more integration and equality of opportunity but other leading practitioners like Dr Helen Boyle maintained a separatist approach at the Lady Chichester Hospital until 1930.[20] This chapter uses the careers of Dr Isabel Emslie Hutton (1887–1960) and Dr Helen Boyle (1869–1957) to illustrate the non-asylum approach in mental health care and also to highlight the battles for equal rights in the workplace and the profession. Hutton adopted a very different model of practice than Boyle, who might be characterized as a separatist pioneer, but both were second-generation medical women who were at the forefront of professional resistance to the large institutions for acute, temporary, recoverable mental cases.[21]

Helen Boyle created a unique framework for the treatment of mental deficiency and nervous disorders. She pioneered a distinctly separatist approach and achieved more professional recognition than Isabel Hutton, becoming the first woman president of the Royal Medico-Psychological Association in 1939. Throughout her career she was a pioneer of the early treatment of nervous disorders, a firm advocate of mental out-patients, and a founder member of the Guardianship Society, which organized community care for the mentally defective.[22] Boyle qualified in 1893 after studying at the Royal Free Hospital School of Medicine. She never married and single-mindedly pursued her career, first as an MO at the London County Council (LCC) asylum at Claybury and then at the

Canning Town Medical Mission in London. It was here that she observed patients suffering from the early signs of mental disorder with no hope of treatment until they were consigned to the asylum.[23] Prophylactic treatment without certification and the treatment of women by women were Boyle's main goals.

Boyle followed the separatist example of the Royal Free medical school in opening her dispensary for women and girls, which had an all-female committee. The work at the dispensary subsequently lead to the founding of a hospital in 1905 which eventually became known as the Lady Chichester Hospital for Nervous Disorders, treating women and children with temporary acute mental disorders as in-patients and out-patients.[24] This pioneering approach set her in opposition to the Lunacy Commission, which after 1913 became the Board of Control.[25] Boyle absolutely refused to work with the Board of Control which she viewed as autocratic and unresponsive to progressive treatments, arguing that her patients were 'early nervous' and 'borderland' and as such did not come under its jurisdiction. The Hospital appointed women doctors from many different specialisms and highlighted their gender using first names or the prefix 'Mrs' or 'Miss' if they did not have the title 'Dr'.[26] This can be seen as a clear attempt to encourage more women to seek help.

In 1905 Boyle embarked on a trip to Scotland and Germany to observe the care and treatment of non-certifiable mental disorders. She visited clinics in Glasgow, Berlin, Göttingen and Munich and subsequently provided evidence for reform of the asylum system in England.[27] The lunacy laws were different in Scotland and Dr John Carswell in Glasgow had an observation ward at the Barnhill Hospital for patients described as 'doubtful and temporary non-certified cases'.[28] During the 1880s a voluntary admission system for non-certified cases of insanity evolved in Scotland and there were also community guardianship schemes; neither were available in England at this time and asylum care was the only option for rate-aided mental patients who could not be treated in a general hospital or in a convalescent home.[29] Boyle greatly admired the German system of care because psychiatric polyclinics (out-patient facilities) had been established at most universities during the 1890s and early 1900s, which Engstrom states enabled psychiatric expertise to 'reach patients and relatives without resorting to formal institutionalization'.[30] It was in Rasumühle near Göttingen that Boyle saw the ideal clinic, which was run by Professor August Cramer (1860–1912). It was maintained by public funds, built small and homely for lower class patients and provided a source of acute, non-certifiable mental disorders for medical students. Cramer called his clinic 'Nerven-Klinik' to encourage attendance and also to differentiate it from the local asylum.[31] The treatment and care in Glasgow and Germany influenced Boyle's approach to mental disorders, but her work at the Lady Chichester Hospital was essentially illegal under the lunacy laws, which she believed needed radical reform.[32] There was a voluntary admission system under the 1930 Mental Treatment Act but reformers were unimpressed because of the difficult procedure for voluntary discharge.[33] However, the 1930 Act empowered local authorities to set up mental outpatient clinics, which gave patients with mental disorders more choice for treatment outside the large mental institutions.

Marriage, exclusion and the battle for equal rights

Dr Isabel Emslie passed her medical examinations with distinction in Edinburgh in 1910. She then worked at the Stirling District Mental Hospital and researched the Wasserman reaction for syphilis on 800 patients for her M.D.[34] In 1912 Dr Isabel Emslie was appointed the first woman physician in charge of women at the Morningside Asylum.[35] She was at this time interested in the uniquely Scottish system of voluntary admissions.[36] Dr Isabel Emslie joined the Scottish Women's Hospitals in 1915 and had a distinguished war record with service in France and Serbia. She returned to Morningside, following a period of study in Vienna, in January 1921 but her career plans were frustrated by her marriage to Major Tom Hutton in 1922 and her consequent move to London. Hutton met Sir Frederick Mott while attending a series of lectures at the Maudsley Hospital and he asked her to undertake a year's research on General Paralysis of the Insane (GPI). The Board of Control provided 100 pounds for this temporary position with the London County Council (LCC) and although Hutton was a married woman they agreed to her appointment. After a year in the laboratory Hutton was once again looking for work and discovered to her horror that most appointments were subject to the marriage bar. Towards the end of 1922 she was offered a full-time salaried, non-residential appointment at the Maudsley as third Medical Officer, which was ideal for a childless married woman, but as she was considering the offer it was withdrawn because of her marital status. A letter from Dr Mapother to Dr Campbell at the Stirling District Asylum explained why she had not been appointed:

> I should have been very pleased if her appointment had been possible; it was however decided that no exception could be made in her favour to the general rule of the LCC prohibiting the appointment of married women.[37]

Her next application was for a Junior Commissioner's position at the Board of Control and they showed keen interest until she told them of her marital status. Hutton later wrote that the manner of the Board's Secretary changed dramatically to 'frigid politeness' and she was reminded of the absolute bar on married women in government service.[38]

The early realization that the marriage bar excluded her from salaried appointments shaped Hutton's career because she began writing for publication to improve her income.[39] Her first book was published in 1923 and that year she accepted honorary (unpaid) appointments at the West End Hospital and the Maudsley and began a private practice. In 1925 Hutton was offered an honorary appointment at the British Hospital for Nervous Disorders.[40] Although Sir Frederick Mott and Dr Mapother at the Maudsley both advised against taking the position because the hospital was unorthodox, almost unknown and without prestige, she accepted and later recorded that

> it was at this hospital, which I left with great reluctance some thirty years later, that I found work that was preventative, far-reaching in its effects and an inestimable boon to patients and relatives.[41]

It was not unusual for new doctors to take honorary appointments at the start of their career, because it assisted their private practice and the move towards a paid appointment. However for married women these appointments were usually long term because they could get nothing else. A situation bitterly resented by Hutton who had travelled widely and observed that medical women in other countries were receiving large salaries and achieving highly prestigious appointments, particularly in America. Her comments in letters and journals illustrate the injustice and lack of opportunities for women doctors in Britain and she soon became embroiled in a heated debate on the absurdity of the marriage bar.

In 1928 Hutton responded to a leading article in *The Times* by Sir James Purves Stewart who stated that 50 per cent of medical women, often the most brilliant, relinquished the profession in order to marry.[42] Hutton widened the debate by comparing the treatment of women medical students in Britain with those in Europe. She claimed that

> Women students are not barred from the great medical schools such as those of Vienna or Paris and married medical women are allowed to hold public appointments in many foreign countries, even the most primitive.[43]

Hutton also wrote to the *Daily Telegraph* stating that

> in the first place, we find that on marriage medical women are dismissed from every public appointment without exception, and married medical women are ineligible for any such appointments irrespective of their qualifications, age or experience. Whole branches of the profession, such for instance as the treatment of the insane or mentally defective, are closed to medical women after marriage, as are also such special lines of work as school inspections, ante-natal and maternity work and child welfare. This is the action of the public authorities.[44]

Significantly the marriage bar had been relaxed during the First World War but was revived and strengthened afterwards. Pre-war marriage bars had more of an impact on women teachers and civil servants than female doctors but it now threatened to exclude women from the expanding specialisms in medicine. The 1919 Sex Disqualification (Removal) Act stated that

> A person shall not be disqualified by sex or marriage from the exercise of any public function or from being appointed or holding any civil or judicial office or post or from entering or assuming or carrying on any civil profession or vocation.[45]

The government described the Act as a 'Charter for Freedom' providing women with 'equal opportunities, equal chances and equal rights with men'.[46] Crucially however the Act allowed an exemption for the Civil Service and in effect gave local authorities the power to impose a marriage bar if they desired. The LCC revived theirs in 1919. The Medical Women's Federation (MWF) responded by passing a resolution stating that marriage should not disqualify women from medical appointments and unsuccessfully lobbied the LCC to reverse this decision.[47]

In 1921 the MWF surveyed the range of the marriage bar, which was extensive but not absolute throughout Britain.[48] Exclusion was more common in London where competition for the best medical positions was fierce and the dominant employers were government departments, such as the Ministry of Health, and the LCC.[49] The *Evening Standard* reported Hutton as saying that women had no choice but to leave medicine upon marriage because

> they are dismissed from every public appointment on marriage. I have known some extremely clever women doctors who have had to go... the whole thing is just too silly for words. It is a pity that London, of all places in the world, is so parochial in its outlook.[50]

Campaigners like Hutton were extremely angry about the marriage bar policy but men made the rules and broke the rules as it suited them, which can be seen in the exceptions that were made if the appointment was perceived as menial and low paid.

While Hutton was understandably concerned about her own career prospects, her campaign addressed much wider issues. She strongly argued first, that women as taxpayers and subscribers to hospitals should be represented in their management; second, that as patients they should have the choice of being treated by women doctors; and finally, that women students should have training facilities as good as those for men. Here Hutton was particularly critical of the London Medical Schools who had barred women in the 1920s, following a short period of admission. The

Evening Standard, encouraged by an interview with Hutton, took the women's side on the issue and reported the recommendations of the Senate of the University of London, which had investigated the exclusion policy of the London teaching hospitals. In another interview by the same newspaper Hutton said that

> the attitude towards women students has made us the laughing stock of Europe, nowhere else is there such an absurd system ... the objections against the woman student are very amusing.[51]

These objections focused on the 'embarrassing facts', which were required in the training of medical students.

Sir James Purves Stewart noted the contribution of some women doctors, but questioned the value of training more women when 'Fifty per cent of medical women, often the most accomplished, forsake the profession to marry'.[52] Hutton countered this argument with the claim that it was the profession that had forsaken women after marriage not the other way around. A hospital secretary was asked about this issue and rather astutely commented that 'the whole thing has arisen largely through the natural anxiety of the men to protect their own interests'.[53] The debate continued for nearly a year and a letter to the *Manchester Guardian* signed by Eleanor Rathbone, Ray Strachey, Ellen Wilkinson and Isabel Hutton emphasized the problems of the marriage bar and demanded freedom and equal opportunities. This letter also outlined the 1929 conclusions of the University of London's subcommittee on the medical education of women undergraduates, which found no valid arguments 'against the provision of co-education in medicine' and also dismissed the idea that a medical education was wasted on women because of marriage.[54]

Hutton recorded some of her ideas about women doctors and psychiatry during a visit to America in 1932. The trip was designed to promote a book deal with an American publisher and also allow her to meet other psychiatrists. Hutton noted the superior facilities, and better conditions for staff, evident at the new and 'gloriously furnished' medical centre at Cornell Hospital.[55] She was disappointed, however, that the care was very old-fashioned with no open-air nursing, no wards and locked rooms and bars everywhere. Hutton concluded that the clinic was 'to all intent and purpose an asylum'.[56] Hutton later visited Dr Adolf Meyer (1866–1950) at the Phipps clinic. Meyer was a pupil of Kraepelin but he was more optimistic in his approach to schizophrenia and particularly challenged the idea of a heredity factor in mental disorders.[57] Hutton found the outpatient department interesting because there was a great deal of teaching going on with medical students and social workers discussing cases. She also wrote that the head of teaching, Dr Esther Richards, was quite junior and although she had only been in the work for eight years she is an Associate Professor and has a splendid salary easy hours and private consulting work – many women have good posts – one on the staff Dr Baker a nice girl has only been five years a doctor and has an enormous salary.[58]

At the end of the day Hutton wrote despairingly in her journal 'quelle chance d'avoir une poste pareille!'[59] She did, however, find her work in England at two charitable facilities very satisfying according to her diaries and letters. These facilities were the British Hospital, a poor out-patient facility for mental disorders in London, and the Ellen Terry Home for blind mentally defective children, a very small home in Reigate with wealthy benefactors. They were both alternatives to the large state-run institutions and treated rate-aided patients but Hutton continued to apply for other positions in an effort to expand her work.

In 1934 Hutton made one final attempt at a paid position by applying for a part-time appointment at the St Marylebone Institution, stating that she would consider doing honorary work 'provided there was scope for treatment and research'. The reply from the LCC stated that

> Eligibility for appointment to the Council's service is restricted so far as married women are concerned, to those whose husbands are totally or permanently incapacitated by reason of physical or mental disability from supporting them, and in certain cases, those who have been deserted by their husbands.[60]

Hutton replied that 'fortunately I do not come under the category of the deserted wife or one who has a dependent husband'.[61] Shortly after this rejection she visited the Marylebone Institution while researching the possibility and value of adding a few in-patient beds to the British Hospital's clinic. She was not impressed by the superintendent Dr Spurgin, recording that 'I could see at that first glance that he was not the least bit interested in the patient, it was just a job for him'.[62] Hutton was concerned about misdiagnosed cases, the use of padded cells and the practice of sending home observation cases without treatment. She noted 'what a wonderful little teaching centre that could be and what good work could be done there among these so-called observation cases from hysteria right up to pre-senility' but her offer of help was again rejected.[63] This denied Hutton's skills, experience and enthusiasm to the Marylebone Institution patients but reaffirmed her commitment to the British Hospital and her desire to expand a model of 'early treatment' into in-patient care within the framework of the new Mental Treatment Act.

The British Hospital: 'this shabby one, with which I had been advised not to associate myself'[64]

The work of the British Hospital illustrates the difficulties of treating mental disorders in the poor outside the public asylum system prior to the 1930 Mental Treatment Act. Hutton's decision to work at the British Hospital in 1925 was a brave one because the hospital, founded in 1890, had a poor reputation, but it had been gradually improving since the early 1920s. Dr Lyttleton Stewart Forbes Winslow originally opened an out-patient clinic in Euston Road, London in February 1890 and it became known as the British Hospital for Functional Nervous Disorders.[65] Winslow also owned two small private asylums, had a private practice, worked at the West End Hospital and was planning to have a convalescent home for poor patients and pedagogical facilities. In 1891 the *New York Sun* reported on Winslow's 'great work among London's poor' and explained that the hospital only treated the indigent poor who were afflicted with mental disorders.[66] Winslow stated in this interview that he wanted to 'get at the poor people in that early stage of derangement' and also to treat children of the poorer class.[67]

The British Hospital was similar to the 'dispensary', which had developed from the middle of the eighteenth century to treat physical ailments. A dispensary had no wards, no in-patient facilities and treated patients exclusively on an out-patient basis.[68] Dispensaries for mental disorders were, however, new to the nineteenth century and towards the end of the century a few asylums and general hospitals had them but they were a rarity outside London.[69] At the start of the twentieth century dispensaries became known as 'clinics' and in London there were two for 'early mental cases', one at St. Thomas's Hospital and the other at the Charing Cross Hospital.[70] Winslow's facility was therefore a useful addition to the other clinics in the capital but the problems running this clinic without public funds were immense. First, there was no provision under the Lunacy Acts of 1890 and 1891 for a charitable facility, with no beds, to treat mental disorders. Second, the term 'hospital' was reserved exclusively for a foundation supported by endowment or subscription. Finally, because the hospital was actually a clinic and did not have beds it was ineligible for support from most trusts and charities. These burdens threatened to destroy Winslow's project before it got off the ground although Waddington argues that even the established hospitals in the 1890s had 'fatally deficient' sources of income.[71]

Winslow was however determined to gain and maintain the confidence of his patients by treating them outside of the asylum system and therefore had to rely on voluntary contributions and private donations to fund the hospital. All donors were given out-patient letters and each patient had to have a letter from a governor, a subscriber, a minister of religion, a magistrate or a medical practitioner confirming that the patient was deserving of free treatment, which was the usual practice for charitable facilities.[72] If wealthier persons wished to attend they were charged a small sum and encouraged to make a donation. The British Hospital saw patients in the evening, which was not only convenient for doctors working at other hospitals but also for the working poor.[73] These measures were fairly standard and could have ensured that a pioneering approach to mental health care would flourish, but Winslow's entrepreneurial approach to fundraising and cavalier attitude to record keeping tended to discredit the facility he created. In 1893 it was reported that the British Hospital had treated 15,000 patients over three years and that patients were placed in private homes with the incidental expenses paid for by the Samaritan Fund. Little detail is given in the annual reports of this practice but it appears similar to the Scottish guardianship schemes. The 1893 figures for attendance are remarkable if compared with the attendance of other clinics after the First World War and therefore have to be treated with some scepticism.[74] The few surviving financial records of this hospital also show that the Samaritan Fund was not viable and therefore this aspect of the work may also have been exaggerated.[75] The financial statement of 1892 showed that the donation boxes, patient contributions and annual subscriptions amounted to £526. This is a considerable sum if it is compared with Dr Helen Boyle's income for her dispensary in Brighton from 1899–1901, which was £152 3s 9d.[76]

Appeal pamphlets for the British Hospital used alarming statistics and emotive language as evidence of the urgent need to curb the increase in insanity and it was not long before the fundraising practices of Winslow's hospital were brought to the attention of the Charity Organization Society (COS). The COS was established in 1869 and Rose states that 'it might seem to epitomize all that was worst in the Victorian attitude to the poor' because it persistently criticized charities that were perceived as amateur and uncritical of the poor.[77] The work of the COS was based firmly on the principles of individualism and self-help and the poor were categorized into those deserving and undeserving of charitable help. The COS's attention was drawn to the fundraising activities of the British Hospital when a woman approached them for help stating that her only source of income was a third of her collections for the hospital. It was common practice to use street collectors for charities at this time but not so common to pay them. Winslow became aware that the COS was investigating the hospital and took legal advice. In 1892 a letter was sent to the COS chairman, Charles Loch, which accused it of being an 'irresponsible self-asserting society' and demanded an apology for the slanderous allegations based on 'pure malice'.[78] The antagonism between Loch and Winslow continued until 1913 and the hospital lost a great deal of revenue because of this unresolved, and very public, conflict.

There were serious problems with the administration of the British Hospital and the COS was quick to exploit this, writing in 1904 that

> There is still no improvement in the administration, and the financial defects still remain. The hospital ... has not been allowed to participate in the proceeds of either the Hospital Sunday or King Edward's Hospital Fund. Its methods of raising money by collections in the streets and at railway stations is highly objectionable. On these grounds I am still unable to recommend the hospital for charitable support.[79]

However, the COS was also guilty of misrepresentation because the King Edward's Hospital Fund did not support the treatment of mental disorders or out-patient clinics.[80] The COS had a hard line approach to mental disorders believing that the asylum was the only place for care and treatment. It also believed that many patients were responsible for their own illness because they did not work or abused alcohol and were therefore part of the 'undeserving' poor. The 1913–14 hospital Annual Report, after Winslow's death and the resignation of Charles Loch, highlights that the COS was now supporting the need for out-patient clinics for mental disorders, which was a considerable change in approach.[81] Outside medical practitioners were called upon to assist the hospital after Winslow's death and it was reported in December 1913 that Dr Hollander had resigned because he was opposed to the administrative practices of the hospital because it left it open to 'the aspersion that it was not being kept up for the benefit of the patients, but for the benefit of those who draw the salaries and commissions from the funds collected'.[82] However, by 1922 Dr Hollander had returned to the hospital stating that the defects in the administration had been remedied.[83]

The hospital gradually improved its administrative and financial systems but when Isabel Hutton joined in 1925 it was still struggling with a poor reputation despite the apparent value of its approach to care. Four years later Hutton extolled the virtues of out-patient treatment for mental and nervous disorders and wrote that:

> there exists in North London a small clinic which helps men and women to carry on their ordinary lives while still being treated for nervous or mental disease ... from four to five hundred new patients are dealt with each year, and the total attendances for that period are over four thousand.[84]

The article explained that originally the patients had not been charged but now wherever possible they paid one shilling and a small sum for medicine. Hutton also wrote that:

> they occasionally come with a doctor's card, and this we naturally prefer, much more often, however, they have not seen a doctor, but come having seen the board, or are brought by a friend for whom the clinic 'has done wonders'.[85]

Hutton emphasized the success of cases treated at the clinic, which were judged by the ability to prevent further attacks.

The British Hospital clearly did not have a separatist approach to medicine as it had male doctors and patients of both sexes but it was on the fringe of medical practice because of earlier scandals. Hutton certainly achieved a degree of clinical freedom at the institution and, in common with other leading female doctors like Helen Boyle, sought to create a distinct niche for herself by drawing attention to women's issues. Hutton highlighted the problems of the over-anxious mother and argued that successful treatment depended on helping other members of the family, especially the children. These ideas were behind the development of child guidance clinics from the late 1920s and echoed the wider aspirations of health and welfare professionals who were increasingly drawn to the casework approach. Hutton believed that neuroses in women could be caused by sexual difficulties, diet, sepsis or other diseases while poverty, poor housing, overwork and too many children also contributed to their nervous disorders. The consultations at the clinic involved a painstaking gathering of personal histories and a very wide range of mental and physical disorders were treated. This approach was very similar to Dr Helen Boyle's work at the Lady Chichester Hospital.[86] The work with children at the British Hospital complemented Hutton's experience with the mentally defective children at the Ellen Terry Home which clearly gave her a great deal of satisfaction.

Ellen Terry and a home for the blind mentally defective child[87]

The Theosophists opened the home for blind mentally defective children in 1926 at Reigate and named it after Ellen Terry (1847–1928), a Victorian actress whose eyesight had failed as she grew older. Terry supported work with blind children, giving her time and money generously.[88] The Servers of the Blind League were involved with the Ellen Terry Home (ETH) and organized fundraising; one leaflet stated that this was the first home to deal with these two conditions in children under sixteen.[89] The Theosophist Society ran the home during the first few months providing the children with a vegetarian diet and alternative therapies, but the Board of Control and the Board of Education intervened to ensure that the children were cared for in a more orthodox manner. Dr John Carswell was appointed visiting physician by the Board of Control, but he resigned after a few months and recommended Isabel Hutton as his replacement.[90] Hutton's appointment at the ETH is another example of the Board's inconsistency in relation to the marriage bar.

Hutton's experiences had led her to adopt a fairly optimistic approach to the problem of mental deficiency. She remained convinced of the value of training and education at a time when many practitioners were both pessimistic in outlook and custodial in approach. She also wrote that many 'backward' children were in fact suffering from a gland disorder and with treatment could improve a great deal. The regime at the ETH placed great emphasis on training, improvement and education. While most mental deficiency institutions were undergoing significant expansion to facilitate a more custodial approach, the ETH strived to maintain a small, homely atmosphere with a maximum of thirty children in residence. Only half of the children were certified 'mental defectives' and subject to the jurisdiction of the Board of Control, the others came under the Board of Education as being in need of special training. Training concentrated on the acquisition of clean bodily habits and good table manners, instruction on household tasks, and the training of the senses. The gramophone was used for listening, singing, dancing and exercising and occupational therapy developed handicraft skills and dexterity. The education syllabus emphasized sound and touch and Braille was taught to the more able minority who then borrowed books from the National Library for the Blind and read to the other children. Speech training was seen as a priority because the level of effective speech was believed to indicate the level of mental ability. Hutton made several visits to the home each week and observed the children while they worked, sang and played and she wrote that

> their reactions to training, their various unpredictable illnesses, their progress and temporary regressions and in some cases their degeneration, were most interesting and proceeded in a manner which I had not anticipated.[91]

It soon became apparent that the benefit to the child was greater if the training regime began as early as possible.[92] Hutton wrote that very young blind children were not diagnosed early because they 'were not examined by psychiatrists until they reached school age' and so she began to assess very young children at the Servers of the Blind League in London.[93] Hutton's observations on the children at the ETH illustrates the mental and physical progress of many of the children but she acknowledged that 'the mental deficiency of such children may be entirely due to their blindness, since they are thus cut off from so many external influences.'[94]

This interpretation of mental deficiency, caused by sensory deprivation and countered by efforts to reawaken the child's mind through specialist training, echoes the care and treatment offered by the original five English voluntary idiot asylums in the nineteenth century. This has been the subject of considerable recent research and it is generally agreed that in the twentieth century there was less emphasis on 'improvement and an increasing discourse on containment'.[95] This approach created some problems for the ETH as there is no evidence of Board of Control funding in the few remaining annual reports.[96] Instead the responsible local authority made a contribution towards a child's upkeep but this did not cover the full cost of the care. In 1933 local authorities contributed £2,606 4s 6d and £3,800 was raised from charitable sources; the total expenditure that year was £5,511 4s 4d for the care of thirty children – £184 per child per annum or approximately £3 13s per week. Fundraising was the main source of income for the home and the intensive care and training was very expensive if it is compared with alternatives available at the time. In 1932 the cost of keeping a person at the Stoke Park Colony (for epileptics) was between 18s 8d and 22s 2d per week depending on the grade of the case. In 1933 other institutions for those defined as mentally defective charged the following: Chailey £1 15s, Cuckfield £1 16s and Steyning £1 17s.[97] At Dungates Farm, run by the Brighton Guardianship Society, the charges from January 1934 were 20s per head per week.[98] This type of care was however different because the boys contributed to their own upkeep by working on and outside the farm and the medical involvement was far less than at the ETH. The Guardianship Society was run on a very tight budget and often had a deficit at the end of a year. However, in 1933–34, a time of national economic hardship, the ETH finished the year with £955 'excess of Income over expenditure'.[99] Hutton was presiding over a regime that was financially sound and while it remained a marginal provider of beds it offered a real alternative to conventional mental deficiency work.

Conclusion

This chapter uses the careers of two medical women to outline the difficulties single and married women faced when trying to develop a medical career and the strategies they used to work in their chosen speciality. It attempts to fill a gap in the history of psychiatry where both women doctors and out-patient care have been neglected, and further argues that women struggling to enter the profession often adopted radical approaches towards care and treatment that served to 'normalize' provision for the mentally ill.[100] Hutton faced problems in her career because of her marital status. She worked in and around London, which meant she was excluded from the full-time lucrative paid positions, but she was determined to be financially independent. She received approximately £250 per annum for her work at the Ellen Terry Home and the rest of her income came from her private practice and her publications. Dr Isabel Hutton's career in London battling against prejudice, patriarchy and the marriage bar was frustrating, fragmented and outside mainstream psychiatry which meant she had very little power to effect radical change in the treatment of mental disorders nationally. Dr Helen Boyle, on the other hand, took a separatist approach in Brighton which provided her with work and a career on her own terms alongside a network of female doctors but this work was also outside mainstream psychiatry and she too had very little influence on the direction of mental health care. Her evidence to the Royal Commission on Lunacy and Mental Disorder in 1925 contained many innovative ideas for change but they were largely ignored in the subsequent 1930 Mental Treatment Act.

Hutton battled against the unequal opportunities in medicine, only achieving a senior consultant's post when the British Hospital was taken over by the National Health Service (NHS) in 1948 before being compulsorily retired in 1953. Hutton complained that NHS appointments had serious drawbacks for doctors used to working long hours voluntarily and wrote bitterly, 'I begged to be allowed to continue working at the clinic in an honorary capacity but I found that in no circumstances is such service accepted.'[101] Dr Hutton's place in the history of medicine is assured because of her war service with the Scottish Women's Hospitals but she also made a valuable contribution to medicine through her early work on GPI, as a writer of lay medical books and as a firm supporter of outpatient care for the mentally disordered poor. Her campaign for equal rights in medicine also deserves a place in feminist history.

Dyhouse notes that the question of whether or not medical training was wasted on women continued to be argued through the 1960s and beyond.[102] The restrictive quotas for women medical students was only abandoned in 1973, two years before the Sex Discrimination Act was passed, because the view prevailed that women's contribution to the profession would be less because of their domestic commitments.[103] Recent research into the career choices of newly qualified doctors (1993) shows that psychiatry is the least popular speciality with only 4 per cent of men and women stating it as a first preference.[104] Psychiatry was not a popular specialism at the start of the twentieth century either but Boyle and Hutton both made a positive choice to work in a medical sphere where radical change was desperately needed. Both were committed to outpatient prophylactic care, which was the antithesis of the asylum system at the time, and both battled against patriarchy in the government agencies and the profession generally.

Research in 1997 showed that women doctors believe that medicine is still male dominated and that 'they have to work harder to compete, have less status, get passed over for promotion, and find it difficult to get a GP partnership'.[105] Women have accounted for half of medical school graduates since 1991 but as recently as 2001 a report by the Royal College of Physicians concluded that hospital medical specialities 'remain a male dominated profession', largely because of the inflexible working practices, and made recommendations for more job-shares and part-time opportunities for those specialists with family commitments.[106] For campaigners like Hutton, who believed women as doctors had much to offer patients, especially female ones, by pioneering new ways of working, this would have been a particularly depressing conclusion. Although in 1960 Dr Letitia Fairfield wrote that Isabel Hutton had 'steadily refused to let the most obstinate prejudice get her down' and that she made the most of the opportunities that came her way.[107]

Notes

1 J. Oppenheim, *Shattered Nerves: Doctors, Patients and Depression in Victorian England*, Oxford: Oxford University Press, 1991; P. Chesler, *Women and Madness*, London: Doubleday, 1972; S. Poirier, 'The Weir Mitchell Rest Cure: Doctor and Patients', *Women's Studies* 10, 1983, pp. 15–40; B. Sicherman, 'The Uses of a Diagnosis: Doctors, Patients and Neurasthenia', *Journal of the History of Medicine*, 32(1), 1977, pp. 33–54; G. E. Berrios and H. Freeman (eds), *150 Years of British Psychiatry, 1841–1991*, London: Gaskell and Royal College of Psychiatrists, 1991; W. F. Bynum, R. Porter and M. Shepherd (eds), *The Anatomy of Madness* (vols I, II & III), London: Tavistock, 1985 and London: Routledge, 1988; J. Andrews, A. Briggs, R. Porter, P. Tucker and K. Waddington, *The History of Bethlem*, London: Routledge, 1997; A. Digby, *Madness, Morality and Medicine: A Study of the York Retreat, 1796–1914*, Cambridge: Cambridge University Press, 1985.
2 L. Westwood, 'Avoiding the Asylum: Pioneering Work in Mental Health Care, 1890–1939' (unpublished DPhil, University of Sussex, 1999); S. Cherry, *Mental Health Care in Modern England: The Norfolk Lunatic Asylum/St Andrew's Hospital c.1810–1998*, Woodbridge: Boydell Press, 2003.
3 Chesler, *Women and Madness*; E. Showalter, *The Female Malady: Women, Madness and English Culture, 1830–1980*, London: Virago, 1987. For recent research see L. Bird, *The Fundamental Facts … all the Latest Facts and Figures on Mental Illness*, London: The Mental Health Foundation, 1999.
4 See W. L. Parry-Jones, *The Trade in Lunacy: A Study of Private Madhouses in the Eighteenth and Nineteenth Centuries*, London: Routledge, 1972; C. McKenzie, 'Women and Psychiatric Professionalization, 1780–1914', in The London Feminist Group (eds), *The Sexual Dynamics of History: Men's Power, Women's Resistance*, London: Pluto Press, 1983, pp. 107–119.
5 M. Elston, 'Women Doctors in a Changing Profession: The Case of Britain', in E. Riska and K. Wegar (eds), *Gender, Work and Medicine: Women and the Medical Division of Labour*, London: Sage, 1993, pp. 27–61, see p. 29.
6 L. Walker, '"Conservative Pioneers": The Formation of the South African Society of Medical Women', *Social History of Medicine*, 14(3), 2001, pp. 483–505. Walker acknowledges the influence of A. Witz, *Professions and Patriarchy*, London: Routledge, 1992, and her challenge to previous accounts that had tended to portray women doctors simply as victims of a patriarchal profession.
7 Witz, *Professions and Patriarchy*, pp. 75 and 83.
8 See C. Blake, *The Charge of the Parasols: Women's Entry to the Medical Profession*, London: The Women's Press, 1990.
9 C. Dyhouse, *No Distinction of sex? Women in British Universities 1870–1939*, London: UCL Press, 1995, pp. 12–13; C. Dyhouse, 'Driving Ambition: Women in Pursuit of a Medical Education, 1890–1939', *Women's History Review*, 7, 1998, pp. 321–341.
10 Witz, *Professions and Patriarchy*, pp. 73–92.
11 Elston, 'Women Doctors in a Changing Profession', p. 29.
12 A. Helen Boyle, 'Watchman What of the Night'? (Presidential Address), *Journal of Mental Science*, LXX (358), September 1939; C. McKenzie, 'Women and Psychiatric Professionalization, 1780–1914', p. 117.
13 M. A. C. Elston, *Women Doctors in the British Health Services: A Sociological Study of their Careers and Opportunities* (unpublished PhD thesis, University of Leeds, 1986), Chapter 6, also see Fig. 7.1, figures taken from the *Englishwoman's Yearbook: Medical Directory*.
14 Contemporary Medical Archives Centre at the Wellcome Trust for the History of Medicine (CMAC) SA/GC archives of Dr Letitia Fairfield.

15 CMAC, SA/MWF/D11. 'The Work of Women Medical Officers in Mental Hospitals', *Journal Of Mental Science*, October 1927, Reprint.

16 Archival material relating to these organizations is held at the Women's Library, Old Castle Street, London, E1 7NT.

17 Alison Oram has identified women teachers as a group severely affected by the marriage bar but this exclusionary policy is never mentioned in relation to women doctors. A. Oram, 'Serving Two Masters? The Introduction of a Marriage Bar in Teaching in the 1920s', in *The Sexual Dynamics of History*, pp. 134–148.

18 L. McCarthy, 'Idealists or Pragmatists? Progressives and Separatists among Australian Medical Women, 1900–1940', *Social History of Medicine*, 16(2), 2003, pp. 263–282; Private Papers of Dr Isabel Hutton (hereafter PP Hutton).

19 McCarthy, 'Idealists or Pragmatists?', pp. 270–271.

20 She was concerned that government approval of her hospital for early nervous disorders, via the regulating authority on lunacy, would lead to interference from a male-dominated intransigent organization.

21 G. Eyre Woodhead, the founder of the Brighton Guardianship Society, is a good example of this. Records held at the East Sussex Record Office in Lewes. See L. Westwood, 'Avoiding the Asylum'.

22 For more on Boyle's involvement in the Guardianship Society see Westwood, 'Avoiding the Asylum'.

23 C. L. Hingston and C. Vince, 'Death of a Pioneer', *Medical Women's Federation Journal*, 58, 1958, pp. 58–67; Obituary of Dr Helen Boyle, *BMJ*, 30 November 1957, p. 1310.

24 See L. Westwood, 'A Quiet Revolution in Brighton: Dr Helen Boyle's Pioneering Approach to Mental Health Care, 1899–1939', *Social History of Medicine*, 14, 2001, pp. 439–457.

25 Thomson argues that the Board of Control was cautious about supporting innovative practice such as care in the community because poor public relations placed it in a defensive position. M. Thomson, *The Problem of Mental Deficiency: Eugenics, Democracy and Social Policy in Britain c.1870–1959*, Oxford: Clarendon Press, 1998, pp. 80–81.

26 Westwood, 'A Quiet Revolution in Brighton', p. 443.

27 H. Boyle, 'Some Points in the Early Treatment of Mental and Nervous Cases (With Special Reference to the Poor)', *Journal of Mental Science*, 51, October 1905, pp. 676–710.

28 J. Carswell, 'The History of an Experiment in Dealing with the Reported Cases of Insanity Occurring in the Barony Parish of Glasgow', *Journal of Mental Science*, 40, July 1894, pp. 394–475. See also H. Sturdy and W. Parry-Jones, 'Boarding-out Insane Patients: The Significance of the Scottish System 1857–1913' in P. Bartlett and D. Wright (eds), *Outside the Walls of the Asylum: The History of Care in the Community 1750–2000*, London: Athlone Press, 1999.

29 See Carswell, 'History of an Experiment'; Sturdy and Parry-Jones, 'Boarding-out Insane Patients'.

30 E. J. Engstrom, 'The Birth of Clinical Psychiatry: Power, Knowledge and Professionalization in Germany, 1867–1914' (unpublished PhD thesis, University of North Carolina at Chapel Hill, 1997), pp. 286–287.

31 Engstrom, 'The Birth of Clinical Psychiatry', p. 298.

32 Memorandum of evidence given on behalf of the Lady Chichester Hospital to the Royal Commission on Lunacy and Mental Disorder, 20 May 1925 (CMAC) SA/MWF/21. Records of the Lady Chichester Hospital held at the East Sussex Record Office (ESRO) in Lewes. The patient records have survived from the early 1920s. A project supported by a grant from the Wellcome Trust to catalogue and preserve these papers has just begun.

33 Mental Treatment Act (20 & 21 Geo. (P.P., 1930, V)).

34 PP Hutton, held by her niece, details withheld on request, undated resume and obituary, *The Times*, 12 January 1960.

35 For a brief history of this asylum see A. Beveridge, 'Life in the Asylum: Patients' Letters from Morningside, 1873–1908', *History of Psychiatry*, IX, 1998, pp. 431–469.

36 See Carswell, 'The History of an Experiment'; Sturdy and Parry-Jones, 'Boarding-out Insane Patients'.

37 PP Hutton, Letter dated 27 December 1922.

38 I. Hutton, *Memories of a Doctor in War & Peace*, London: Heinemann, 1960, p. 213.

39 I. E. Hutton, *The Hygiene of Marriage*, London: Heinemann, 1923; *With a Woman's Unit in Serbia, Salonika and Sebastapol*, London: Williams & Norgate, 1928; *The Sex Technique in Marriage*, New York: Emerson, 1932; *The Last Taboo: Mental Disorders in Modern Life*, London: Heinemann, 1934; *The Hygiene of the Change of Life*, London: Heinemann, 1936.

40 PP Hutton, Diary from 22 September to 6 November 1925.

41 Hutton, *Memories of a Doctor*, p. 220.

42 PP Hutton, 23 March 1928.

43 I. Hutton, *The Times*, 'Women Medical Students', 26 March 1928.

44 I. Hutton, *Daily Telegraph*, 'Women in the Medical Profession, should Marriage be a Bar?', 26 March 1928.

45 A. M. Oram, 'Serving two masters? The introduction of a marriage bar in teaching in the 1920s', *The Sexual Dynamics of History*, pp. 136–137.

46 D. Spender, *Time and Tide Wait for No Man*, London: Pandora Press, 1984, p. 129.

47 CMAC. SA/MWF/B2. Quarterly newsletters, September 1920.

48 CMAC. MWF newsletters, July 1921, pp. 9–10. The Public Health Department in Manchester employed several married women and eight married medical women held posts under the corporations in Manchester and Salford. The Chief MO in charge of Maternity and Child Welfare for the County of Durham was a married woman and Northumberland and Newcastle had no rules against the employment of married women.

49 CMAC. MWF newsletters, July 1921, p. 9. When challenged by the MWF the MoH explained that its medical jobs were often arduous, exacting and required extensive travel and were therefore unsuitable for women with home ties. Another argument used was that female civil servants had to be unmarried and to treat medical women differently would be unfair and impractical.

50 PP Hutton, *Evening Standard*, undated, late 1928?

51 PP Hutton, *Evening Standard*, 7 January 1929.

52 PP Hutton, *The Times*, 'Women Medical Students', 26 March 1928.

53 PP Hutton, *Evening Standard*, 7 January 1929.

54 PP Hutton, *Manchester Guardian*, 2 March 1929.

55 PP Hutton, American Journal, 6 October 1932.

56 PP Hutton,

57 See M. Gelder 'Introduction: Adolf Meyer and his influence on British Psychiatry', *History of Psychiatry*, 14,4,56, December 2003, pp. 475–493.

58 PP Hutton, American Journal, 17 October 1932, Hotel Belvedere, Baltimore.

59 PP Hutton, American Journal, 'What luck to have a position like that!'

60 PP Hutton, 8 March 1934.

61 PP Hutton, 9 March 1934.

62 PP Hutton, Report on visit to Marylebone Institution, 15 May 1934.

63 PP Hutton, Report on visit to Marylebone Institution, 15 May 1934.

64   Hutton, *Memories of a Doctor*, p. 258.
65   The hospital was originally called The Forbes Winslow Memorial Hospital after Forbes Benignus Winslow, a well-known alienist and father of the founder, who died in 1874.
66   For more on the British Hospital see Westwood, 'Avoiding the Asylum'.
67   London Metropolitan Archive (LMA). A/FWA/C/D198/1–2, March 1891.
68   I. S. I. Loudon, 'Origins and Growth of the Dispensary Movement in England', *Bulletin of The History of Medicine*, 55(3), 1981, pp. 322–342.
69   Anonymous, 'Out-patient Department at the Wakefield Asylum', *Journal of Mental Science*, 36, October 1890, pp. 529–530.
70   A. Helen Boyle 'The Early Treatment of the Psychoses and Psychoneuroses', *BMJ*, 24, November 1928, pp. 923–926.
71   K. Waddington, 'Finance, Philanthropy and the Hospital: Metropolitan Hospitals 1850–1898' (unpublished PhD thesis, University College London, 1995), p. 336.
72   See Harold W. Hart 'Some Notes on the Sponsoring of Patients for Hospital Treatment under the Voluntary System', *Medical History*, 1980, pp. 447–460.
73   LMA. A/FWA/C/D198/1, *Organised Philanthropy*, 2 September 1891.
74   Westwood, 'Avoiding the Asylum', pp. 179–184.
75   St. Mary's Hospital Archive (SMHA) Praed Street, London. A few annual reports and other documents are held here.
76   ESRO. HB63/1 – Annual Report.
77   M. E. Rose, *The Relief of Poverty 1834–1914*, London: Macmillan, 1972, p. 25; R. Humphries, *Sin, Organised Charity and the Poor Law in Victorian England*, London: Macmillan, 1995.
78   LMA. A/FWA/C/D198/1–2. Letter from Winslow's solicitor, 1 October 1894.
79   LMA. A/FWA/C/D198/1–2. Letter to the Duchess of Grafton 1904.
80   F. K. Prochaska, *Philanthropy and the Hospitals of London: The King's Fund 1897–1990*, London: Clarendon Press, 1992, see appendices II and III.
81   SMHA. Annual Report.
82   LMA, *Truth*, December 1913.
83   LMA, *Truth*, June 1922.
84   PP Hutton, 'Mental and Nervous Outpatients' by a Woman Physician, *Service*, XII(2), 1929 (Written anonymously but found among Hutton's private papers.)
85   PP Hutton, 'Mental and Nervous Outpatients'.
86   Westwood, 'A Quiet Revolution'.
87   For the history of the care and control of the mentally defective see D. Wright and A. Digby (eds), *From Idiocy to Mental Deficiency: Historical Perspectives on People with Learning Disabilities*, London: Routledge, 1996 and Thomson, *The Problem of Mental Deficiency*.
88   The Theosophist Society was founded in 1875. It claimed to be derived from the sacred writings of Brahmanism and Buddhism but denied the existence of any personal god.
89   Material courtesy of the National Trust Ellen Terry House, Smallhythe Place. Undated leaflet from The Braille and Servers of the Blind League.
90   Hutton, 'Memories of a Doctor', pp. 247–254.
91   Hutton, 'Memories of a Doctor', pp. 247–254.
92   PP Hutton, 'The Blind Mentally Defective Child – As Observed in a Group of One Hundred and Twenty Cases', December 1926 to 1938, 30,000 word unpublished paper not completed until 1952, hereafter known as 'Observations'.
93   'Observations'.
94   'Observations'.

95 D. Gladstone, 'The Changing Dynamics of Institutional Care: The Western Counties Idiot Asylum 1864–1914', in D. Wright and A. Digby (eds), *From Idiocy to Mental Deficiency*, pp. 134–160. See also essays in that volume by M. Thomson, D. Wright and M. Jackson.

96 National Trust, Smallhythe Place (NTSP), Annual report 1933–34.

97 ESRO – C/C/11/50/2 East Sussex Mental Deficiency Committee Minute Book.

98 ESRO. GUA 32/8, 32/10, 13/1–10, 14/1–14. Dungates and Tubwell Farms' records.

99 NTSP. Annual Report 1933–34.

100 Over the last twenty years Showalter, Jalland and McKenzie have attempted to raise the profile of women in the psychiatric profession prior to the Second World War. See Showalter, *The Female Malady*; P. Jalland, *Octavia Wilberforce: The Autobiography of a Pioneer Woman Doctor*, London: Cassell, 1989; McKenzie, 'Psychiatric and Professionalization'.

101 Hutton, *Memories of a Doctor*, p. 232.

102 C. A. Dyhouse, 'Women Students and the London Medical Schools, 1914–1939: The Anatomy of a Masculine Culture', *Gender and History*, 10(1), April 1998, pp. 110–132, p. 111.

103 Elston, 'Women Doctors in a Changing Profession', p. 34.

104 Lambert, Goldacre, Edwards and Parkhouse 'Career Preferences of Doctors who Qualified in the United Kingdom in 1993 Compared with those of Doctors Qualifying in 1974, 1977,1980, 1983', *BMJ*, 313, 6 July 1996, pp. 19–24.

105 R. Dobson, 'Women Doctors Believe Medicine is Male Dominated', *BMJ*, 315, 12 July 1997, p. 80.

106 Royal College of Physicians Working Party Report, 2001, www.rcplondon.ac.uk/pubs/wp_womeninmed_summary.htm (accessed 1 November 2005).

107 Obituary, *The Lancet*, 23 January 1960, p. 231.

6 Family, gender and class in psychiatric patient care during the 1930s

The 1930 Mental Treatment Act and the Devon Mental Hospital

David Pearce

It has appeared in practice that there is among a great number of the less enlightened of London's population extreme reluctance on the part of husbands, for example, to 'sign away' their wives, as they put it. If mental hospital care is necessary the husband will reluctantly acquiesce; but if it is put to him that he should himself take an active step in the matter and sign a formal application for his wife's admission to mental hospital care he will refuse point blank, even in the face of tactful explanation and persuasion ... Ignorance and prejudice die extremely hard, and it will take a long time to educate the average East End Londoner, let us say, to take an enlightened view of what is really his duty to his wife stuporose and confused after childbirth.[1]

(Curtis, 1938)

Introduction: the historical significance of the 1930 Mental Treatment Act

The commentary quoted above illustrates one psychiatrist's view that the certification of an individual often began with an assessment of the prospective patient's behaviour by members of their own family who were usually responsible for alerting medical professionals to the predicament of those suffering mental illness. This doctor was writing a few years after the passage of the important Mental Treatment Act of 1930. This legislation was designed to remedy some of the problems which were perceived to have arisen after the passage of the important 1890 Lunacy Act, which had provided for the certification of lunatic paupers and their admission to a public asylum, their compulsory entry into the institution being usually arranged by a local Relieving Officer of the Poor Law. It was clearly assumed that the certified person was seriously disordered and unable to consent to their own treatment. The new Act introduced in 1930 amended rather than replaced its predecessor of 1890, though significant reforms in the terms on which persons could be treated were introduced. In addition to the formal certification and compulsory admission of an insane person to an approved institution, the 1930 Act introduced two new classes of patient: first, the voluntary patient could gain admission to a mental hospital by written application, which clearly expressed their wish for treatment; second, the class of temporary patients were those considered by medical doctors as having a relatively brief illness with good prospects for recovery but who were incapable of accepting or refusing admission to a hospital. The temporary patients were subject to involuntary treatment for a maximum of six months in the first instance, though with two further extensions (of three months each) possible without the need for formal certification by a magistrate.

The impact of the 1930 Mental Treatment Act on the care of patients has attracted relatively little scholarly attention, though the literature includes various assessments which indicate that the impact of the measure was to increase the choices available to families as much as individuals in deciding on treatment and that the provisions for voluntary stays in hospital would be likely to encourage greater use by the middle classes of public institutions. The quotation given above suggests that, even in the mid-twentieth century, how the family of prospective patients were likely to respond to the risks and benefits of admission would depend on the information available to them and on the persistence of ignorance and prejudice in regard to mental illness. Even where the consent of the individual was necessary prior to any admission, as in the case of voluntary patients admitted under the 1930 legislation, scholars such as McGarry and Chodoff argue that some element of persuasion and even coercion might be present, ranging from gentle persuasion to more forceful pressure, which meant that the agreement of individuals to such treatment should be understood as points on a 'spectrum of assent' in which family members often contributed to decisions made by individuals.[2] This chapter seeks to address the question of the influence of gender, families and social class on the admission, treatment and discharge of patients admitted to the Devon Mental Hospital at Exminster during the years 1931–38. All admissions, amounting to some 3,000 in total, were examined, covering the different categories of patient established under the 1930 legislation.

The role of families in the committal and discharge of individuals to the publicly funded asylum in England and Wales has been the subject of some debate in recent studies, with scholars such as Prestwich, Suzuki and Wright arguing for the central role of families in the confinement and release of the insane from institutional care.[3] In his earlier study of discharges from Buckinghamshire County Pauper Lunatic Asylum in the Victorian period, Wright argued that the decision to discharge a patient depended on 'a consideration of the ability and willingness of the inmate's family to receive the person back into the household' as well as the availability of space in the asylum, the concern of magistrates for public safety and the preferences of the guardians of the Poor Law who sent individuals to the asylum.[4] Adair *et al.* showed in their study of the Devon County Lunatic Asylum (the predecessor of the Devon Mental Hospital sited at Exminster) in the period 1845–1914 that the unmarried were disproportionately represented among the inmates of the Victorian asylum and that the willingness of families to accept the return of a family member was one factor in the decision to discharge those who were deemed to have recovered, or shown 'relief' from their symptoms.[5] Until we have more detailed information on decision-making within kinship groups and the negotiations between relatives and officials, it is difficult to reach any firm conclusions on the role of families in the admission and discharge of patients and very little research has been completed on the period 1914–48 which would enable scholars to assess the impact of changing legislation on the influence exerted by family members as responsibility for the care of the insane steadily passed from the Poor Law to local government and the direct influence of county magistrates diminished during the twentieth century.

The scope for some family influence in the passage of individuals to and from the asylum and mental hospital should not obscure the impact of social class and status in the institutional committal, treatment and discharge of mental patients. Andrew Scull has described the expansion of the psychiatric in-patient population in the nineteenth century as being 'substantially an expansion of the pauper sector', though there remains some question as to whether those entering the public asylum should be considered paupers.[6] A number of scholars have noted the limited asylum provision made for those groups, such as the governess, whose social rank discouraged an approach to the Poor Law authorities but whose modest means often precluded access to the more expensive private institutions.[7] The new legislation of 1930 introduced significant legal reforms to the admission and detention of mental patients, including a category of voluntary patient who did not require the consent of the asylum authorities to secure their discharge. Temporary admissions were also permitted for the first time, allowing committal to the mental hospital for a period of six to twelve months. The terms on which the consent of patients was secured remains a matter for further enquiry. McGarry and Chodoff argued that voluntary patients frequently experienced some degree of pressure or persuasion from family, friends or the medical profession and we should place the admission of such individuals on a 'spectrum of assent' rather than imposing a sharp distinction between the compulsory and the voluntary entry into institutional care.[8] The evidence from both the Devon Asylum and the later Mental Hospital indicates that the medical staff of the institution and more particularly the Superintendent continued to exercise considerable sway over the treatment and release if not the admission of patients to Exminster and that the discretionary power of psychiatrists should not be underestimated even as the role of external agencies is acknowledged.[9] At the same time it appears that an important consequence of the new legislation was to encourage greater use of the public mental hospitals by more affluent groups, including lower middle class salaried employees.

There is now a formidable mass of recent research on the Victorian asylum and the various ways in which the insane were diagnosed during the nineteenth century. Relatively few of the symptoms and conditions identified by general practitioners and asylum medical staff in the later years of the nineteenth century can be readily aligned with the neuroses familiar to modern psychiatry.[10] One interesting feature of research on mental patients in the later twentieth century is the finding that those compelled to enter a mental hospital were primarily of a lower social class, and also less likely to display neurotic illness than higher social groups.[11] The research undertaken on the Devon Mental Hospital in the 1930s was designed, in part, to address the question of the relationship between diagnosis, terms of admission and social class among the intake.

Reformers who championed a reform of the Lunacy Act of 1890 frequently argued that mental illness was a progressive disease and prospects for recovery were better when a sufferer received early treatment. To facilitate this, they advocated measures that reduced the threat of compulsion and encouraged people to accept early voluntary treatment. In the debates on the proposed legislation which became the Mental Treatment Act of 1930, Labour spokespeople such as McShane and Lawrence (the latter being Parliamentary Secretary to the Minister of Health 1929–31) argued that working class mothers in particular would benefit from a period of rest and respite from the strains of managing the family household and should receive the specialist treatment which trained psychiatrists could provide.[12]

This chapter argues that the legislation of 1930 marked an important change in the ways in which people were admitted to, and treated within, Britain's mental hospitals, though it is fair to say that the Mental Treatment Act amended rather than swept away the provisions of the 1890 lunacy legislation. An obvious change can be found in the provision of a legal right for patients to enter rate-aided mental hospitals by expressing their wish (in writing) to do so. Admission on a voluntary basis required a clear decision by the individual to accept residential treatment. It was not sufficient to demonstrate an absence of resistance to such care. Temporary patients on the other hand were persons who were deemed by their doctors to be incapable of giving such clear consent but who were considered to have good prospects of early recovery. These patients were committed to a mental hospital for an initial period not exceeding six months, though with the possibility of two three-month extensions, without the requirement for compulsory detention on the orders of a magistrate. Under the terms of the 1930 legislation voluntary patients had the power to discharge themselves by giving seventy-two hours notice while

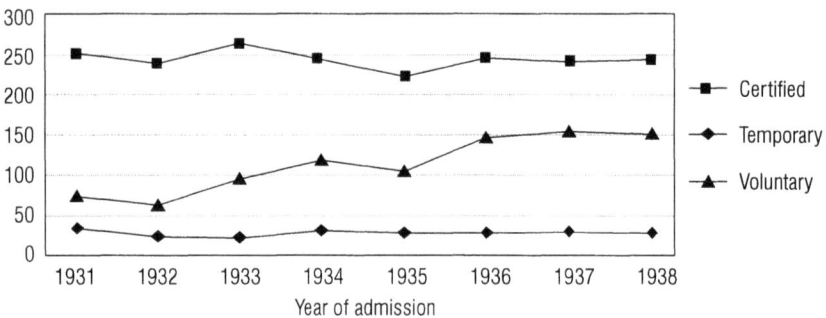

Figure 6.1   Admission of patients by legal status to Devon Mental Hospital, 1931–38.

the temporary patient was detained until their period of committal expired or their release was agreed by the medical authorities.

The graph (Figure 6.1) indicates the numbers admitted in the different categories to the Devon Mental Hospital grouped by legal status in the years following the introduction of the Act.

The admission registers show a substantial, fairly stable number of certified patients admitted to the Devon Hospital during this period, alongside a smaller but rapidly growing number of voluntary patients entering Exminster. The absence of any clear substitution of volunteers for the certified suggests that the voluntary group were a fresh and perhaps different constituency of patients from those who were sent on the order of a magistrate. The patients admitted on a voluntary basis differed from the certified group in certain respects. They were noticeably younger than the average for the inmate population as a whole while certified patients were significantly older than the average. The smaller group of temporary patients did not differ in their age from the mean for the asylum intake as a whole. The following section considers the influences of family, gender and social class which are discernible in the admissions.

The influence of family, gender and social class in the Devon Hospital admissions

The distinct groups of admissions to the Devon Hospital during the 1930s indicate variations in the marital status and family relationships of those entering the Exminster facility in these years. Taken as a whole, the Exminster patients were less likely to be married than the wider Devon population recorded in the census of 1931, though the involuntary (certified) group had a much higher proportion of unmarried people than did the voluntary patients. The role of family members in the committal of the patients also appears to have been affected by the terms of the 1930 legislation. Although the terms of the Act stipulated that the individual should clearly consent to treatment prior to entry on a voluntary basis, the evidence from the Devon Hospital indicates that relatives played an influential role in such admissions. In comparing the persons identified on the admission forms with those to be contacted in the event of death, we find only a limited number of patients were unable or unwilling to record a near relative. Such individuals were much more likely to be compulsory than voluntary admissions, though a number of married males also gave their closest male relative rather than their wife as the person to be contacted.

Attempting to understand the importance of family and kinship ties from such sources is not an easy task. It seems likely that families would have calculated the costs and benefits of admission prior to any committal of their productive and unproductive members to the Devon Hospital. The greater visibility of close relatives among the voluntary patients may indicate that concerned relatives were able to persuade family members to enter hospital at an earlier stage in their illness while more isolated people would have deteriorated to a state which caused concerned neighbours or the authorities to intervene. Scholars of the Victorian asylum have long recognized that the existence of domestic support figured in the decisions of medical staff to commit and/or release individuals to/from closed institutions. The evidence from this period shows that unmarried patients were significantly more likely to die in the Devon Mental Hospital than their married counterparts. Marital status continued to figure in the distinctive experience of mental patients in the mid-twentieth century.

The influence of gender on the identification and treatment of mental illness has attracted considerable discussion in the recent historiography of insanity and mental disability.[13] In her analysis of the impact of the 1930 Act, Busfield has argued that in the years following the introduction of voluntary status under this legislation, persons with 'diagnoses falling in the psycho-neurotic range' were admitted in increasing numbers and that such diagnoses were 'predominantly female'.[14] The suggestion that the Mental Treatment Act disproportionately extended the number of women in the voluntary class is not apparent in the Devon case, where, though the numbers do not quite reach statistical significance, females predominate more markedly in the temporary and certified groups of admissions during the 1930s (Table 6.1). Nor were female patients unequally represented among those diagnosed as suffering from neuroses. The diagnostic groups with the heaviest proportion of women were those of confusional psychosis, mania and melancholia. The excess number of females in these three categories more than accounted for the superiority of female over male admissions.

One of the most interesting features of the Devon intake is the greater preponderance of women over men among the 'temporary' patients admitted in the 1930s. Contemporary experts frequently commented that the psychiatric illnesses affecting females were more likely to remove their

Table 6.1 Sex of patients compared to legal class in the Devon Mental Hospital

Sex	Total	Certified	Temporary	Voluntary
Female	1,507 (57.8%)	1,050 (58.4%)	46 (67.6%)	411 (54.7%)
Male	1,111 (42.2%)	748 (41.6%)	22 (32.4%)	341 (45.3%)

capacity for volition, disqualifying their entrance on a voluntary basis. Marshall's study of 3,000 direct admissions to Bexley Mental Hospital showed almost one-fifth of women were given diagnoses suitable for temporary residence, as compared to little more than a tenth of men. Since these diagnoses were in practice descriptions of behaviour rather than rigorous categories, including delirium and gross confusion, stupor (including severe depression), and apathy, it is perhaps not surprising that females were more likely to be placed under these diagnostic headings, whereas 'general paralysis' and 'recent mania' were the only terms used primarily for males at Bexley.[15] The assessment offered by Busfield and others appears to be more relevant to the group of temporary rather than voluntary patients admitted after 1930, since it is difficult to avoid the conclusion that the diagnoses of such patients were influenced by the gendered perceptions of women among contemporary, primarily male, doctors responsible for the examination of these individuals.

The social and occupational profile of those admitted to the Devon Hospital in the period cannot be attributed to the expansion of what Scull refers to as the 'pauper section' of the English population in explaining the growth of nineteenth-century asylums.[16] It was noted earlier that the impetus for growth came from the voluntary patients. The evidence from the Devon case suggests that there were clear social class differences in the background of the different categories of patient and whereas 'labourers' were noticeably more likely to enter Exminster as certified patients, clerks and similar salaried employees were more evident among the voluntary intake. These occupational variations are also apparent in the diagnoses given to the patients. Approximately one in three male clerks were given a diagnosis of neurosis, compared to about one in thirty male labourers. Since no female clerical workers were said to be suffering from neurosis, it is unlikely that such variations were due to sex differences among the intake to the Hospital. Socio-demographic factors also appear to have influenced the outcome of residence at Exminster, with male clerks noticeably more likely to be discharged than labourers (Table 6.2), though the main features of Hospital releases are discussed below.

Registrations made at the Devon Mental Hospital during these years clearly suggest that voluntary status and a diagnosis of 'neurosis' was more strongly associated with 'white-collar' rather than 'blue-collar' employment in the contemporary labour force. The factors which led to greater voluntary admissions among non-manual staff employees have not been

Table 6.2 Outcome of certified male clerks and labourers in the Devon Mental Hospital

Occupation	Died	Discharged
Labourers	90	58
Clerks	0	15

the subject of extensive, detailed historical research and any interpretation of the Devon statistics must remain speculative. It appears likely that such individuals were more likely to understand the opportunities presented by the fresh legislation in 1930, and have reserves of savings which would tide their families over during their absence in hospital. Such an explanation lays stress on the demand for mental health services, though it is also likely that doctors and the Poor Law officers who continued to have some role in the admission process were more likely to suggest the option of voluntary treatment for higher-income individuals. The first point to make in this regard is that neuroses were now more readily understood and identified as a male as well as a female mental illness. Doody *et al.* used a retrospective classification of diagnoses to one Scottish asylum in the last quarter of the nineteenth century and found that only 1 per cent of patients could be identified, in modern psychiatric terms, as suffering from neuroses.[17] The corresponding figure for the Devon Mental Hospital in our period was 6 per cent, indicating a clear increase in the use of the diagnosis by the 1930s. Porter among others has emphasized the significance of the shell-shock 'epidemic' during the First World War, together with a popularization of scientific and psycho-analytic literature, in altering public perceptions of psychiatry in the early twentieth century. The growing scientific literacy of the middle classes may have contributed to a greater readiness to admit more educated individuals to public mental hospitals as voluntary admissions.

The records of admissions to the Devon Mental Hospital provide us with glimpses of the interplay of class background and medical perception rather than conclusive evidence of how social status and diagnostic classification were entwined. Voluntary patients were significantly more likely to be privately funded, though the increase in their admission to Exminster during these years was primarily due to the influx of rate-aided patients. The proportion of fee-payers hardly altered in this period. There do appear to have been subtle differences in their relationship with the Poor Law as well as medical staff outside and inside the Hospital. Since these patients were more likely to be identified as suffering from milder, 'neurotic-type' illnesses, there were better prospects for recovery than for the certified admissions, which were drawn largely from poorer social groups. Although the Relieving Officer of the Poor Law would be contacted in regard to the financial means of the voluntary as well as the compulsory admission, inflicting some stigma on the higher-income employees and their families, it appears that in most voluntary cases these officials were not directly involved prior to admission to Exminster.

Class bias is also apparent in the diagnosis and certification of patients in contemporary sources such as Henderson and Gillespie's *Text-book of Psychiatry* (1936), which recommended that certification was undesirable 'where the patient occupies an important public position, e.g. director of company, partnership, etc'.[18] The clear implication was that the social status of higher income patients was a fragile asset which could be easily damaged by compulsory admission to a mental hospital when other options were available. The same authors advised doctors to consider certification of patients where 'no adequate accommodation' was available in the individual's family home or in special nursing accommodation, or 'where money is a consideration'.[19] Such differences in the socio-demographic profile of the voluntary and certified patients appear to be remarkably similar to those recorded by Riecher-Rossler and Rossler in their survey of several studies of western countries published between 1958 and 1982. They found that patients who were committed on a compulsory basis were more likely to be drawn from the most vulnerable groups in society.[20] Such individuals were primarily older, unmarried males who were living alone. These findings can be compared with contemporary commentaries during the 1930s, such as that by Perk, who reported that the social origins of the voluntary admissions which followed the 1930 legislation were mainly from 'a higher social status' than the certified patients.[21]

The relatively small group of people admitted as temporary patients in these years again reveal some interesting characteristics. This group was most clearly associated with private status, half being funded in this way, though such patients were more likely than were rate-aided individuals to be reclassified as certified, compulsory residents at a later period in their stay at the Devon Hospital. One possible explanation for this surprising result may be that families of a higher social status and income wished to avoid the stigma of certification under the terms of the 1930 legislation, therefore securing their committal on a temporary fee-assisted basis. Whether it was the clear evidence of continued illness or the lesser stigma of reclassification as a certified resident later in the patient's career, the transfer to more permanent detention in the Hospital was fairly common. Private hospitals utilized this provision of the 1930 Act as well as public amenities. The Board of Control responsible for the regulation of mental hospitals noted in 1933 that only 2 per cent of temporary admissions were recorded in the previous year, though the proportion was higher 'in places to which only private patients are admitted'.[22] Other commentators also emphasized the limited use made of temporary admission under the Mental Treatment law for the benefit of rate-aided patients.[23]

The negotiation of admission status frequently involved delicate relationships of family connections as well as considerations of class and gender. One husband agreed to the admission of his wife to the Devon Hospital as a private patient only on the condition that she entered on a temporary order. Her residence was extended to the permitted maximum of one year, though she continued to actively resist her detention throughout that period. Rather than allow her to be certified and reclassified within Exminster, the husband successfully secured her release at the end of the year even though the medical staff believed that her condition had not significantly improved since her original admission.[24] Such episodes of admission and discharge suggest that the social origins and connections of the Devon patients figured in the terms on which different social groups approached the Mental Hospital and the conditions under which they were permitted to depart from it. The greater use made of both voluntary and temporary admissions by more affluent groups may be contrasted with the concern expressed by the Board of Control in its annual report for 1928, where it was argued that 'the poorer classes' should not be denied facilities for voluntary treatment 'in the early and hopeful stages of mental disorder which are open to those more fortunately circumstanced'.[25] The evidence from admissions to Exminster suggests that the unequal access to non-certified care continued in the years following the passage of the 1930 Act.

The impact of societal relationships on the pattern of admissions and discharges recorded during the nineteenth and twentieth centuries has attracted considerable scholarly attention in recent years. We know rather less about the influence of such connections on the treatment provided within such institutions.

Patient relationships and treatment at the Devon Hospital

In parallel to the changes in the legislative framework, the therapeutic options for doctors treating psychiatric patients were being transformed in the 1930s. At a time when patients were given greater legal rights to accept or reject psychiatric treatment, fresh and distinctly unpleasant treatments were being introduced to assist in their cure. The introduction of these new approaches raised expectations of curative treatment, in keeping with the nomenclature of the new Act of 1930. An examination of the treatment provided at the Devon Mental Hospital in the 1930s allows the examination of these new and frequently hazardous therapies which were developed for patients. These included Malaria Fever Therapy (MFT), which was developed as a treatment for the syphilis which attacked the central nervous system, identified as the 'general paralysis of the insane' (GPI) during the nineteenth century. The method of treatment involved the inoculation of patients with the malarial parasite, encouraging the development of malaria which led to a rise in blood temperature and the death of syphilitic organisms. With the assistance of quinine to control the malarial fever, this was held to be an effective if unpleasant means of controlling an otherwise incurable brain disease which invariably resulted in the paralysis and death of the sufferer. Another important attempt to cure psychiatric illness by the induction of physical reaction was the use of Cardiazol Shock Therapy (CST). This pre-dated the extensive use of Electro-Convulsive Therapy (ECT). Where CST was adopted, the patient was injected with a noxious chemical, Pentamethylenetrazol, with the intention of provoking a form of epileptic fit. It was believed that epileptics were unable to develop schizophrenia and such convulsions might counteract its symptoms. This treatment was again not without a degree of risk.

The influence of the sexual and social characteristics of the patients on the kind of treatment offered to them requires some discussion. Ussher and Showalter have emphasized the importance of gender in regard to treatment. Showalter in particular suggesting that the administration of insulin, electrical currents and surgical lobotomy were more common among women and also represented as more likely.[26] One important question concerns the nature of consent for treatment under the 1930 legislation. In English law no person may consent to medical treatment for another adult, though in practice mental hospitals usually requested the permission of nearest relatives before embarking on such procedures. The influence of family members can therefore be detected in the approval of treatment as well as its impact on patients of different sex. The records of the Devon Hospital indicate that in all cases involving MFT and CST, relatives were asked to give their consent by letter, though the stigma attached to the condition of syphilis appears to have affected the information provided by the Hospital.

The relatives of the Devon patients, and more particularly male relatives of females, not infrequently wrote to the medical staff of the institution to request or suggest physical treatments for their family members. MFT was largely confined to male patients who suffered from GPI, while Cardiazol Shock Therapy was introduced at Devon only at the end of our study period, being used sparingly and applied to only fifty-six patients, usually those who were recently admitted. The husband of a female patient, not suffering from GPI, requested a report on his wife's condition from the Medical Superintendent in 1933, adding that he wished her 'to be put under Malaria Treatment'.[27] The response of the Medical Superintendent, Dr Richard Eager, to this rather bizarre request is illuminating, in that he did not dismiss the efficacy of the treatment for the patient concerned but chose to advise the husband that her doctors saw no reason why she should receive malaria therapy, but promised to 'further consider this matter'.[28] The staff was clearly concerned to reassure such relatives that they would actively consider any suggestion made in regard to treatment, even when it was clearly seen to be inappropriate.

There is also evidence that male relatives were anxious to pursue the possibility of shock therapy being applied to their female relatives, often in response to press or other media reports. The following letter was written to Eager by a father just after the end of the study period:

> Dear Sir
> I am enclosing a cutting from the 'Evening Standard' of the 21st instant regarding the curing of mental patients by electric shock. Will you kindly inform me if you think either of my two daughters has the kind of mental infirmity in which such treatment might be of benefit. I quite understand that it is difficult to give any opinion without having had experience of what has happened to other cases of similar character to that of my daughters. No harm will be done by my bringing the information to your notice.[29]

While the relatives contacting the Devon Hospital were almost invariably males, particularly in regard to the progress of female patients, there is little indication that such pressure contributed to a disproportionate use of the new physical treatments to the women being treated at the institution. MFT was largely confined to men and men were equally likely to receive CST therapy as were women.

In some cases, family members were directly requested to consent to malarial treatment for GPI, while in others this stigmatized illness was referred to merely as a 'grave nervous disorder'.[30] The evidence suggests that the voluntary patients were more likely to be advised of the nature and risks of the new physical therapies, though it is almost impossible to ascertain the degree to which they could give informed consent. While Malaria Fever Therapy was unpleasant and not without its dangers, voluntary patients were equally likely to receive this form of treatment. Among the 1938 hospital intake voluntary patients were more likely to be recommended CST as other groups of patients who were eligible for this treatment (Table 6.3). This is remarkable given that the voluntary patients had a much higher proportion of those diagnosed as having neurotic illnesses which were not believed to be suitable for CST. Not only did the voluntary patients benefit from better facilities and more relaxed supervision but they had greater access to what were undoubtedly unpleasant physical therapies available at this period.

The readiness of medical staff to offer the physical therapies to the non-certified patients cannot be wholly explained in terms of the greater

Table 6.3 Intended use of Cardiazol Shock Therapy – 1938 admissions

Legal status	Number of patients	Intention to treat with cardiazol shock therapy
Certified and temporary	233	9 (3.9%)
Voluntary	130	16 (12.3%)

purchasing power of these patients. In the case of the private patients, the fees did not cover the cost of special treatments, for which an additional charge was made. Private patients were no more likely than rate-aided individuals to receive such treatments. It is possible that the medical staff were more cautious in administering such therapies to those who could not withhold their consent, though the evidence suggests that even where such staff were enthusiastic about the efficacy of physical shock therapy they rarely provided full and accurate information on which patients or relatives could provide informed consent. The central Board of Control certainly endorsed the application of these treatments, without favouring the voluntary over the certified groups.

A more persuasive explanation for the unequal use of these therapies during the 1930s may be found in the legal rights of the different groups and the need for psychiatric doctors to form 'therapeutic alliances' with patients, relatives and others. Since the tenure of voluntary (and temporary) patients was much less certain than that of the certified majority, the medical staff appears to have believed that they needed to effect an early cure of their patients. Dr Richard Eager confided in his nursing textbook in 1939 that the more 'active treatment' the voluntary patients received, 'the smaller will be the number of cases who wish to leave before "recommended"'.[31] The medical staff sought to maintain a delicate balance of consent and control over the patients who could, in strict legal terms, discharge themselves without the agreement of their physicians. Paradoxically, this involved offering this group greater access to the less pleasant and more hazardous, though apparently more effective, physical treatments which promised an earlier relief or resolution of their illness.

The efforts of the staff at the Devon Hospital did not always achieve the results anticipated. Almost half of those admitted as voluntary patients discharged themselves against the advice of the staff. This was a much higher proportion than among the certified group, though in the latter case an individual could only be discharged if a relative could demonstrate that they had arranged adequate care outside the institution. Even in this instance the Superintendent was empowered to issue a 'Barring Certificate', preventing the action of the relatives, though this power was never used. In the last instance the Visiting Committee could decide the fate of the individual patient, though they appear to have rarely intervened in such matters by the 1930s. The following section considers the pattern of discharges from the Devon Hospital.

Discharges from the Devon Mental Hospital, 1931–38

The discharge of patients from the Victorian asylum has attracted considerable comment since the research of Walton and Scull was published more than two decades ago, though there is much less research on the role of relatives and friends in persuading the physicians and the Visiting Committee of asylums and mental hospitals to discharge patients in the mid-twentieth century.[32] The most striking parallel between the Victorian inmates and the patient population surveyed in this study is the significant number of those compulsorily admitted who were to die within the wards of Exminster. During the 1930s we find only one third of the certified group were discharged on the order of the Visitors, compared to 45 per cent who died in the institution. There are several possible reasons for the failure of medical treatment to provide sufficient relief for the release of such a substantial number of certified patients in the study period. Their illnesses and their prognoses are likely to have varied from the non-certified groups, in that those compelled to enter Exminster were usually diagnosed as more severely ill than those who entered on a voluntary or temporary basis. Such individuals were also less likely to have close relatives outside the hospital to offer care and support for those who could have been maintained outside, particularly if they continued to suffer from chronic mental illness. Married patients who entered with certificates were significantly more likely to be discharged and less likely to die in hospital than their unmarried counterparts. Although the readiness of families to receive patients back into their care may have influenced the decision of the hospital authorities to release patients, the evidence indicates a range of possible circumstances which affected the departure of Hospital residents. A number of studies have linked poor prognosis in psychiatric illness to unmarried status.[33] The unmarried were generally older (in the case of the widowed) and younger (the single patients) than the main constituency of married patients who were certified.[34]

In assessing the pattern of discharges from mental hospitals at this period the social assumptions as well as professional judgement of the medical staff should be recognized. Doctors appear to have been more willing to discharge involuntary patients who had relatives and the readiness of these family members to communicate with the institution in regard to admission, diagnosis and treatment would probably have been taken as an indication of their continuing concern. The expectations which the medical staff had of the certified group appear to have been lower than the voluntary patients, who (as we have seen) were much more likely to have received the active physical treatments which were being developed at this time. Such staff may have rationalized this approach in terms of the need to effect rapid improvements to sustain the therapeutic alliances which they had formed with the voluntary entrants and their relatives. The fact that the more consensual patients were also of a rather higher social group may also have figured where doctors assumed that more affluent families could provide resources for the care of their members, including private help and medical assistance.

Further evidence that medical staff were sensitive to the financial circumstances and class status of such patients is provided in contemporary accounts such as that of McRae, who noted the difficulties presented to families which faced not only the loss of income from members admitted to mental hospital but also the consequent invalidation of their signature for legal and financial documents. He also reassured his readers that discharged patients usually faced little difficulty in regaining their former employment. Yet his most pointed comment was reserved for the relatives of those who discovered ways of playing public funds to their pecuniary advantage, as he explained the motives of those dispatching and retrieving family members to mental hospitals.

> There is a flagrant practice nowadays that, in rate-aided cases where N.H. insurance benefit has been accumulating for months or even years, the relatives press to have the patient discharged to their care to enable them to have payment of the sum accrued – as much as £40 to £50 in some cases – and when this is spent the patient is re-certified and returned to the asylum till a further accumulation makes a repetition of the procedure worthwhile.[35]

Such accounts indicate that contemporary medical opinion could be affected by sceptical views of the motives which guided families whose financial needs made such strategies an acceptable form of sustaining the household after the loss of its members to mental hospitals. Poorer families were clearly capable of making these strategic calculations when faced with the costs and benefits of mental illness. Observers such as McRae framed the doctor's dilemma in terms of assessing the motives of relatives as well as the medical prospects of his patient.

Conclusions

In a recent review of the new physical treatments developed in the mid-twentieth century, Andrew Scull wondered, 'what is it that appears to make the mentally ill so vulnerable to therapeutic experimentation?'[36] This chapter has placed the progress of the new treatments in a legal, institutional and social context which explains their uneven application in the years following the important Mental Treatment Act of 1930. Particular attention has been paid to the influence of family, gender and class in interpreting the pattern of admissions, treatment and discharges from the Devon Mental Hospital before 1938. Such a case study cannot offer a comprehensive assessment of the impact of legislation, which requires a detailed analysis of those individuals who were examined under the terms of the 1930 Act but not admitted as well as those who entered the institution. Nor do the available sources permit a direct insight into the complex range of decisions, concerns and motives which guided patients and their relatives. Even the expectations of the medical staff have been largely derived from fragmentary comments which survive in the Hospital records and a scattering of archival and published materials.

Within these constraints, this chapter has provided a response to some of the questions raised by Scull and other historians of mental illness. My first concern has been to rephrase Scull's discussion of the new physical therapies by considering not only the enthusiasm with which some of these treatments were applied by medical personnel (sanctioned by regulatory authorities such as the Board of Control), but also their uneven application. In contrast to the impression given in Scull's survey, the evidence from Devon suggests that it was not the certified patients who formed the prime target of experimentation but rather the voluntary group. The latter represented a new and distinctive social constituency for the mental hospital in these years and their personal status and resources, as well as those of their relatives, appear to have endowed them with a discretionary power over their entry, treatment and exit which was not possessed by those certified for detention and treatment.

In common with other studies it was found that there was a strong correlation between marital status and prospects for recovery and release from the establishment, though considerable care is needed in the interpretation of the various possible factors which figured in the condition of the unmarried or widowed patient. The substantial proportion of women in the 'temporary' category of patient appear to have fared least well in terms of their tenure at the Hospital, often entering as private cases but frequently reallocated to the certified majority after a limited period. More generally, the evidence discussed in this chapter does not support the views expressed by scholars such as Busfield, Showalter and Ussher, that female patients were a particular subject of the new treatments, or even of diagnoses of neuroses. There are clearly instances where male relatives pressed for the application of shock therapies to such patients, though the (primarily male) medical staff resisted where the appeals did not confirm their own treatment models.

This chapter has argued that we should understand the influence of families and of gender in relation to a wider social nexus of class and status. The reform of mental health law in 1930 and the introduction of the categories of voluntary and temporary patient appear to have expanded the scope for family relatives to influence the passage of individuals to and from the hospital, as well as the treatment provided by the medical staff. Again, there is rather more evidence of therapeutic alliances being formed among the voluntary group than those compelled to enter and remain in the custody of the superintendent. Doctors evidently felt under greater pressure to alleviate or remove the symptoms of mental illness, which would help to explain their readiness to apply both malarial and cardiazol treatment to the voluntary group. In acknowledging the presence of family influence in regard to the care of patients it is also appropriate, therefore, to note the unequal resources possessed by relatives in the different social groups.

The study also indicates some of the limits on this influence over medical personnel in the Devon case. The senior medical staff continued to exercise decisive influence over the choice of treatment as well as the judgement of its impact on the individual patient. The entrepreneurial talents and professional ambitions of the medical staff can be traced in the concern of Eager and his colleagues to secure a reputation for the early use of the new therapies, as well as the later publicity given to the use of occupational therapy at the Devon Hospital. In offering the unpleasant and more hazardous shock therapies to patients whom they perceived as having better prospects of improvement, the physicians were also responding to the pressure of the central Board of Control which promoted the new treatments in the 1930s.

Finally, this study has suggested that the relations of gender and family as well as the influence of doctors and relatives should be understood within a political and social context where the values of class and status influenced perceptions of mental illness. In advocating the introduction of the reforms to permit voluntary and temporary use of public mental health institutions, the Board of Control and a variety of political and humanitarian commentators emphasized the benefits of early respite and treatment for groups such as working class mothers who faced the strain of managing the family household with sparse resources. Yet there was also a large number of salaried, lower-middle and middle class employees who had struggled to fund private psychiatric care since the Victorian years and who were even more sensitive to the stigma of Poor Law medical provision than the working class family. The evidence from Devon suggests that the 1930 Act achieved its purpose in providing hospital treatment to a larger number of people who had not previously resorted to certification of their relatives, though it did not fulfil the expectations of Labour parliamentarians that the main beneficiaries would be working people in the early stages of mental illness. Admissions to the Devon Hospital indicate that it was the better-educated, more affluent and higher-status families which took greatest advantage of the provisions of the Mental Treatment Act to place their disordered members in residential care where professional psychiatrists were employed by local ratepayers. Voluntary admissions could be made through local physicians without the degrading requirement to approach the Relieving Officer in the first instance. Many of the smaller group of temporary patients were admitted as private patients, which involved no contact with the workhouse authorities, only to join the majority of certified patients with poorer prospects of treatment and recovery in later years.

The writings of contemporary psychiatrists and hospital doctors reveal the strong humanitarian impulses of many among the medical staff who cared for the patients of the institutions supervised by the central Board of Control. Whether from a concern to alleviate the suffering of patients who displayed neurotic as well as psychotic symptoms, or in response to the pleas of concerned relatives, physicians such as Eager were anxious to achieve improvements long before the psychotropic medicines of the

1950s became available. Their perceptions and their humane initiatives were clearly framed, however, within the circumstances of institutional and social power. In bemoaning the unenlightened attitudes of the 'average East End Londoner', psychiatrists such as Curtis were depicting the ignorance of the working class labourer rather than the white-collared man on the Clapham Omnibus. We can find echoes of such social discrimination in the treatment offered to patients at the Devon Hospital as well as in the negotiations which their doctors conducted with their relatives.

Notes

1 R. H. Curtis, 'Some Developments in Mental Treatment', *Journal of Mental Science*, September 1938, pp. 183–202, p. 189.
2 L. McGarry and P. Chodoff, 'The Ethics of Involuntary Hospitalization', in S. Bloch and P. Chodoff (eds), *Psychiatric Ethics*, Oxford: Oxford University Press, 1981, pp. 203–219, p. 210.
3 The essays by P. E. Prestwich, A. Suzuki and Wright, Moran and Douglas in R. Porter and D. Wright (eds), *The Confinement of the Insane: International Perspectives, 1800–1965*, Cambridge: Cambridge University Press, 2003, for example. An early contribution to this debate was J. Walton, 'Casting Out and Bringing Back in Victorian England: Pauper Lunatics 1840–1870', in W. F. Bynum, R. Porter and M. Shepherd (eds), *The Anatomy of Madness: Essays in the History of Psychiatry, vol. II*, London: Tavistock, 1985, pp. 132–146.
4 D. Wright, 'The Discharge of Pauper Lunatics from County Asylums in mid-Victorian England: the Case of Buckinghamshire, 1853–1872', in J. Melling and B. Forsythe (eds), *Insanity, Institutions and Society, 1800–1914: A Social History of Madness in Comparative Perspective*, London: Routledge, 1999, pp. 93–112.
5 R. Adair, J. Melling and B. Forsythe, 'Migration, Family Structure and Pauper Lunacy in Victorian England: Admissions to Devon County Pauper Lunatic Asylum, 1845–1900', *Continuity and Change*, 12, 1997, pp. 373–401, p. 389.
6 A. Scull, 'Madness and Segregative Control: The Rise of the Insane Asylum', in P. Brown (ed.), *Mental Health Care and Social Policy*, London: Routledge and Kegan Paul, 1985, pp. 17–40, p. 34.
7 See Chapter 4 in this book.
8 McGarry and P. Chodoff, 'The Ethics of Involuntary Hospitalization', p. 210.
9 J. Melling, B. Forsythe and R. Adair, 'Families, Communities and the Legal Regulation of Lunacy in Victorian England: Assessments of Crime, Violence and Welfare in Admissions to the Devon Asylum, 1845–1914', in P. Barlett and D. Wright (eds), *Outside the Walls of the Asylum: The History of Care in the Community 1750–2000*, London: Athlone Press, 1999, pp. 153–180.
10 G. A. Doody, A. Beveridge and E. C. Johnstone, 'Poor and Mad: a Study of Patients Admitted to the Fife and Kinross District Asylum between 1874 and 1899', *Psychological Medicine*, 26, 1996, pp. 887–897, p. 891. Doody *et al.* claim that only 1 per cent of the patients admitted to this Scottish asylum in the late nineteenth century were diagnosed in terms that could be categorized as neurotic conditions.
11 A. Riecher-Rossler and W. Rossler, 'Compulsory Admission of Psychiatric Patients – an International Comparison', *Acta Psychiatr Scand*, 87, 1993, pp. 231–236, p. 234.
12 *Hansard*, 11 April 1930.
13 J. Andrews and A. Digby (eds), *Sex and Seclusion, Class and Custody:*

Perspectives on Gender and Class in the History of British and Irish Psychiatry, Amsterdam: Rodopi, 2004.

14 J. Busfield, *Men, Women and Madness: Understanding Gender and Mental Disorder*, Basingstoke: Macmillan, 1996, p. 134.

15 J. K. Marshall, 'A Note on the Potential Use of Temporary Treatment', *Journal of Mental Science*, January 1936, pp. 43–46, p. 44. Eighteen per cent of females and 11 per cent of males were given diagnoses considered suitable for temporary status. Females predominated in every diagnostic group except general paralysis and recent mania.

16 A. T. Scull, *Museums of Madness: The Social Organization of Insanity in Nineteenth-Century England*, London: Allen Lane, 1979, p. 242, p. 34.

17 Doody, Beveridge and Johnstone, 'Poor and Mad'.

18 D. K. Henderson and R. D. Gillespie, *A Text-book of Psychiatry for Students and Practitioners*, Oxford: Oxford University Press, 1936, p. 562; D. Perk, 'Some Reflections on the Mental Treatment Act', *Journal of Mental Science*, July 1935, pp. 740–744, p. 740.

19 Henderson and Gillespie, *A Text-book of Psychiatry*, p. 562.

20 Riecher-Rossler and Rossler, 'Compulsory Admission of Psychiatric Patients – an International Comparison'.

21 Perk, 'Some Reflections on the Mental Treatment Act', p. 740.

22 Board of Control Annual Report, 1933, British Library, MFR 2446, p. 24.

23 Dr Robinson writing in the *Journal of Mental Science*, January 1935, p. 245 recorded in the Minutes of a RMPA Quarterly Meeting.

24 Patient 19413, Devon Record Office (hereafter DRO) file 3769A H2/164.

25 Board of Control Annual Report, 1928, British Library, DSC 1114.460000, p. 1.

26 J. M. Ussher, *Women's Madness: Misogyny or Mental Illness?*, London: Harvester Wheatsheaf, 1991, p. 175; E. Showalter, *The Female Malady: Women, Madness and English Culture 1830–1980*, London: Virago Press, 1987, p. 205.

27 Female patient E. B. E., letter dated 10 September 1933, DRO file 2769A H2/140.

28 Dr Richard Eager's notes written on the above letter. The original statement made by Eager in an earlier draft promised the husband that 'if we think it would be beneficial to her it shall be done'. This was struck out and amended as quoted.

29 Case notes for patient M. O. R., letter dated 21 May 1940, Wonford Hospital, basement store.

30 Case notes for male patient G. H., letter dated 14 April 1932, DRO file 3769A H2/138.

31 Richard Eager, *Hints to Probationer Nurses in Mental Hospitals*, 3rd edition, London: H. K. Lewis, 1939, p. 210.

32 Walton, 'Casting Out and Bringing Back in Victorian England'; Scull, *Museums of Madness*.

33 For example see A. B. Goodman, 'Paranoid Schizophrenia: Prognosis Under DSM-II and DSM-III-R', *Comprehensive Psychiatry*, 30(3), 1989, pp. 259–266.

34 The average age of those certified patients that were married was 51.8 (789 patients), compared with 42.4 for the single (711 patients) and 65.9 for the widowed (227 patients). Data from Admission Registers, DRO 3769A H5/3 to 3769A H5/5.

35 D. McRae, 'Some Observations on the Care of the Insane', *Journal of Mental Science*, September 1937, pp. 491–504, p. 499.

36 A. Scull, 'Somatic Treatments and the Historiography of Psychiatry', *History of Psychiatry*, V, 1994, pp. 1–12, p. 12.

7   The 'manufacture' of mental defectives

Why the number of mental defectives increased in Scotland, 1857–1939

Matt Egan

Introduction

In 1923, a letter was published in the *Glasgow Herald* under the headline 'The "Making" of Defective Children'. It was written by John Grimmond, a disgruntled member of Glasgow's local education authority.[1] In the letter, Grimmond accused Glasgow's educational establishment of developing what he considered to be an unhealthy enthusiasm for transferring pupils from 'ordinary' school classes into special classes for so-called 'feeble-minded' or 'educable' mental defectives. Grimmond simply did not accept that all the children being sent to special classes were mentally defective. He contended that many of the children being transferred may well have been 'backward' in their studies, but not to such a degree that they should be certified by a school medical officer and separated from their peers. According to Grimmond, '[f]rom the cases which I have investigated it might be urged that the present policy tends to manufacture mental defectives'.

Grimmond's letter questioned the scientific validity of mental deficiency diagnoses, rather than challenging the status of science itself, so it would be a mistake to give his views the anachronistic label of 'postmodern'. Nonetheless there are parallels between his letter and the arguments put forward in some of the recent histories of mental deficiency.[2] Indeed the title of two monographs on the subject, Mark Jackson's *The Borderland of Imbecility: Medicine, Society and the Fabrication of the Feeble Mind*[3] and James W. Trent's *Inventing the Feeble Mind: A History of Mental Retardation in the United States*,[4] seem to unconsciously paraphrase the *Glasgow Herald*'s headline. To varying degrees, many modern commentators have allowed the scepticism associated with postmodernism and social constructionism to influence their approach to the history of mental deficiency. In the introduction to his history of mental deficiency in England and Wales, Mathew Thomson makes clear his belief that mental defectives were 'socially, politically, ideologically and linguistically constituted'. Nonetheless, he criticizes the 'dogmatic social constructionist position which denies the existence of individuals with disabilities altogether' and refuses to involve himself in the 'sterile battle over the reality of mental illness'.[5]

The number of 'defectives' certainly increased during the late nineteenth and early twentieth centuries. The question of whether or not the increase in mental deficiency was due to the 'manufacture' of cases, or simply the result of more rigorous identification, or an actual increase in the number of people affected by mental deficiency is more than just a sterile debate. This chapter will show that Grimmond was just one of a number of well-placed contemporaries in the early twentieth century who suggested that the increase in mental deficiency was either partly or wholly a 'fiction' caused by changing definitions and diagnoses.[6] None of these historical figures was a dogmatic social constructionist, indeed some were doctors who specialized in mental impairment. The reasons behind the increase are important both to those whose lives were changed dramatically by Scotland's mental deficiency administration, and to modern policy-makers and others with an interest in learning disability. The number of people being labelled and treated differently by the state on account of apparently low levels of intelligence is still on the increase, yet this phenomenon and its implications are largely unquestioned by policy-makers.[7]

Some historians have chosen to explore in more detail the changing social contexts within which historical actors constructed mental deficiency, although few focus on developments in Scotland.[8] Within the English historiography, Mark Jackson has provided a particularly insightful account of the origins of feeble-mindedness. He argues that the sub-category was

the product not only of diverse cognitive developments in the emerging fields of psychiatry, anthropology, criminology, and education, but also of shifting administrative practices and experiences in asylums, schools, prisons, workhouses, and courtrooms.[9]

Taking a purely qualitative approach, he focuses on changing ideas and practices but does not attempt to measure the extent to which the 'borderland' of mental deficiency was extended in terms of the number of people labelled.

A quantitative account of the increase in mental deficiency will allow us to better understand the impact of the social and cognitive shifts described by Jackson, and pinpoint more accurately where and when the expansion of mental deficiency took place. Fortunately, the Scottish archives have retained sufficient quantitative evidence from surveys and governmental reports to permit such an analysis. Furthermore, as this chapter will discuss, the similarities between Scottish and English approaches to mental deficiency provision at that time mean that the Scottish data can also provide insights into developments that occurred beyond its borders.

Scotland and England

Historians often separate Scottish history from English history and many supposedly 'British' studies often omit or marginalize accounts of Scottish developments. Mathew Thomson's *Problem of Mental Deficiency: Eugenics, Democracy, and Social Policy in Britain* (emphasis added) exemplifies a 'British' history that focuses almost exclusively on England. Scottish historians often object to this trend, and in turn produce histories that emphasize the distinctiveness of the Scottish experience. Scotland's separate political, legal, and educational institutions and numerous distinct cultural traditions are often emphasized in such histories. This is frequently justifiable, but it needs to be recognized that the modern history of Scotland is closely tied to that of England: politically, culturally and economically. Some practitioners based in England were keen to learn from, and copy, best-practice in Scotland,[10] and vice versa. Hence, it is appropriate for historians from both sides of the border to explore the connections as well as the differences between Scottish and English history.

Scotland had a separate mental deficiency administration to England, but the similarities heavily outweighed the differences.[11] There is evidence that distinctions between mental abnormalities arising from birth or childhood (termed 'idiocy') and mental abnormalities occurring later in life ('lunacy') have been made in legal and medical discourses in both Scotland and England since the middle-ages, although definitions were often vague and inconsistent.[12] Around the mid-nineteenth century, a number of institutions had opened both north and south of the border that were specifically intended for so-called 'idiots'. The larger institutions tended to accommodate a mixture of private, charitable and (increasingly) 'rate-aided' pauper cases. Some experts preferred to call their patients 'imbeciles' or 'mental defectives' and over time idiocy came to denote a more severe category of mental deficiency than imbecility, whilst mental deficiency became a generic term for all categories.

In Scotland, the most prominent institution was the Scottish National Institution for Imbeciles at Larbert in Stirlingshire, which first opened in 1863. Its importance lay partly in its size, accommodating over 250 patients by the end of the century, and partly in the international standing of one of its earliest superintendents, Dr William W. Ireland. Ireland was superintendent between 1871 and 1881, during which time he published what is often regarded as Britain's first comprehensive textbook on idiocy and imbecility.[13]

Special classes for mentally defective pupils in day schools appeared in England and then Scotland from the late nineteenth century and were governed by local education authorities.[14] These special day classes were designed to cater for a newly created category of 'feeble-minded' or 'educable' mental defective.[15] These children were deemed more mentally able than idiots and imbeciles, but still defective in the sense that teachers and doctors judged them to be incapable of benefiting from teaching in what became known as the 'ordinary' classrooms. The earliest special classes tended to appear in major urban centres like London and Glasgow. English and Scottish legislation on special education was permissive until 1913 (Scotland) and 1914 (England and Wales). After that time, education authorities were obliged to ensure educable mental defectives received special education, but in practice, many local authorities were slow to commit resources to this area.

Scotland had another type of state provision for mental defectives besides institutions and special schools. The practice of 'boarding-out' defectives to foster-guardians situated in rural areas has long been characterized as a particularly unique feature of the Scottish mental deficiency administration that was used throughout the period studied here. However, boarding-out to foster-guardians was also practised to a more limited degree south of the border, whilst even in Scotland the vast majority of certified mental defectives were not boarded-out in this way. Instead, defectives either remained under the care of their own families (who sometimes received financial assistance through the state's policy of 'familial guardianship'), attended special day classes, or resided in institutions.[16]

Scottish legislation on the institutionalization and boarding-out of mental defectives was brief and permissive until the passing of the Mental Deficiency and Lunacy (Scotland) Act, 1913.[17] This was based on English legislation passed the same year, save for some technical details that took account of the parochial basis of Scotland's Poor Law administration. The Scottish Act did establish a separate authority, the General Board of Control for Scotland (GBCS), to oversee implementation at a national level. The GBCS had powers of compulsory detention similar to those of the English Board of Control.

After 1913, Scottish legislation gave local authorities more choice than their English counterparts as to whether or not they established their own local services for mental defectives, or contracted-out to other local authorities (e.g. by paying for institutional beds or special school places in other areas). However, regardless of which side of the border one chooses to examine, a similar pattern of local authority engagement emerges. Urban local authorities usually took a more active role in administering provision for mental defectives than rural authorities in both England and Scotland.[18] In other words, the most important differences between mental deficiency administrations occurred at local rather than national level.

Nonetheless, over time and to different degrees, both urban and rural authorities increased their provision for mental defectives throughout Britain. This development occurred alongside increases in the proportion of the British population identified as being mentally defective. Despite the similarities between Scotland and England in this regard, statistics and other data on the 'manufacture' of mental defectives were collected and archived separately (often in ways that do not readily allow for the data to be combined). For this reason Scotland, rather than Britain, is the unit of analysis for this chapter.

Measuring the increase in mental deficiency prior to 1913

Quantitative data on mental deficiency often came from surveys conducted by government officials and/or medical experts. They are extremely problematic if one (foolishly) attempts to use the figures to make anachronistic observations on the 'true' incidence of learning disability in the population at any one time. Officials attempting to count the number of mental defectives in Scotland needed to decide how to distinguish them from 'lunatics', and from people who were considered 'ordinary' but 'dull or backward'. Such distinctions were governed by changing criteria that were subjective and contextual.

Distinctions between mental defectives and lunatics could be contentious, although the late nineteenth and early twentieth centuries witnessed a growing consensus within medico-legal discourse on this point. Since the 1860s, institutional developments and legal changes began to reflect a tendency amongst medical specialists, officials and philanthropists in this field to emphasize idiocy as distinct from other mental health problems. Initially, mental deficiency was regarded as a special sub-category of lunacy, but by 1913 it was formally separated from lunacy in Scottish law.[19] In each case, the definition of mental deficiency centred on individuals showing signs of mental impairment from an early age.

More problematic was the lack of agreement over the criteria that marked mental defectives from 'ordinary' people. From the writings of doctors specializing in mental deficiency in the nineteenth century, the diagnostic criteria that occurred most frequently included: specific intellectual characteristics of the patient (such as attention, imagination and abstract thought); the age at which a child learned to sit up, walk and speak; ability to communicate; mobility; the degree to which the patient could protect him/herself from external dangers; knowledge of everyday facts such as family names, days of the week and currency; moral behaviour and hygiene.[20] By the late nineteenth century, physical signs of deficiency (referred to as 'stigmata') were also assuming a greater importance in diagnoses, as medical practitioners applied the theories of criminal anthropologists and alienists (such as Cesare Lombroso and Benedict A. Morel) who linked a variety of physical defects with various forms of 'degeneracy'.[21] Stigmata featured prominently in the influential work of William W. Ireland.[22]

Doctors therefore identified mental defectives on the basis of a mixed bag of symptoms and characteristics, evaluated and prioritized largely at the discretion of each individual examiner. Hence, personal judgements played a significant role in identifying mental defectives. The problem of standardizing diagnostic criteria became particularly evident during large-scale surveys aimed at counting the number of mental defectives, because such surveys generally relied on the judgement of a number of people, including doctors and people without medical training.

This problem was recognized at the time and the Scottish Lunacy Commission qualified the results of its own 1857 survey, *Report on Lunatic Asylums in Scotland*, by saying that its statistics 'can only be regarded as a vague approximation of the truth'.[23] According to the report, there were 2,603 'congenital idiots and imbeciles' (0.9 per 1,000) in the Scottish population.[24] The number of lunatics reported was roughly twice that figure. Whilst the Commission took into account institutionalized and boarded-out people considered by the authorities to be insane, the figures also included the results of a survey in which police constables, sheriff-officers and clergymen were asked to send details of insane people living in their local communities. Many of those identified by the survey had not undergone a medical examination. When the Commission received the returns, it found that figures varied widely from one locality to the next, leading the report to conclude that there had been no standardization in the way information had been collected.[25]

The problems caused by varying standards were magnified in the case of decennial census returns. Census enumerators did attempt to find out the number of idiots and imbeciles (and in later years feeble-minded persons) in Scotland, but their results were dependent on designated heads of household being willing to describe household members in this way. William W. Ireland believed that the results of such enquiries underestimated what he considered to be the true incidence of idiocy and imbecility, as heads of household would often be unwilling to admit that family members fell into these categories. Writing of census returns in 1898 he states, diplomatically, that: '[i]n no other country is this difficulty of getting at the whole truth about the prevalence of idiocy greater than in Scotland, from the proud, cautious, and reserved character of the people.'[26] In contrast, the Census enumerators believed their figures might over-represent the number of mental defectives, because they included people who had obviously developed mental impairments late on in their life (and should therefore be classed as lunatic rather than defective):

> For instance, the list of those returned as 'imbecile' or 'feeble-minded' includes an officer of the Royal Navy, two ministers of the Established Church of Scotland, an advocate, two sick nurses, a school mistress, and a very considerable number with other occupations requiring skill and technical knowledge.[27]

Scottish Census Commissioners stopped collecting returns on mental defectives after 1911 on grounds of unreliability. However, the returns are interesting to historians as they give some indication of lay opinion in Scotland, or to be more precise, they tell us the number of people described to the enumerators as mental defectives by heads of households. Between 1871 and 1911, the census returns showed an average of 1.5 per 1,000 (just over 6,000 in total) of the Scottish population were described as mentally defective by the general public (see Table 7.1). This is lower than the estimated incidence of 2 per 1,000 suggested by William W. Ireland in 1898.[28] An English investigation carried out by the Charity Organisation Society (COS) in 1876–77 suggested that the figure 29,452 (1.3 per 1,000) given in the 1871 census for England and Wales similarly underestimated the number of mental defectives. In line with William W. Ireland's later comments, the COS ascribed this alleged under-representation to 'the prevailing ignorance on the subject and the natural desire to conceal the existence of idiocy in families'.[29] English Commissioners ceased including mental deficiency in the census after 1891.

The advent of universal state education in the late nineteenth century provided an alternative means to the census for scrutinizing a large section of the population. Furthermore, following the work of London-based school surveyors such as Francis Warner and George E. Shuttleworth, doctors and teachers in the 1890s began to employ the concept of feeble-mindedness to explain relatively high rates of educational failure in state schools. In 1898, a Departmental Committee on Defective and Epileptic Children took a rough average of many widely varying estimates made by witnesses with a background in special education and reported that approximately 10 per 1,000 of the school-aged population was feeble-minded in England and Wales.[30] The Committee did not concern itself as to whether this figure could also be applied to the adult population, but then, from the start feeble-mindedness was primarily bound to the issue of education.

Table 7.1 Proportion of the Scottish population regarded as mentally defective[a] by heads of household in the decennial censuses of Scotland, 1871–1911

Date	Number of people labelled mentally defective	Per 1,000 of Scottish population labelled mentally defective
1871	4,621	1.4
1881	5,991	1.6
1891	5,017	1.2
1901	6,623	1.5
1911	7,911	1.7

Sources: Census of Scotland, 1871–1911.

Note

a The censuses of 1871, 1881 and 1891 refer only to 'imbeciles' and 'idiots', whilst the censuses of 1901 and 1911 also refer to the 'feeble-minded'.

It was another ten years before state officials attempted to ascertain the number of mental defectives in the entire population with a definition that included idiots, imbeciles and feeble-minded people. The Royal Commission on the Care and Control of the Feeble-Minded reported in 1908 that 4.6 per 1,000 of the total population of England and Wales were mentally defective. The report suggested that the incidence of mental deficiency was proportionally highest amongst the school-age population[31] but, as in 1898, attempts to quantify the issue were hindered by lack of agreement: '[w]e have thus variations in estimate from 0.25 per cent, 0.5, 0.8 to 1 per cent, and even 2 per cent'.[32] The Commissioners finally decided that 35,662 mentally defective children were currently denied the special education they needed. Adding these to the 9,082 pupils already accommodated in special classes at that time would indicate that 7.4 per 1,000 of the pupils on school registers in England and Wales should, according to the Royal Commission, be placed in special classes for the feeble-minded.[33]

The Royal Commission's investigation into mental deficiency in Scotland came up with different figures to those in England, but again the incidence was markedly higher amongst the school-aged population compared to the general population. Commissioners focused on Glasgow in their Scottish survey because its school board had both a number of special day classes, and employed a part-time school medical officer with a background in psychiatry, named John Carswell, to diagnose mental defectives. Carswell conducted a survey for the Royal Commission that could justifiably be called the most thorough local investigation into the incidence of mental deficiency that Scotland witnessed during the entire period examined here. He was assisted by Archibald K. Chalmers, Glasgow's Medical Officer of Health, and Landel Rose Oswald, Physician Superintendent at the local asylum at Gartnavel.

Following the specifications laid down by the Commission, Carswell, Chalmers and Oswald's survey of Glasgow included both state schools and state-funded (generally Roman Catholic) 'voluntary' schools, in addition to defectives kept at home or placed in institutions. They identified 634 mentally defective children in schools. They also identified ninety children not attending school and cared for at home. Finally, from their report, at least another 109 defective children can be identified from Poor Law or charitable institutions and at Larbert.[34] This comes to 833, or 7.2 per 1,000 of the school-aged population in the city. The survey failed to find anywhere near as many adult mental defectives as it had children. Consequently, after searching for mental defectives of all age-groups with the assistance of Poor Law inspectors, charitable workers, institutional staff and general practitioners they reported that 2.5 per 1,000 of Glasgow's total population (all age-groups) was mentally defective. The feeble-minded label proved less applicable to adults, partly because it was largely understood within an educational context, and partly because adults living in the community were better able to avoid the kind of medical surveillance children experienced at school.[35]

Nonetheless, the figure of 2.5 per 1,000 still surpassed that given by Scotland's decennial censuses and William W. Ireland's estimate. The increase reflected Carswell's greater willingness to apply the 'feeble-minded' label to children who appeared to be struggling in the ordinary classrooms. This was something he was quite open about, as his comments in Glasgow School Board's school medical officer's report for 1910 testify:

> it would be wrong to limit our conception of the function of Special Schools to providing for children whose deficiency is essentially similar to that of the imbecile child, though less in degree ... the distinction between mere backwardness on the one hand and imbecility on the other can be made, but the term mental defect should be *elastic*.[36] [emphasis added]

William W. Ireland, on the other hand, had been wary of this practice. Indeed a few years earlier, the *Journal of Mental Science* reported a confrontation between Ireland and Carswell in which Ireland told of his 'considerable suspicion' regarding special education in day schools, protesting that 'it would be an outrage to those backward children if they were sent in among imbecile children. Many children were bright enough in the playground, although they were stupid at their lessons'.[37] Ireland's objection to special education in day schools was characteristic of many institution superintendents at that time. In his English study of education for imbeciles in the nineteenth century, Michael Barrett discusses the vested interests behind this debate,[38] suggesting that special education for the feeble-minded was a particular concern for institution superintendents (like Ireland) who might fear a loss of business if day schools labelled the more able imbeciles as feeble-minded and sent them to special day classes rather than institutions.

As a school medical officer specializing in mental deficiency, Carswell obviously supported both special education in day schools and the legitimacy of the feeble-minded category. Unlike Ireland, Carswell was also much more willing to shift the somewhat opaque boundary that distinguished feeble-minded defectives from pupils who were considered 'ordinary but backward'. Consequently, within five years of Carswell's 1905 survey, the number of mentally defective children identified in Glasgow was 1,001, over four-fifths of whom were on the school roll.[39] This is notably more than the 833 defective children identified in Glasgow's schools, homes and institutions in 1905, despite the fact that the 1905 survey was much more thorough and wide-ranging than Carswell's subsequent work. Carswell's identification of mental defectives on Glasgow's school roll after 1905 relied heavily on teachers notifying suspected mental defectives to Carswell (through their headmasters), rather than Carswell, Chalmers and Oswald enlisting Poor Law Officers, doctors, police and teachers to identify every school-aged child in the city as they did in 1905.

The rise in the number of mental defectives between 1905 and 1910 is therefore not explained by more rigorous medical surveillance in the later years. It is explicable in terms of Carswell broadening his definition of mental deficiency over time to include more pupils of higher ability.

However, Carswell was not solely responsible for stretching the definition of mental deficiency to include more children of higher abilities. Teaching staff and headmasters embraced Carswell's 'elastic' definition, and became increasingly willing to notify Carswell about difficult pupils considered to be in need of a special medical examination. Robert S. Allan, the Chairman of Glasgow School Board, told the Royal Commission on the Feeble-Minded in 1906 that this trend reflected a new enlightenment amongst headmasters, who had 'been taking more interest in the matter lately, and they understand better what was wanted'.[40] Whether the headmasters' interest was inspired by a desire to assist struggling children or to remove a perceived source of difficulty from the ordinary classrooms is debatable. The evidence suggests that both motives were present.

In the years that followed, Carswell found that the number of suspected mental defectives notified to him by teachers continually grew. For the most part, he concurred with the opinions of the teachers. For example, during the school year 1909–10, he was called upon to examine 302 pupils suspected by teachers of being mentally defective. Of this number, Carswell certified 215 as 'mentally defective', sixty-two as 'doubtful mental defect' and twenty-five as 'not mental defective'. In cases of 'doubtful mental defect' Carswell still insisted on taking them out of the ordinary classes 'and placing them in a Special School for a specified probationary period of a year'.[41] He justified this action with the following argument:

> I think probationary care, training and observation which those children require are best secured in a Special School; indeed, it would be a useless proceeding to leave them in the ordinary schools, because it is on account of their absolute failure to profit by training there that they are brought forward for medical inspection.[42]

The broadening of mental deficiency was achieved with the approval of Glasgow's school board, even though there was no direct financial incentive for the board to back the corresponding expansion of special education. Even with additional Treasury assistance to special classes, the cost incurred by ratepayers for the special education of a mentally defective pupil averaged £1 12s in 1906, as opposed to £1 6s 9d for a pupil in an ordinary class.[43] However, when the Royal Commission asked Carswell to justify the additional expense, he replied, 'I think it is a humane and proper thing to do and a scientific thing to do, and I do not think the expense is so very great that the ratepayers need complain of it.'[44] R. S. Allan, on the other hand, focused on benefits to the ordinary classes that he believed resulted from the removal of difficult pupils. The Chairman of

Glasgow School Board told the Royal Commission that it was 'a great relief to the ordinary schools to have these children dealt with separately'.[45]

Encouraged by teachers wishing to remove struggling children from the ordinary classes, Carswell developed an increasingly 'elastic' definition of mental deficiency. This was how mental defectives were 'manufactured' in Glasgow. The special education system was consequently able to expand: ordinary teachers were able to remove difficult pupils, and the medical officer maintained his official position in charge of referrals to special classes despite the fact that his decisions were largely prompted by educational rather than medical concerns. The special class teachers, the ordinary teachers and the school doctors all benefited and in their opinion the pupils benefited too. Unfortunately surviving archival sources from the school board do not provide first hand accounts of the pupils' (or indeed their parents') views on this matter.[46]

Measuring the increase in mental deficiency 1913–39

Following the Mental Deficiency Act (Scotland), 1913 and the Education (Scotland) Act, 1918, national government statistics show that the number of mental defectives receiving special provision grew as the government committed more resources to this area.[47] The large-scale surveys of mental deficiency conducted during the 1920s were organized by the Scottish Office authorities responsible for mental defectives under these Acts (i.e. the General Board of Control for Scotland and the Scottish Education Department).

Most surveys in the inter-war period concentrated on children of school age because the education system provided an ideal arena for medical officers or psychologists to examine large numbers of the population. In 1921, the Scottish Education Department (SED) conducted a national survey based on returns from school medical officers and found that around 5,000 (approximately 5 per 1,000) of the school population of Scotland were mentally defective. A disproportionately high number of these came from Glasgow as a result of the city's more developed special education system. According to a circular drafted (but never distributed) by the SED in 1926, 5 per 1,000 was regarded as an underestimate, with officials preferring the figure of 8.6 per 1,000 put forward by Sir George Newman, Chief Medical Officer for the English Board of Education and Board of Health.[48]

The GBCS's *Annual Report* for 1925 gave details of the only major survey of the period to include all age-groups. It presented figures from the SED alongside the results of its own inquiry conducted by medical officers working for parish councils and district boards of control. Although the report admitted that there 'may have been slight overlapping in some cases', the various returns suggested that there were 12,969 defectives throughout Scotland.[49] From the total population of Scotland given in the census of 1921, this would give a figure of 2.6 per 1,000 of the population. The number of mentally defective children was placed at 6.6 per 1,000 of the school-aged population.

In the 1930s, Scottish psychologists conducted a major survey on the intelligence of children using psychological tests (commonly referred to as intelligent quotient or IQ tests). This was in contrast to the SED and GBCS enquiries in the 1920s, which were conducted by local medical officers, who mostly continued to rely on traditional diagnostic methods. During this period, psychologists were still in the process of establishing themselves as a profession with a role to play in identifying mental defectives. Their chief tools were mental tests, inspired by those developed by the French psychologists Alfred Binet and Theodore Simon in 1905. The tests were intended to measure innate intelligence (as opposed to acquired knowledge) against the age of each child tested. The tests could be applied orally to individuals or, following the work of psychologists such as Lewis Terman in the US, and then Cyril Burt and Godfrey Thomson in the UK, they could also be turned into written and pictorial tests in order to measure the IQ of larger numbers of people simultaneously.

In 1925, Godfrey Thomson was appointed to the Chair of Education at Edinburgh University and became a key figure in the Scottish Council for Research in Education, founded five years later. It was largely as a result of his influence that the Council chose as its first major undertaking a comprehensive survey aiming to measure the intelligence of every single eleven-year-old child in Scotland in 1932. Approximately 90,000 children were examined using a group test developed by Thomson which became known as the Moray House Test. Uneducable children and children residing in institutions were included in the inquiry. A sample of 1,000 children were also tested individually.[50]

The Council's final report defined mental deficiency in terms of the rule of thumb commonly used by psychologists that anyone with an IQ below seventy was likely to be mentally defective (an IQ of 100 was considered representative of average intelligence). The Council found that, '[i]f 70 I.Q. be taken as the boundary line separating the dull from the "mentally defective", it appears that not fewer than $1\frac{1}{2}$ and not more than 3 per cent of children born in 1921 fall within this category'.[51]

This noticeably vague estimate reflected the Council's uncertainty regarding the Moray House Test's accuracy in measuring intelligence at the lowest end of the IQ scale. The authors qualified their findings by saying that 'it would be rash in the extreme to assume that the "mental defectives" in Scotland represent as many as 2 per cent [i.e. 20 per 1,000] of the school population'.[52] The council went on to revise this figure further following a re-analysis of the data by Agnes Miller Macmeeken, from the psychology department of Edinburgh University.[53] The results of this analysis were published in 1939 and concluded that 1.26 per cent (i.e.

12.6 per 1,000) of Scottish children were mentally defective, having an IQ below seventy.[54]

Between 1921 and 1939, Scotland's large-scale surveys showed a distinct rise in the proportion of the population regarded as mentally defective, although the picture was complicated by doubts expressed by those who conducted the surveys. Despite these complexities, it is clear that the figures presented in the 1930s were significantly higher than those presented in the 1920s (see Table 7.2).

State provision for Scotland's mental defectives

The national estimates and large-scale surveys referred to above provide only one indication of how the mental deficiency label came to be applied to an increasing proportion of the population. Estimates and surveys often had limited direct impact on people's lives. No individual became regarded as a mental defective as a result of a general estimate. Even when medical professionals and psychologists conducted large-scale surveys of school pupils, the medical examinations or mental tests did not necessarily lead to certification or the provision of special services for the pupils involved. Some children labelled mentally defective for the purposes of a specific survey could continue being treated as ordinary, albeit backward, once the examination was completed.

Scotland's increase in mental deficiency can also be measured by looking at the number of certified individuals in receipt of special education, institutional care or private guardianship for mental defectives. The chief advantage of this method is that by taking into account every certified individual in receipt of some form of special provision, the historian is able to focus on people who regularly experienced the effects of being labelled mentally defective. That is, children segregated within the education system, people removed from their family home and sent to live in institutions or boarded-out to foster-guardians, or registered mental defectives remaining with families who received additional state assistance and supervision. The number of people receiving special provision was always less than the number of mental defectives in the population estimated from the larger surveys, but both sets of figures kept on rising throughout the period.

The number of individuals in receipt of specialized state provision for mental defectives rose dramatically in Scotland during the inter-war period (see Figure 7.1). SED statistics show that the proportion of Scottish pupils on the school roll in receipt of special education more than doubled from 2.8 per 1,000 in the school year 1919–20 to 6.2 per 1,000 in 1937–38 (2,482 pupils in 1929–30 to 4,800 in 1937–38, against a slight overall decline in the Scottish population).[55] The total number of people in Scotland (combining SED and GBCS statistics) receiving any form of special provision also doubled from 4,259 in 1919 to 9,782 in 1938.[56] Approximately 0.9

Table 7.2 Summary of surveys showing incidence of mental deficiency within the Scottish population during the inter-war period

Date	Survey by	Population	No. of mental defectives per 1,000 of the surveyed population
1921	SED	School-aged population	5 (actual found) 8.6 (estimated figure)
1925	GBCS	School-aged population	6.6
1925	GBCS	Total population (children and adults)	2.6
1932	Scottish Council for Research in Education	Every 11-year-old in Scotland	15–30 (but probably less then 20)
1939	Scottish Council for Research in Education	Recalibration of 1932 survey based on approx. 1,000 new tests	12.6

Sources: NAS ED 28/230, draft SED circular (6 December 1926); HMSO, Annual Report of GBCS 1925, p. lvii; Scottish Council for Research in Education, The Intelligence of Scottish Children, p. 123; A. M. Macmeeken, The Intelligence of a Representaiive Group of Scottish Children, p. 138.

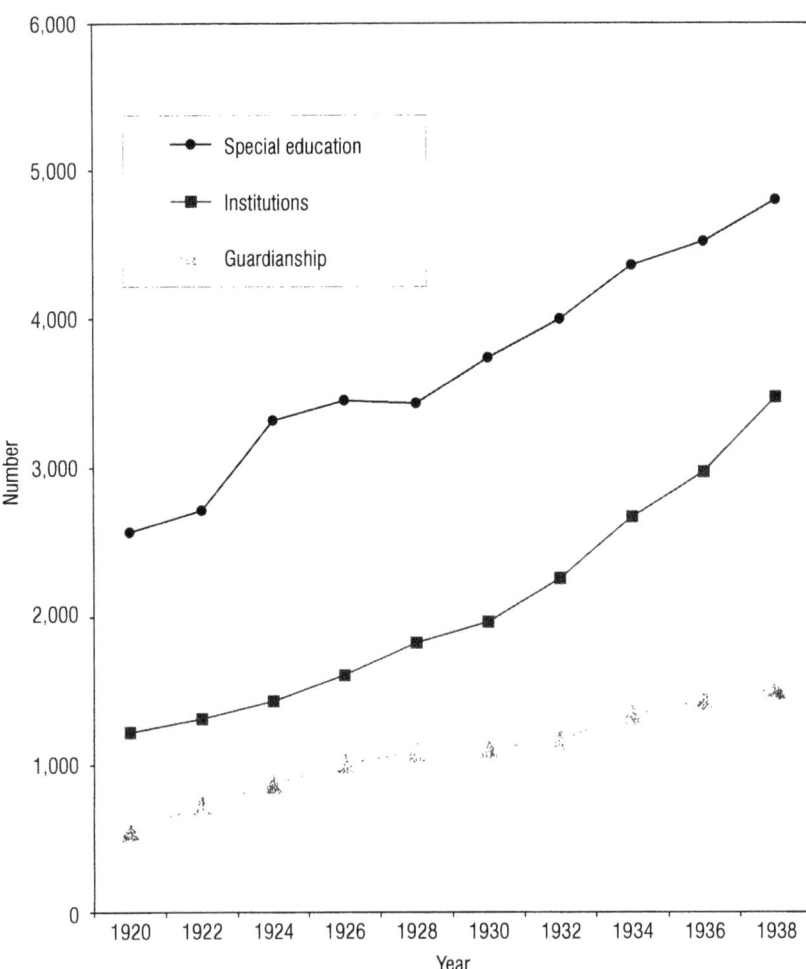

Figure 7.1 Number of mental defectives in receipt of special education, institutional provision or under private guardianship in Scotland (all ages).
(sources: Annual Reports of GBCS 1920–38; NAS ED 55, SED
Annual Statistics 1919–20 to 1937–38).

per 1,000 of Scotland's population were being treated as mentally defective by the authorities in 1919, compared to 2.0 per 1,000 in 1938.

This rise can partly be explained on administrative grounds. As more
local authorities began to fulfil their obligations under the Mental Deficiency Act, more people came to be certified as mentally defective. For
instance, in the school year 1919–20 only a third of Scotland's education
authorities had their own special schools and classes for mental defectives.

By 1937–38 the figure was close to two-thirds.[57] Not surprisingly, the number of mentally defective pupils in Scotland nearly doubled during the same period that the proportion of local education authorities holding special classes similarly expanded.

But the increase in the number of people labelled mentally defective was not simply caused by new local authorities taking an interest in this kind of provision. Rather, throughout the inter-war period, teachers, doctors and officials continued to broaden their definition of mental deficiency to include people with higher grades of ability. For this reason, the proportion of the population labelled mentally defective grew even in those areas that already had well-established special services. For instance, Glasgow's education authority had been administering its special education system since the late nineteenth century. Yet, the proportion of the city's school children labelled defective during the inter-war period still rose dramatically from 8 per 1,000 pupils on the city's school roll in 1919–20 to 14 per 1,000 in 1937–38.[58] Nor was this rise simply a cumulative increase over time. Although a new 'batch' of pupils who would become certified as mentally defective entered Glasgow's school system at the start of each school year, an old 'batch' (i.e. final year pupils) left the schools each year and were no longer recorded in the SED's statistics. The increase occurred because each year, children of higher mental ability were certified and segregated.

Contemporaries were aware that the criteria by which individuals were identified as being mentally defective were continuing to broaden during this period. For instance, Dr R. D. Clarkson, then Medical Superintendent of Larbert, told a government committee on Scottish health services in 1935 that 'the number of mental defectives is increasing very largely' but 'this is due to different diagnosis. Forty years ago almost half of the cases that are now being certified as mentally defective would not have been so certified'.[59]

Not every local authority encouraged this expansion in labelling. Certain school medical officers, particularly those working in the close-knit rural communities of the Highlands, felt that the feeble-minded label unnecessarily stigmatized children with low educational attainment. One SED inspector, Allan L. Rodger, described the situation as follows:

> [a]nother obstacle to progress in matters relating to the care and educ[ation] of MD children is the stigma which many people, unfortunately attach to the condition. Because of this attitude (not confined entirely to the man-in-the-street), some doctors are reluctant to say that a child is MD and many teachers refrain from directing the doctor's attention to possible cases and a few parents resist the verdict.[60]

Even within Glasgow's education authority, Scotland's flagship authority where special education was concerned, there was contention. John Grimmond's letter to the *Glasgow Herald* in 1923 illustrates how some contemporaries involved in educational policy contested the increased use of the mental deficiency label. Grimmond, it will be recalled, complained that 'the present policy tends to manufacture mental defectives'.[61]

Surprisingly, Grimmond's verdict was to be substantiated by the education authority's own school medical officer responsible for mental deficiency. Dr Robert Marshall was appointed to the post after Carswell changed jobs to become a medical commissioner for the GBCS in 1914. Marshall had been assistant superintendent at Gartnavel Asylum and his appointment to the school board was made on the recommendation of Gartnavel's Chief Medical Superintendent, Landel Rose Oswald.[62] Judging from his journal publications, Marshall's real interest lay in insanity rather than mental deficiency[63] but as 'Consulting Neurologist' to Glasgow Education Authority it is extremely probable that he diagnosed more mentally defective children in the first twenty years following the Mental Deficiency Act than any other individual doctor in Scotland. Marshall made clear that his criteria for distinguishing between imbeciles, feeble-minded children and ordinary children was 'purely a scholastic one'.[64] The majority of mental defectives he diagnosed were feeble-minded children, destined for special education, which makes it all the more remarkable that in 1931 the *Scottish Educational Journal* reported a speech delivered by Marshall to the Scottish Association for Mental Welfare, in which the school medical officer specializing in mental deficiency informed his audience that:

[f]eeble-mindedness was a legal fiction, and not a disease.[65]

Marshall viewed the medical diagnosis and certification of feeble-minded children as little more than bureaucratic procedures made necessary by law for transferring pupils with poor educational ability into special classes. The *SEJ*'s reporter described his speech as 'interesting' and little else was said on the matter, suggesting that neither the journal's editorial staff, nor its readership found Marshall's comments particularly controversial.

Who were the mental defectives?

The fact that most mental defectives were children, diagnosed primarily on scholastic criteria and segregated by the education system, illustrates that the historiography of mental deficiency suffers from its frequent omission or marginalization of special education. By concentrating on colonies and institutions, historians such as Jackson and Thomson not only fail to tell the whole story but may not even cover half of it.

Figure 7.1 has already demonstrated that Scotland's mental deficiency administrators were primarily concerned with young people, as it is evident that the majority of mental defectives received special education in day schools. This is despite the fact that according to the 1931 census, less than 20 per cent of the Scottish population were between the ages of five and sixteen.

GBCS statistics show that Scotland's institutions were also geared towards accommodating younger patients. The GBCS usually placed juveniles (under eighteen years old) in separate institutions from adult defectives. During the inter-war period the ratio of adult to juvenile institutional patients averaged at 2:3. Again, it should be born in mind that the general population of Scotland contained many more adults than juveniles, which serves to emphasize the degree to which young people were targeted.[66] Private guardianship (which includes boarding-out) was the only form of provision that, judging from the annual rate of admissions, was more geared to adult defectives.[67] This is because whilst private guardianship was supervised by the GBCS, children living at home tended to be dealt with by the education authorities.

A gender analysis of the Scottish institutional inmates generally supports Mathew Thomson's argument that the mental deficiency authorities used institutions to target males while they were young, whilst females were more likely to remain a concern throughout their adult life (reflecting contemporary anxiety over criminality amongst male youths and sexual activity amongst adult females). However, the pattern is not as consistent when it comes to private guardianship in Scotland.[68]

Within the special education system a gender ratio of three boys for every two girls remained fairly constant throughout the period.[69] Again, this corroborates Thomson's arguments that where youths were concerned, the authorities were more interested in males than females. However, it would be problematic to assume that this simply reflected the view that young males were more likely to engage in criminal activity. Within the school system, educational ability rather than propensity to crime appeared to be the most important factor in determining whether a child should attend a special school or not.

Provision for mental defectives was primarily an activity engaged in by urban local authorities. At the start of the inter-war period there were roughly five mentally defective pupils receiving special education in burgh schools for every one mentally defective pupil receiving special education in a county school (2,074 burgh special pupils, compared to 408 county special pupils in 1919–20). By 1937–38 the ratio had shifted to 2:1 (3,221 burgh special pupils to 1,579 county special pupils). The counties had therefore begun to make ground, but it should be born in mind that throughout the period the overall school population in the counties (ordinary and defective pupils) was over 50 per cent greater than that of the burghs.[70] Burgh authorities were therefore segregating a significantly higher proportion of their school population than county authorities. GBCS statistics on institutions and guardianship demonstrate a similar tendency towards burgh authorities.[71]

The annual statistics of the SED and GBCS give information about age, gender and locality, but they are less forthcoming on the subject of social class, doubtless because of the difficulties involved with obtaining statistics on this subject. Glasgow's school medical officers periodically looked at the housing conditions of its pupils, taking into account the number of residents and the number of rooms in each household. The results indicate that mentally defective pupils lived in more crowded households than the average school pupil. However, their homes are not as crowded as the homes of pupils from Roman Catholic schools or physical defectives, many of whom had deficiencies such as rickets that were directly related to poor living standards.

There are problems in assuming that household size and family size can give an accurate representation of social class. Perhaps the most persuasive evidence to support the argument that mental deficiency administrators targeted the poorer sections of society can be found not from statistical evidence but within the Mental Deficiency Act itself. The Act specifically directed officials to provide for neglected or abandoned children, criminals and adults claiming poor relief. GBCS statistics show that close to 100 per cent of defectives accommodated in institutions or under private guardianship throughout the period were rate-aided rather than private.

Conclusion

In 2000 the Scottish Executive published a report on policies and services for people with learning difficulties in Scotland.[72] Its title, *The Same As You?*, and many of its recommendations owed much to the 'equal rights' and 'social inclusion' discourses of its time. It stands in contrast with some of the harsher rhetoric of the early twentieth century, perhaps best encapsulated in the title of the British government's 1908 Royal Commission on the 'Care and Control of the Feeble-Minded'. However, both reports sought to emphasize the importance of their recommendations by pointing to the increasing number of people affected. *The Same As You?* estimated that 23 or 24 per 1,000 people in Scotland have either a mild, moderate, profound or multiple learning disability.[73] The authors also stated that 'the number of people with learning disabilities will continue to grow by 1% a year over the next 10 years'. The Scottish figure for the year 2000 was therefore roughly ten times that given in 1908. It was over twenty-five times the figure given by the Lunacy Commission in 1857, and twice the size of the figure given for Scottish children in 1939. The gap is predicted to widen.

During the nineteenth and twentieth centuries, there have been many changes. Medico-legal labels have been altered, and so have some of the definitions associated with them. New diagnostic techniques have been introduced, particularly in association with the development and consolidation of the psychology profession. There have also been broader changes to the way mental defectives received specialized state provision, and in the discourse that surrounded them. Yet amongst all these changes, the increase in the number of people being singled out for special treatment because they are judged to have low intelligence remains a continuous feature. Indeed many of the changes contributed to that increase.

Continuing a trend begun in Glasgow in the late nineteenth century, the expansion of special provision in Scotland occurred alongside an increase in the number of people labelled mentally defective. The increase in labelling occurred partly because more local authorities began identifying mental defectives but also because the borderline between defective and ordinary intelligence continued to be raised, with the result that people with higher levels of abilities were now being regarded as mentally defective. Some contemporaries publicly questioned the assumption that all of those labelled actually had a medical disorder. However, scepticism regarding the medical basis of certification did not necessarily constitute an attack on segregated provision per se. As Marshall demonstrates, it was possible to view feeble-mindedness as a purely legal category yet still actively support special education.

Andrew Scull has suggested in his work on insanity in the late nineteenth century that historians do not have to belittle the 'devastating character of the losses sustained by this form of communicative breakdown'[74] in order to argue that professionals encouraged 'an expansion of the boundaries of what constituted mental illness'.[75] Likewise, this chapter does not suggest that theories of mental deficiency bore no relationship to the genuine difficulty that some people experience acquiring socially valued skills or the discrimination they often face. It does, however, assume that the decision to mark one person out as 'defective' and another as 'normal' was problematic, contested and embedded within wider considerations such as institutional management, government policy, medical theories, behavioural norms and relations between state officials, professionals and the public.

Whilst these wider considerations have been described in more detail elsewhere,[76] this chapter has sought to highlight the importance of educational issues. It was in Scotland's schools that most mental defectives were identified and segregated. The alleged benefits of special education promoted by those doctors and teachers responsible for its administration allowed teachers in the ordinary classes to become increasingly intolerant of educational failure. They became more willing to notify struggling children to school doctors, who certified them mentally defective. This explanation might seem more prosaic than theories of national efficiency, citizenship, social control and eugenics (although it does not exclude such theories), but the day-to-day practice of labelling within the education system was conducted by local doctors and teachers, not politicians and social theorists, and the work itself was prosaic.

Notes

1 *Glasgow Herald*, 19 December 1923.
2 D. Barker, 'How to Curb the Fertility of the Unfit: The Feeble-minded in Edwardian Britain', *Oxford Review of Education*, 9, 1983, pp. 198–199; D. Barker, 'The Biology of Stupidity: Genetics, Eugenics and Mental Deficiency in the Inter-war Years', *British Journal for the History of Science*, 22, 1989, pp. 247–275; G. E. Berrios and R. Porter, *A History of Clinical Psychiatry: The Origin and History of Psychiatric Disorders*, London: Athlone Press, 1995; E. J. Larson, 'The Rhetoric of Eugenics: Expert Authority and the Mental Deficiency Bill', *British Journal for the History of Science*, 24, 1991, p. 59; P. Potts, 'Medicine, Morals and Mental Deficiency', *Oxford Review of Education*, 9(3), 1983, pp. 181–196; M. A. Barrett, 'From Education to Segregation' (PhD thesis, University of Lancaster, 1987); D. Wright, 'The National Asylum for Idiots, Earlswood, 1847–1886' (DPhil thesis, University of Oxford, 1993); S. Watson, '"The Moral Imbecile": A Study of the Relations Between Penal Practice and Psychiatric Knowledge of the Habitual Offender' (PhD thesis, University of Lancaster, 1988); D. Wright, '"Childlike in his Innocence": Lay Attitudes to "Idiots" and "Imbeciles" in Victorian England', in D. Wright and A. Digby (eds), *From Idiocy to Mental Deficiency: Historical Perspectives on People with Learning Disabilities*, London: Routledge, 1996, pp. 118–133.
3 M. Jackson, *The Borderland of Imbecility: Medicine, Society and the Fabrication of the Feeble Mind in Late Victorian and Edwardian England*, Manchester: Manchester University Press, 2000.
4 J. W. Trent Jr., *Inventing the Feeble Mind: A History of Mental Retardation in the United States*, Berkeley: University of California Press, 1994.
5 M. Thomson, *The Problem of Mental Deficiency: Eugenics, Democracy, and Social Policy in Britain, c.1870–1959*, Oxford: Clarendon Press, 1998, p. 9.
6 *Scottish Educational Journal*, 14, 1931, p. 606.
7 Scottish Executive, *The Same as You? A Review of Services for People with Learning Disabilities*, 2000.
8 Examples of historical studies that shed light on mental deficiency in Scotland include H. Sturdy, 'Boarding-Out the Insane, 1857–1913' (PhD thesis, University of Glasgow, 1996); H. Sturdy and W. Parry-Jones, 'Boarding-out Insane Patients: The Significance of the Scottish System 1857–1913', in P. Bartlett and D. Wright, *Outside the Walls of the Asylum: The History of Care in the Community 1750–2000*, London: Athlone Press, 1999, pp. 86–114; Lachlan Macmillan, 'Origins and Evolution of Special Education for Children with Intellectual Disabilities in Greater Glasgow 1862–1962' (PhD thesis, University of Strathclyde, 1998); G. O. B. Thomson, 'Legislation and Provision for the Mentally Handicapped Child in Scotland since 1906', *Oxford Review of Education*, 9, 1983, pp. 233–230; N. Anderson and A. Langa, 'The Development of Institutional Care for "Idiots and Imbeciles" in Scotland', *History of Psychiatry*, viii, 1997, pp. 243–266.
9 Jackson, *Borderland of Imbecility*, p. 22.
10 In this volume (Chapter 5) Louise Westwood explores the influence traditional 'boarding-out' had on early community care schemes before and after the 1930 Mental Treatment Act.
11 M. Egan, 'The "Manufacture" of Mental Defectives in Late Nineteenth and Early Twentieth Century Scotland' (PhD thesis, University of Glasgow, 2001), pp. 274–275.
12 R. Neugebauer, 'Treatment of the Mentally Ill in Medieval and Early Modern England', *Journal of History of Behavioural Sciences*, 14, 1978, pp. 158–169; R. Neugebauer, 'Mental Handicap in Medieval and Early Modern England:

Criteria, Measurement and Care', in Wright and Digby (eds), *From Idiocy to Mental Deficiency*, pp. 22–43; J. Andrews, 'Begging the Question of Idiocy: The Definition and Socio-cultural Meaning of Idiocy in Early Modern Britain: Part 1', *History of Psychiatry*, 9, 1998, pp. 65–95.

13 Anderson and Langa, 'Development of Institutional Care', p. 255; K. Day and J. Jancar, 'Mental Handicap and the Royal Medico-Psychological Association: A Historical Association, 1841–1891', in G. E. Berrios and H. Freeman, *150 Years of British Psychiatry 1841–1991*, London: Gaskell, 1991, pp. 268–278, p. 274; W. W. Ireland, *On Idiocy and Imbecility*, London: J. & A. Churchill, 1877.

14 G. Sutherland, *Ability, Merit and Measurement*, Oxford: Clarendon Press, 1984, pp. 5–24; Egan 'The "Manufacture" of Mental Defectives', p. 78.

15 Early twentieth century legal definitions of 'educable' and 'feeble-minded' defectives differed slightly. Although this attracted some comment in England, I have found no evidence of it troubling Scottish officials who treated the terms synonymously. The category of 'moral imbecile' also became widely used at this time, but in practice few defectives were ever certified as such in Scotland.

16 G. Gibson, 'The Boarding-out System in Scotland', *Journal of Mental Science*, 71, 1925, pp. 253–264; Sturdy and Parry-Jones, 'Boarding-out Insane patients', in Bartlett and Wright, *Outside the Walls of the Asylum*, pp. 86–114; L. Abrams, *The Orphan Country: Children of Scotland's Broken Homes from 1845 to the Present Day*, Edinburgh: John Donald, 1998; Egan, 'The "Manufacture" of Mental Defectives', pp. 273–274.

17 Mental Deficiency and Lunacy (Scotland) Act, 1913 (3 & 4 Geo. 5, c. 38).

18 Egan, 'The "Manufacture" of Mental Defectives', pp. 158–201; M. Thomson, *Problem of Mental Deficiency*, pp. 206–238.

19 Mental Deficiency and Lunacy (Scotland) Act, 1913 (3 & 4 Geo. 5, c. 38).

20 G. E. Berrios, 'Mental Retardation: Clinical Section – Part II', in Berrios and Porter, *A History of Clinical Psychiatry*, pp. 225–238; Jackson, *Borderland of Imbecility*, p. 112.

21 D. Pick, *Faces of Degeneration: a European Disorder c.1848–c.1918*, pp. 44–59; Jackson, *Borderland of Imbecility*, pp. 89–128.

22 W. W. Ireland, 'On Idiocy, especially in its Physical Aspects', *Edinburgh Medical Journal*, 19(2), January to June 1874, pp. 593–610 and pp. 689–702.

23 HMSO, *Scottish Lunacy Commission Report on Lunatic Asylums in Scotland*, I, 1857 (2148), p. 37.

24 *Report on Lunatic Asylums in Scotland*, I, p. 37.

25 *Report on Lunatic Asylums in Scotland*, I, p. 36.

26 W. W. Ireland, *The Mental Affections of Children: Idiocy, Imbecility and Insanity*, London: J. & A. Churchill, 1898, p. 4.

27 *Census of Scotland* I, 1911, xviii.

28 Ireland, *Mental Affections*, p. 7.

29 Quoted in Jackson, *Borderland of Imbecility*, p. 34.

30 HMSO, *Departmental Committee on Defective and Epileptic Children*, I, p. 5.

31 HMSO, *Royal Commission on the Care and Control of the Feeble-Minded*, VIII (Cd. 4202, 1908), p. 6.

32 *Royal Commission on the Feeble-Minded*, VIII, p. 90.

33 *Royal Commission on the Feeble-Minded*, III, p. 88 and p. 91.

34 HMSO, *Royal Commission on the Care and Control of the Feeble-Minded* III (Cd. 4217, 1908), pp. 369–405.

35 *Royal Commission on the Feeble-Minded*, VIII, p. 398.

36 GCA D-ED 9/1/33, School Board of Glasgow, *Annual Report on Medical Inspection of Children* 1910, p. 51.

37 J. Carswell, 'The Care and Education of Weak-minded and Imbecile Children in Relation to Pauper Lunacy', *Journal of Mental Science*, 44, 1898, p. 484.

38 Barrett, 'From Education to Segregation', pp. 237–246.
39 GCA D-ED 9/1/33 *Annual Report of the School Board of Glasgow*, 1909–10.
40 HMSO, *Royal Commission on the Feeble-Minded*, III, p. 269.
41 *Annual Report on Medical Inspection of Children* 1910, p. 51.
42 *Annual Report on Medical Inspection of Children* 1910, p. 51.
43 HMSO, *Royal Commission on the Feeble-Minded*, III, p. 269.
44 *Royal Commission on the Feeble-Minded*, III, p. 65.
45 *Royal Commission on the Feeble-Minded*, III, p. 269.
46 An oral history would be best suited for examining their views but the resources for such a study were unavailable to me.
47 Egan, 'The "Manufacture" of Mental Defectives', pp. 158–201.
48 NAS ED 28/230, draft SED circular, 6 December 1926.
49 HMSO, *GBCS Annual Report* 1925, Cmd. 2737, 1926, lvii.
50 Sutherland, *Ability, Merit and Measurement*, pp. 128–144.
51 Sutherland, *Ability, Merit and Measurement*, p. 123.
52 Sutherland, *Ability, Merit and Measurement*.
53 A. M. Macmeeken, *Intelligence of a Representative Group of Scottish Children*, London: University of London Press, 1939, pp. 2–13.
54 Ibid., p. 138.
55 Egan, 'The "Manufacture" of Mental Defectives', pp. 202–227.
56 GBCS figures taken from HMSO, *GBCS Annual Report* 1938, p. 41.
57 NAS ED 28/231, *SED Circular No. 105*, 1 September 1937.
58 Egan, 'The "Manufacture" of Mental Defectives', pp. 202–227.
59 HMSO, *Report of Department of Health for Scotland's Committee on Scottish Health Services* 1936 (Cmd. 5204), 1935–36, p. 60.
60 NAS ED 28/228, Departmental Committee on the Scottish Lunacy and Mental Deficiency Laws: private memo by A. L. Rodger, 2 May 1938.
61 *Glasgow Herald*, 19 December 1923, p. 7.
62 GCA D-ED 1/1/1/17 *Minutes of School Board of Glasgow*, 4 March 1914, pp. 645–646.
63 Marshall's publications included: 'Intra-Cranial Tumour with Mental Symptoms', *Journal of Mental Science*, 1909, pp. 310–321; 'Periodic Attacks of Excitement and Depression in the Chronic Insane', *Journal of Mental Science*, 1911, pp. 74–85; 'Differential Diagnosis of Manic Depressive Insanity and Dementia', *Glasgow Medical Journal*, LXXX, 1913, pp. 185–192.
64 *Scottish Educational Journal*, 14, 1931, p. 606.
65 *Scottish Educational Journal*, 14, 1931, p. 606.
66 HMSO, *GBCS Annual Reports* 1920–39.
67 *GBCS Annual Reports* 1920–39.
68 Egan, 'The "Manufacture" of Mental Defectives', pp. 221–222.
69 Egan, 'The "Manufacture" of Mental Defectives'.
70 Egan, 'The "Manufacture" of Mental Defectives', pp. 223–224.
71 HMSO, *GBCS Annual Reports* 1920–39.
72 Scottish Executive, *The Same as You? A Review of Services for People with Learning Disabilities*, 2000.
73 The estimate for England and Wales is closer to 30 per 1,000: HMSO, Department of Health, *Valuing People: A New Strategy for Learning Disability for the 21st Century* (Cm 5086), 2001, pp. 14–16.
74 A. Scull, 'Reflections on the Historical Sociology of Psychiatry', in A. Scull, *Social Order/Mental Disorder*, London: Routledge, 1989, p. 9.
75 A. Scull, 'Was Insanity Increasing?', in A. Scull, *Social Order/Mental Disorder*, p. 243.
76 Egan, 'The "Manufacture" of Mental Defectives'.

8 Tension in the voluntary–statutory alliance

'Lay professionals' and the planning and delivery of mental deficiency services, 1917–45

Pamela Dale

Introduction

The development of mental deficiency services has attracted much attention in recent years after a period of comparative neglect. This work has started to re-evaluate the relationship between provision for the mentally ill and long-term care for people who we would now regard as having a learning disability. This group was a visible, but minority, presence in most pauper lunatic asylums.[1] Late nineteenth-century reformers, concerned to restore the therapeutic potential of the asylum, and make other institutions more efficient and effective, insisted that the days of the mixed asylum had to end.[2] This necessitated the creation of new services for mental deficiency cases. The trajectories of provision for mental illness and mental deficiency were thus encouraged to diverge. The former became positively associated with legal reforms bolstered by therapeutic advances that required and facilitated early treatment, community care and finally decarceration programmes.[3] The latter was more problematically enmeshed in debates about the merits of permanent segregation, even eugenic sterilization.

It is however important to acknowledge that both the mental health and mental deficiency sectors were affected by similar concerns about both classification and questions of funding and entitlement. It is misleading to overstate either advances in the therapeutic management of mental illness or to suggest that mental deficiency services provided a new backwater for hopeless cases. There was much dynamism in the mental deficiency sector and the ideological as well as practical complexities of provision created new partnerships that were often in advance of arrangements for mental health. As Mathew Thomson points out the mental deficiency sector pioneered experiments in community care, new designs for institutions, the involvement of diverse professional groups, new partnerships with the voluntary sector and political alliances that crossed class and gender boundaries in a way that encouraged radical new solutions to long-standing social problems.[4] This chapter does not foreground either the difficulties or potential benefits accruing to service-users from these developments but instead focuses on the emergence of new loci of care, the power struggles of professional groups with a traditional and new interest in the problem, the expansion of municipal and voluntary sector provision and the potential for a distinct feminization as well as medicalization of service delivery.

This analysis engages with John Welshman's work on hostels (see Chapter 10), Vicky Long's chapter exploring the emergence of psychiatric social workers (Chapter 9) and Louise Westwood's argument that female practitioners could create an alternative service culture (see Chapter 5). In particular it endorses Matt Egan's conclusion that it was the work of diverse interest groups concerned with the 'normal' development of schoolchildren that served to 'manufacture' mental deficiency cases (see Chapter 7). Rather than a specific set of criteria that allowed for an uncontested diagnosis of 'deficiency', it was children who presented difficulties when starting, leaving or changing schools who were assessed as potential mental deficiency cases.[5] Particular anxieties surrounding age-appropriate behaviour, with a specific concern with adolescence, were expressed by parents and community figures as well as mental deficiency activists.[6] It was this shared concern that facilitated the operation of the Mental Deficiency Acts (MDAs) in the South West of England but it was the competition between interest groups, and the strategic alliances formed between the different professionals, that determined the detail of mental deficiency services and the fate of individuals consigned to them.

The idea of transition in mental deficiency policy and practice at a local and national level (shaped by funding regimes, access and entitlement issues, legislative reform, scientific and medical advance) echoed concern about the impact of transition in the lives of individuals. Families were seen to require specialist and intensive help as they went through crises in their life cycle. Births, deaths, periods of sickness and unemployment, children starting and leaving school, adolescents starting work or leaving home, the admission of any family members to any form of institutional care were all events that were likely to lead to the admission of a person with a learning disability to a mental deficiency institution.[7] Yet the institution they were admitted to, the planned and actual duration of their stay and where they went afterwards were matters for debate. This was because services in the South West of England were themselves undergoing transition as they responded to the implementation of the MDAs and the transformation of other local and national services directly and indirectly concerned with provision. This was especially true in Devon where the County Council pro-actively re-organized mental deficiency services after 1917.[8] Statutory organizations were however dependent on the voluntary sector to provide institutional and community based services and also relied on co-operation from other statutory and voluntary agencies operating in the fields of health, education, welfare and criminal justice.[9]

Crucial to the operation of all these organizations were emerging groups of 'lay professionals'. The term 'lay professional' is justified because these individuals combined the experience of lay people with specific expertise that is not easily fitted into existing models of care provision. Lay professionals included teachers, social workers, local government officers, charity workers, probation officers and institution managers, together with councillors and lay members of governing bodies and visiting committees. The lay professionals engaged in voluntary work operated on Finlayson's 'moving frontier' and remained active in formulating policy as well as delivering services throughout the inter-war period.[10] The exchange of personnel and ideas between the statutory and voluntary sectors did much to shape the character of mental deficiency policy. Mathew Thomson even talks about a symbiosis at the centre of government between the Board of Control and the Central Association for Mental Welfare (CAMW).[11] This relationship between the statutory and voluntary sectors had a local dimension that was equally important, although competition as well as co-operation characterized mental deficiency work.[12] Lay professionals competed with one another for professional status, control of services and access to funds. Lay professionals also played an important mediating role between families and institutions that determined the development of services and the people who would use them.

The lay professionals were an important dimension to mental deficiency work in the inter-war period but their involvement with the organization and financing of care was by no means a new development. David Wright notes that control over nineteenth-century institutions, including admission and discharge policy, was left to lay boards, Poor Law authorities and County Magistrates.[13] He uses this apparent restriction on the powers of medical superintendents as evidence that families were the key actors in the process of confinement. Yet it seems that both the supply of and demand for nineteenth-century asylum care were managed by a series of lay professionals. As the scope of health, education, welfare and criminal justice work expanded so did the number and variety of lay professionals. As local authority and voluntary sector services developed the lay officials and volunteers they employed self-consciously professionalized their work. This involved co-operation, and also competition, with other groups of lay professionals and medical practitioners.[14] The broad remit of mental deficiency work ensured that a variety of statutory and voluntary agencies as well as different professional groups had to bargain with one another over the disposal of cases and access to funds. This does not preclude the idea that families were able to negotiate with and even manipulate local welfare provision, but there were ranks of lay professionals standing between the family and the institution and they seem to have been in a strong position to determine access to care.

Wright demonstrates that by the late nineteenth century a variety of factors made home care more difficult and the problems of family carers more visible.[15] The proliferation of health and welfare services in the early twentieth century was both a cause and a consequence of a number of related developments that had pushed mental deficiency up the political agenda. Mark Jackson regards the late Victorian and Edwardian periods as critical in the history of people with learning difficulties.[16] These decades certainly witnessed the identification of new categories of mental deficiency and their association with social pathology. Yet although Jackson notes the way these ideas crystallized in a number of physical and ideological sites that were increasingly colonized by doctors, and lay campaigners like Mary Dendy who advocated a medical model of care, it is not clear what the immediate impact of this was.[17] In this period new institutions were created and older ones apparently re-orientated to meet the demands of the new rhetoric of care, but there is no clear chronology for deciding what, if any, was the dominant ideology.

Thomson points to a hegemonic belief that the mentally defective were a major social problem as an explanation for the 1913 Act and its implementation.[18] This apparent hegemony gives a model of a universal problem requiring a national solution although Thomson's model is considerably more subtle. It does however imply a coherent and well-resourced strategy to deal with the problem of mental deficiency that was not consistently delivered. Thomson poses a variety of reasons for this but it may be useful to draw attention to the different agendas and patchy service development that characterized provision before 1913. This had implications for the implementation of the MDA that went beyond questions of resources and political will. Evidence from the South West of England confirms that mental deficiency was perceived to be a major social problem, although it was not understood to be one problem but a whole series of interlinked and overlapping ones. The need to provide care for the severely handicapped was a separate issue from the provision of special education, and the management of criminal and immoral behaviour was an additional if related concern.[19] The neglect and abuse of dependent family members was a cause for intervention that for the most part was distinct from concerns about the behaviour of individual 'defectives' in public spaces. Again the action taken depended on the status of the individual and their personal and family circumstances. Events that superficially had much in common were treated differently depending on whether the people involved were subject to mental deficiency orders, or were suspected cases under investigation, or were already patients in mental deficiency institutions.[20]

These groups fell under the management of diverse agencies offering different permutations of care and control. They had complementary rather than identical philosophies, and while at some level a consensus about mental deficiency policy existed there were many factors acting against combining effort and pooling resources to provide one single unified service.[21] This was despite the centralizing influence of the Board of Control, and the provisions of the MDAs, which encouraged a co-ordinated approach and potentially provided a unifying ideology. Evidence from national and local sources suggests that the Board of Control was quite clear about how mental deficiency services, in the community as well as in institutions, should be run.[22] Yet the delivery of this model of care, which relied heavily on local authority-funded, medically run mental deficiency colonies, was very problematic. In the absence of comprehensive colony provision, existing institutions with distinct models of care arguably exercised disproportionate influence over the future direction of institutional and community care.

A strong consensus on the nature of mental deficiency and the future of mental deficiency services eventually developed within the Devon County Council Medical Department.[23] This medical model of care and control proved attractive to certain other medical practitioners and was deferred to by some groups of lay professionals but never gained universal acceptance. Much literature on the subject of mental deficiency points to a widely held, but fairly weak, consensus on the management of mental deficiency as a social problem in a variety of institutional settings. This apparently explains legislative action on the question of segregation but the continued rejection of a wider eugenic agenda, especially sterilization. In the Devon area however it seems more important that two narrow groups of self-styled mental deficiency experts advocated competing lay and medical solutions to the problem. The idea of a local authority-funded, medically run colony proved popular with members of the statutory authority, whose mental deficiency committee minutes reflect ongoing support for sterilization as well as segregation.[24] The lay organizations, that the local authority funded to provide institutional and community care, continued however to advocate models of care that emphasized education, training and rehabilitation in the community, although not always support for family carers.[25]

This chapter concentrates on two very different types of voluntary organization. The first are the voluntary organizations set up to facilitate the ascertainment of mental deficiency cases and supervise cases under statutory supervision. These organizations were usually affiliated to the CAMW but their work was adapted to meet local requirements, as determined by their sponsoring local authority, and services were far from uniform. The Devon Voluntary Association (DVA) and the Plymouth Voluntary Association (PVA) offer two regional examples with reasonably well preserved records. In the South West of England the major provider of institutional care, the Western, later Royal Western, Counties Institution (RWCI) at Starcross near Exeter in Devon was also under lay control.[26] The MDA had deliberately stimulated voluntary effort to create community services that provided both support and surveillance. The future role of the independent voluntary institutions was more ambiguous. The Board of Control and local councils viewed the beds at Starcross as a useful resource but were suspicious of its commitment to education and training rather than the new priorities for mental deficiency work set out in the 1913 Act. The RWCI, as an independent institution with a distinctive niche market, was crowded out by the expanding boundaries of the local and national state. Thomson stressed this point in his account of the prehistory of mental deficiency, but he neglected to examine the way institutions like the RWCI were able to adopt different strategies in response to the threat of competition.[27] The way that the RWCI sought to influence evolving community care provision to bring 'promising' cases to the institution for rehabilitative training and entry into the Starcross programme of license and discharge was particularly important.[28] It was not until the 1930s that the RWCI had to really confront the new agenda for mental deficiency work outlined by Jackson and Thomson. By this time the institution had successfully initiated its own programmes of community care that provided continuity with a much earlier and more optimistic belief in the potential to rehabilitate the mentally impaired.[29]

When Thomson asserts that what was different about 1930s community care was its scale rather than its essential nature he clearly has in mind the type of community-based services and monitoring facilities described by Walmsley, Atkinson and Rolph.[30] Their description of mental deficiency work in the County of Somerset after 1914 shows that comprehensive community services, backed up by specialist institutional provision, pre-dated the MDA.[31] In Devon this was not the case and competition between lay and medical personnel as well as statutory and voluntary agencies created uncertainty over the future of institutional and community-based mental deficiency services. In 1930, when Thomson notes the Board of Control *Annual Report* first used the term 'community care', there was a fairly comprehensive network of community services in Devon that had been built up over the previous decade.[32] It would be wrong however to attribute the failure to develop provision prior to this as a rejection of community care. Nor did the adoption of such services necessarily signify wholehearted approval of community-based initiatives. Mental deficiency policy in Devon remained in a state of flux and had not yet come to terms with the legacy of service delivery at Starcross. The RWCI was a large provider of institutional care but its long-standing commitment to specialist residential care for children had left a significant gap in the life-time care of people with learning disabilities in Devon.[33]

A commitment to education and training

The RWCI was one of the original five English voluntary idiot asylums, established during the nineteenth century. Founded in 1862, it was explicitly modelled on the pioneering Earlswood Asylum. It was run on similar lines to a voluntary hospital and relied upon subscriptions and donations.[34] Subscribers had an important role in the selection of potential inmates through their entitlement to vote in elections and also influenced policy through the Annual General Meeting. At Starcross these arrangements were undermined by an increasing dependency on Poor Law-funded patients.[35] Although the switch towards pauper cases was influenced by the search for financial stability, given a shortage of subscribers, it was also consistent with the founders' original concern to provide education/training for 'idiot children of the poor'. The financial security flowing from this decision encouraged expansion. After extensions and new building in the 1870s, 1890s and again in the Edwardian period, Starcross could accommodate approximately 300 pupil-patients.

As the institution grew in size and importance the position of superintendent attracted considerable social status. By the inter-war period Captain Charles W. Mayer, Superintendent 1924 to 1946, and successive chairmen of the Managing Committee were working together to oversee the development of the institution. The subscribers, later termed company members, were eased out of the decision-making process which was increasingly controlled by the managers.[36] This term was used by the institution in the inter-war period to cover a range of people who were members or co-opted members of the managing committee and its sub committees. The term apparently embraced the superintendent, who was very much a part of the policy-making process, but crucially excluded all other officers of the institution until 1937.[37] The co-opted members of the managing committee were by the 1920s increasingly drawn from the partner local authorities, and for the first time included women. They demanded more day-to-day control over the institution and this put them at odds with the cadre of traditional company members. This position was finally resolved with the adoption of a structure known as the Joint Committee, allowing members to be more explicit about which interest group or organization they were representing.[38] This became crucial as the breadth of local mental deficiency work increased and the purchaser–provider relationship between the RWCI and its partner local authorities was formalized. The purchaser–provider terminology, borrowed from the twenty-first-century mixed economy of care, gives some clues to the strength of innovative partnerships between the statutory and voluntary sectors, and also some of their inherent tensions.

The original educational ethos of Starcross, outlined by the founders, was protected by successive generations of managers. In the years before 1914, when the MDA came into effect, only reasonably healthy and well-behaved children with evidence of ability to learn were admitted, although some pupil-patients were retained beyond school age. Since an insufficient number of local cases met the criteria a national recruitment strategy was facilitated by agreements with a number of Boards of Guardians across England and Wales. This policy was in complete contrast to the other voluntary idiot asylums where higher proportions of private and charitable cases were maintained.[39] They also accepted more severely handicapped patients and were apparently as concerned with care and treatment as education and training. The RWCI had registered as an Idiot Asylum but only admitted 'high-grade' cases who, after 1914, fell into the category of the 'feeble-minded' but even within this terminology were understood to be at the upper end of the ability spectrum.

The policy of developing the Starcross asylum as a residential special school made the RWCI more vulnerable to the emergence of competition from day special schools than any of the other original idiot asylums. Failure to secure co-operation with Devon County Council over the local implementation of the 1899 Education (Defective and Epileptic Children) Act soured relations between the main provider of institutional care in the county and the new statutory authority even before the MDA. It is apparent from decisions taken in 1914 that the Starcross managers had badly underestimated the impact of this legislation. The changes introduced were understood to be largely administrative and no allowance was made for the new agenda for mental deficiency work embodied in the Act. Comments made at the 1914 Starcross AGM suggest a determination to continue as before.[40] The new Devon County Council Statutory Mental Deficiency Committee was equally enamoured with the idea of creating a comprehensive mental deficiency service independent of Starcross.[41] The outbreak of war saw these schemes shelved, but not abandoned.

It was the Board of Control that finally frustrated these plans.[42] The Board encouraged a rationalization of services by insisting that the RWCI must re-orientate itself from a national to a local catchment area and also blocked schemes for a rival county asylum. This left Starcross with a much smaller pool of 'promising cases' and made the institution dependent on the statutory authority for patients and funds. Initially the new arrangements left the statutory authority with no accommodation under its control but officers and members of the Devon County Council exploited the developing purchaser–provider relationship to gain access to beds and undermine the independent managing committee at Starcross.[43] Groups of patients previously excluded from Starcross on the grounds of severe disability, poor health or behavioural problems were presented for admission. The admission criteria, tightened in the early years of the century to combat competition from day special schools, were relaxed at the insistence of the local authority.[44] Rising costs, staff shortages and bedblocking all resulted from this decision.

The Starcross managers found that they could no longer object to the principle of admitting severely handicapped patients since their institutionalization was a priority for the statutory authority and there was no other suitable accommodation available.[45] This did not however prevent the managers from strictly controlling the size of this inmate population by charging a premium rate for their care and limiting admissions to a number of self-contained annexes. This was meant to provide ease of nursing care but also explicitly protected the lay education and training programmes located in the main building.[46] In the 1920s these programmes were apparently suffering as a result of allowing less able children to be admitted and the managers bemoaned the waste of expensive facilities on what they regarded as unpromising cases.[47] It was only in the 1930s that the training programmes revived as the managers came to realize that groups of very able, but usually older, 'defectives' had been identified as a result of the provisions of the MDAs.[48] For some time the County Council had pressed for the admission of criminal cases, unmarried mothers and neglected children, and they were now cautiously accepted.[49] While there were some disastrous failures that brought unwelcome publicity and official scrutiny, the RWCI was able to claim some expertise in the 'reform and rehabilitation' of challenging patients within its evolving training programmes. These had strong links into the community through employment schemes as well as ongoing contact with patients' families.[50]

The Starcross managers regarded the community care programme as a natural development of the rehabilitative training the institution had traditionally offered. While the managers rejected much of the new agenda for mental deficiency work, and especially its uncomfortable association with eugenically inspired segregation and sterilization schemes, they did accept that it was increasingly difficult to find work for former patients in the open labour market. In the Edwardian period discussions about a farm colony had come to nothing, but the desire to find gainful employment for discharged patients encouraged the search for employers who were willing and able to provide work, accommodation and a degree of supervision. The Starcross managers strongly advocated the idea that training was most effective with younger patients who should be discharged as soon as practicable to ensure the institution was a 'flowing stream not a stagnant pond'.[51]

On several occasions Mayer used his public addresses to suggest that since there were insufficient funds to provide permanent institutional care for the total population of suspected 'defectives' it was more economical and effective to rehabilitate as many as possible through short periods of institutional training.[52] This scheme embraced patients who needed support between community care placements but excluded patients whom the managers believed were too handicapped or dangerous to rehabilitate. The former were directed towards the simpler, and cheaper, facilities provided by workhouses although Mayer had no objection to relatives providing care if they were willing to do so. The state institutions were presented as the natural destination for 'dangerous defectives' although Mayer used local mental hospitals as an outlet for 'difficult' patients who did not meet the criteria for being assessed as 'dangerous'.[53]

A new agenda for mental deficiency work?

This was not the agenda for mental deficiency work that interested the statutory authority. Devon County Council was keen to encourage the development of community-based services but saw their main role being community surveillance rather than provision of care. The local authority was instrumental in reforming the DVA but saw its role as primarily one of ascertaining new cases, and to a lesser extent liaising with families who already had relatives in mental deficiency institutions.[54] At first even limited measures like Guardianship were viewed with suspicion, although later on the DVA developed a range of services that included an occupation centre, a home teaching service, limited respite care and a network of contacts in the education, health, welfare and criminal justice systems.[55] The DVA and, in Plymouth, the PVA employed salaried staff as well as volunteers. They visited patients whose mental status was being assessed and those on the waiting list for institutional care. While the surveillance of, usually working class, communities and families cannot be overlooked the support given to family carers was also important. The DVA workers also visited patients in institutions to check on their progress and supervised licensed and discharged patients in the community.

The growing independence and professionalization of voluntary services in Devon was a crucial determinant of policy and practice towards the mentally defective in the 1920s. The County Council had recreated the DVA in 1917 but the organization secured patrons and funds separate from its arrangements with the local authority.[56] Although the statutory authority had envisaged a fairly limited role for the DVA, in terms of ascertainment work, there was nothing to stop the lady volunteers or the salaried staff asking new questions in new situations. In conversations with the families of prospective patients the voluntary social workers entered the domestic sphere and found out what the burden of care really meant. On a case by case basis efforts were made to understand and relieve the problems faced by family carers. This prompted the development of new services to support carers but it also led to new discourses about the 'problem family' and further stigmatization and condemnation of patients and their relatives.[57]

This re-categorization of families by voluntary social workers had not been anticipated or welcomed by the Starcross managers. In pursuit of young and trainable cases they had not given much thought to the background to each case. The managers believed that the special needs of the mentally defective child could only be met by appropriate institutional care.[58] They approved of families who sought this special care and even evidence of neglect or abuse tended to be regarded as an indication of the difficulty of providing care at home rather than family pathology. By contrast case notes from the voluntary associations suggested that income was not the best guide to the quality of home care. Instead the willingness and ability of family carers to provide suitable care, recognized as a difficult and demanding job, depended on a variety of other factors. These assessments included reference to the social problems that campaigners had long associated with the causes and consequences of mental deficiency; namely pauperism, prostitution, criminality and inebriety. Thus reports focused on the industry, thrift, sobriety and demeanour of the parents as well as the conduct and achievements of all their children, not just the prospective patient.

Emerging from these discussions were concepts of 'good families' and also 'problem families'. For the voluntary social workers 'good families' were not only caring and respectable but also keen to provide home care. They were offered advice and access to services that would facilitate this.[59] Clearly many of the families supported in this way did not seek institutional care even though the Starcross managers viewed their children as a priority for institutional training. What did happen, much to the chagrin of the managers, was that home care continued until the prospective patient, or often their main carer, was too sick for it to continue.[60] Then there was an emergency admission and indefinite stay instead of an organized period of education and training before return to the family home. 'Problem families' were no less challenging for the managers. Here the main difficulty was the co-ordination of effort with the variety of welfare professionals seeking to cope with the spectrum of social problems presented by the family. Voluminous case notes were generated and in many instances the voluntary social workers were able to provide a useful contact point for concerned teachers, charity workers, probation officers, the police and even medical personnel. When working with 'problem families' the voluntary social workers usually recommended institutionalization as a kind of child rescue and it was not unusual for siblings to be presented for admission. The Starcross managers had no problem with this, in fact it not only echoed nineteenth-century rescues documented in the institution's records but also endorsed inter-war claims to 'reform and rehabilitate defectives'.[61] There was some concern about the discharge of patients without a stable family background but these were increasingly channelled through the employment-orientated community care scheme. The Starcross managers found that the voluntary associations usefully bridged the gap between institutional care and community placements. Instead of simply discharging patients, often to distant locations without meaningful aftercare, as the institution had previously done, the network of services and surveillance created by the DVA and PVA provided new opportunities for licensing as well as discharging patients.[62]

The voluntary associations welcomed this new role and the additional funding it generated. While ascertainment work was covered by an annual grant from the statutory authority, the County Council funded the supervision of licensed patients on a case by case basis with additional sums being provided by the Starcross managers. While the relationship between the institution and the voluntary associations was often constrained by the ascertainment priorities of the local authorities, the discharge of patients allowed for more freedom of action.[63] Mayer, somewhat cynically, encouraged the voluntary social workers to provide an assessment of a patient's likely suitability for community care when an application for institutional care was made. Voluntary social workers sought the closest possible co-operation with the statutory authorities and employed a much wider defin-ition of mental deficiency than had traditionally been used at Starcross, but also had some sympathy for the idea that the specialist facilities avail-able at the RWCI should be reserved for a distinct subset of the total insti-tutional population.

Ascertaining and institutionalizing the mentally defective in Devon

When the members of the Devon Statutory Mental Deficiency Committee first met the issues of ascertainment and institutionalization were treated as one and the same. This idea persisted although plans for a comprehen-sive mental deficiency service that would facilitate the incarceration of all known Devon mental deficiency cases in one specialist mental deficiency colony were continually frustrated by financial and organizational dif-ficulties. The obvious location for the mental deficiency colony was Star-cross but it soon became apparent that it was too small and re-development was likely to be ruinously expensive. The proposed colony required funding from all the local authorities in the South West of England and a significant contribution from the institution's own accounts. After extensions in the 1920s the original site accommodated about 500 patients and a similar number of beds were planned at a separate RWCI colony called Langdon Farm. The allocation of the old and new beds as well as agreement on the type of cases to be admitted proved contentious. Protracted negotiations were finally concluded in 1929 but preliminary building work was almost immediately halted by depression-era public expenditure cuts. In the short term this created problems for the RWCI, which was seriously oversubscribed, and the local statutory and voluntary organizations who had to find somewhere else for the prospective patients. The development of community care and partnerships with other institu-tional care providers were seen as temporary solutions to the deferred colony option but came to shape the development of that colony. In a similar way the RWCI, at the centre of a network of increasingly interde-pendent institutions, exerted considerable influence over the development of smaller homes as complementary rather than competing services.[64]

The 1929 colony plan was very much the RWCI plan, envisaging an expanded education programme for children on the original site and a related adult training scheme for former pupils at the new colony. Limited provision was made for sick and/or severely handicapped patients, but no special arrangements were put in place for moderately handicapped patients likely to need long-term care or patients whose mental deficiency was 'discovered' as a result of criminal or immoral behaviour in adoles-cence or early adulthood. Far from meeting the Devon County Council requirement for a comprehensive mental deficiency service this specialist colony relied on a number of other institutions to support its arrangements. Children under the age of seven were placed in a number of small voluntary homes, older children and young adults who failed to respond to training were directed to workhouses while mental hospitals, prisons and state hospitals took other cases excluded from Starcross.

The statutory authority was well aware of the limitations of the original colony plans but had been unable to seize the initiative from the managers who controlled access to the beds at Starcross in a way that encouraged the local authorities to compete against one another. Internal wrangling over policy and severe organizational constraints also beset Devon County Council. In Devon the statutory authority had been slow to ascertain mental defectives before 1920 but then new cases reached a level that threatened to overwhelm the system.[65] In an atmosphere of near panic, as record levels of ascertainment were accompanied by ever gloomier estimates of the likely total population, the statutory committee threatened to become paralyzed by circular debates about the need to ensure government action on the question of sterilization as well as segregation. Mental deficiency work in Devon apparently reached its nadir in the early 1930s. Devon had been one of the areas surveyed on behalf of the Interdepartmental Committee on Mental Deficiency.[66] The resulting Wood Report estimated that at least 5,000 mentally defective persons were resident in the administrative county. Despite strenuous efforts to locate them in the period 1930–35 only 2,621 were discovered. This was a serious setback for an authority that had always sought recognition and approval from the Board of Control. Yet locally the disposal of the 2,621 individuals taxed all the resources of statutory and voluntary agencies in Devon.[67]

A new strategy for mental deficiency work was needed and there was a major re-organization of mental deficiency work in Devon after 1930. This was probably related to new Board of Control regulations, and the requirements of the 1929 Local Government Act and the 1930 Mental Treatment Act, although a change in personnel was also a significant factor. The reorganization of mental deficiency work greatly increased the role of the County Medical Officer of Health (MOH) and his enlarged department. The MOH took the lead in negotiations about the delayed and later revised colony scheme as well as assuming direct control of the Devon County Council institutions and responsibility for ascertaining all new cases in partnership with the DVA.[68] The DVA had sought independence in the 1920s but needed to protect its wide-ranging activities from funding cuts and tried to shelter its services under the umbrella of the medical department. The DVA, through its links to the CAMW, had always favoured the medicalization of mental deficiency work but local medical personnel had not made significant inroads into lay control before 1930. The MOH had been involved in the earliest discussions about statutory mental deficiency work but was unable to secure funds for a mental deficiency specialist and his defence of the rights of private practitioners tended to empower professionalizing lay social workers who selectively chose sympathetic doctors to work with.[69] The voluntary social workers appropriated medical concepts as part of their quest for professional status but tended to defer to the medical profession rather than individual doctors unless there were specific contractual relations.

In the absence of a mental deficiency expert a doctor was assigned to ascertainment work in 1917 but Dr C. A. P. Truman's background as an Assistant School Medical Officer suggested a bias towards work with child cases. He tended to passively wait for cases to be referred to him, and while the DVA brought some cases to his attention most of the referrals originated with the Devon County Council Education Committee. The comment and concern arising from the 'criminal' and 'immoral' cases independently identified by the Board of Control suggest that this was not a routine aspect of ascertainment work despite the oft-stated priorities of the statutory committee.[70] Dr Truman remained in post until his retirement in 1934. His successor, Dr Alice Cox, sought a more active role in the identification and management of mental deficiency as a social problem. She was particularly keen to extend her work into the courts and into institutions thought to harbour large, but often undisclosed, populations of mental defectives.[71]

The medicalization of care: advocates and opponents

Medical control over mental deficiency services was increased but its immediate association with the contentious issues of long-stay patients and cases ascertained as a result of allegations of criminality and immorality threatened to increase the resistance of lay professionals. Over the first twenty years of mental deficiency work in Devon the new, as well as pre-existing, services had developed under lay rather than medical control and the co-operation of lay professionals in a variety of institutional and community-based services had maintained the legitimacy of lay as well as medical claims to expertise. The focus on education and child welfare did much to encourage this. At the same time the medical profession had been weak and divided. Within the local authority the medical department was over-stretched and under-resourced, hence the initial appointment of Dr Truman rather than the desired expert. Lack of medical personnel encouraged the Clerk to the Council to take a lead role in the ascertainment process, bringing his own legal rather than medical bias to the proceedings. Questions tended to focus on settlement issues and the willingness of parents to participate in the certification process rather than any particular medical, or indeed other, needs of prospective patients.[72]

Within the institutions the situation was arguably worse. Across Britain small mental deficiency homes tended to remain under lay management but in Devon the leading provider of institutional care was also firmly under lay control. The part-time and non-resident medical officer (MO) was limited to a general practitioner role at the RWCI. It was the lay superintendent who, at least until the late 1920s, assessed the pupil-patients and made recommendations about admission and discharge to the lay managers. The effectiveness of the MO was also constrained by his own poor health, lack of professional status and other work commitments. There were no treatment facilities at Starcross and this forced the MO to seek co-operation with other hospitals. Some patients were transferred to other institutions but the local mental hospitals were cautious about accepting mental deficiency cases and after the 1930 Mental Treatment Act tried to reverse the flow by presenting many of their chronic cases as good candidates for the mental deficiency sector. Acute services could be obtained from the Royal Devon and Exeter Hospital but the expense involved discouraged exploratory investigations and the assistance of the hospital could not always be relied upon.[73] The local tuberculosis sanatoriums excluded all mental deficiency cases on the grounds of an unacceptable 'double defect', and problems were encountered when admitting patients to the isolation hospital.[74]

It was uncommon for patients to have received specialist medical attention for their condition prior to admission. Doctors played a key role in surveillance/diagnosis but medical personnel working in clinics, hospitals, schools and even prisons tended to pass cases on to the mental deficiency authorities rather than attempt to offer treatment. The voluntary associations then sought the necessary medical certificate allowing for a mental deficiency order but the fate of the individual in terms of their future care depended more on the background social reports than the formal medical diagnosis. This situation persisted even when efforts were made to bring the ascertainment process under the control of the Devon County Council Medical Department. While Alice Cox attempted to monopolize the formal diagnosis of mental deficiency, her work relied on increasingly detailed reports compiled by the DVA, drawing on their relationship with family carers and the contacts they had in the health, education, welfare and criminal justice systems.

Health workers, and in the context of local authority mental deficiency work especially health visitors, had always deferred to medical opinion and now the voluntary social workers found that their position vis-à-vis the other lay professionals was enhanced by the close working relationship established with the medical department. Educationalists were the main losers in the new power structure and lay staff at Starcross and local teachers found themselves at a serious disadvantage. The local trend being reinforced by pressure from Central Government where the Board of Control strongly advocated a medical model of care and the Board of Education unexpectedly withdrew funding from the planned expansion of the RWCI residential special school. The educational methods at Starcross and the apparent dedication of the lay teaching staff had attracted much attention from other service providers.[75] Yet the education on offer was acknowledged to only benefit a fairly narrow group of young and trainable cases. Given the political climate of the time there was no guarantee that the pupils who had been trained would be released from institutional care by their sponsoring local authority and prevailing economic conditions made their employment prospects poor.[76]

The obvious limitations of residential special schooling, coupled with the fear of stigmatizing children by association with adult defectives, had reduced the number of educable pupils at Starcross. This problem was compounded by the development of not just day special schools but innovative arrangements to support children with special needs in elementary schools.[77] These were successful to a point, but could not relieve the problems of home care. Teachers generally accepted that children had to be removed from school and institutionalized when their main carer could no longer cope. The sickness or death of the carer or a deterioration in the health or behaviour of the child were not ideal circumstances for engaging with the Starcross programme. As more patients had care or control needs that dictated lengthy institutional stays there was pressure from local and national government to provide alternatives to the traditional lay model of rehabilitative training. The RWCI finally appointed a resident medical officer and gave him particular responsibility for the management of sick, severely handicapped and disturbed patients.

The appointment of Dr David Prentice in 1937 heralded a new era for the RWCI, and while the results of additional medical care were mixed the trend towards medical control was marked. Prentice was immediately engaged with the problems of the new colony, then under construction. The original plans had long since been abandoned but no new scheme had been agreed upon. The local authorities insisted that the most secure facilities at the main site should hold the most difficult and dangerous patients and since it seemed sensible to retain the existing annexes as a special care unit, it was the young and trainable cases that moved to Langdon. A new hospital block was also constructed on this site while Mayer retained his traditional apartments in the main building. Without many patients to treat at Langdon, or indeed a clearly defined role within the lay hierarchy, Prentice was free to pursue his own research interests. Although the Board of Control and the Devon County MOH had apparently envisaged Prentice taking responsibility for more severely handicapped patients this did not occur. Instead it was the link between high-grade mental deficiency and various types of mental illness that interested Prentice.

The discovery of disturbed as well as delinquent patients drew the RWCI closer to mental health services in the 1940s although this has been overlooked in accounts of both mental health and mental deficiency services. This work, and its obvious links to the allegations of criminal and immoral behaviour that the medical department in Exeter were already investigating, became central to the evolving alliance between the various medical personnel. This advanced the medicalization of care and new ideas about the nature of disability, the limits of family care and the control of institutions. In the new formulations of mental deficiency work lay expertise was down-graded. Local head teachers bitterly complained that their former pupils, incarcerated at Starcross, were not mentally defective at all, but could not secure their release.[78] The certification of a former grammar school boy as a 'moral defective', whilst on remand at Exeter prison, highlights the problematic association of deviancy with notions of defectiveness.[79] It also points to the way medical hegemony over diagnostic tests subordinated traditional measures of intellectual ability and behavioural problems as well as lay claims to expertise in this field. A finding of moral deficiency did not necessarily imply any intellectual defect, only a lack of moral sense, but both were now established as competencies that could only be judged by expert medical opinion.

Lay professionals, medical practitioners and delinquent defectives

Within the mental deficiency sector, doctors appeared to be making significant advances at the expense of lay professionals, yet their role in the management of delinquency was never as straightforward as the control they achieved over the assessment of children or the treatment of severely handicapped patients. Medical domination of local authority mental deficiency work, and the medical model of institutional and community care promoted by the Board of Control, had surprisingly little impact on the working of the criminal justice system. Evidence from the South West of England confirms Pamela Cox's finding that the courts were more interested in determining the innocence or guilt of an alleged offender than making an assessment of the defendant's mental status.[80] In Devon it became practice for the Council Clerk or MOH to give evidence in person to try to secure mental deficiency orders for suspected 'defectives' appearing before the courts. They regularly reported humiliating failures where the courts freed defendants after not guilty verdicts in circumstances that allowed them to evade the surveillance and control of the mental deficiency authorities.[81] It was no consolation that the independently minded magistrates sometimes made unexpected orders in cases previously unknown to the statutory or voluntary agencies concerned with mental deficiency work.[82] This undermined the careful research-gathering exercise that was felt to be essential to support a successful placement within the mental deficiency sector.

Since the courts could not be relied upon to process offenders suspected of being mentally defective within the meaning of the Act, a new policy was devised. The Devon County Council Medical Department tried to encourage families to accept a mental deficiency placement as an alternative to prosecution for certain offences. All cases involving suspected 'defectives' were passed to the DVA for investigation. Family carers were encouraged to co-operate and if they consented to a mental deficiency order the police could usually be persuaded to drop any pending minor charges.[83] Conversely family resistance could be overcome with threatened prosecutions backed up with evidence collected by the DVA.[84] A number of cases were directed to Starcross as an alternative to a court appearance, apparently with the assistance of relatives keen to avoid public disclosure of their care and control problems. It is likely that mental deficiency placements were longer than the sentences usually attached to petty crime but relatives retained more control over the fate of mentally defective offenders by having them processed as ordinary rather than criminal 'defectives'. Crucially 'defectives' institutionalized under most sections of the MDAs were eligible for all local programmes of institutional and community care whereas mentally defective offenders detained under sections eight and nine were subject to additional control and scrutiny by the Board of Control. By working with local statutory and voluntary agencies, family carers were able to influence the incarceration and decarceration of their relatives but were always at a disadvantage in a relationship characterized by unequal access to knowledge and power.

Lay professionals, including social workers, charity workers and even probation officers retained much autonomy and authority in an area where medical influence was limited by the traditions of the courts. Paradoxically the medicalization of delinquency, for a short time at least, also bolstered lay authority at Starcross. Understanding the voluntary social workers' desire to keep reasonably healthy and well-behaved young 'defectives' at home with their approved carers, the managers looked elsewhere to bolster their training programmes. It became necessary to identify cases that the statutory and voluntary agencies directly and indirectly concerned with mental deficiency work were prepared to incarcerate with and without parental consent. Here cases involving criminality, immorality and neglect were all regarded as possibilities, albeit controversial ones. The RWCI was credited with the successful 'reform and rehabilitation' of patients with histories of delinquency and criminality in the mid-1930s although no specialist measures for their reception had been put in place beyond the lay 'moral management' regime.[85] These patients, often classed as 'high-grade', worked within the institution as well as the community care programme, their labour subsidizing the costs of caring for other patient groups.[86] Lay models of rehabilitative training provided a degree of care and control, but ultimately failed to cope as ever more disturbed patients were presented as suitable for admission. Here pressure from the Board of Control to take patients moving from the state hospitals to less secure accommodation was significant but it appears that cases presented for admission from the community were increasingly challenging.

Dangerous, and difficult, patients were in the late 1930s and 1940s passed to the institution's own doctors for investigation. The medical officers were able to offer sophisticated medical diagnoses to explain non-conformity with the lay training programme but did not develop an alternative therapeutic regime. Techniques of medical control, especially restraint and sedation, became more common but patient behaviour took longer to stabilize. As Starcross silted up with long-stay cases the institution became increasingly disengaged from wider developments in health care, education, welfare and criminal justice. The lay professionals bowed out of the management of Starcross but it was not clear that the new medical superintendent had anything new to offer the administration of the RWCI. In fact comparisons with the other four original voluntary idiot asylums in the inter-war period had suggested that Mayer was operating a particularly successful and economical regime that won generous plaudits from his medical colleagues.[87]

Conclusion

There is evidence to suggest that a unique combination of institutional and community care in Devon was successfully meeting the care and control aspirations that lay behind the local working of the MDA, even if arrangements did not conform to national best-practice in the inter-war period. In Devon a broad consensus on mental deficiency work was to some extent shared by a variety of lay professionals and medical practitioners. The level of co-operation achieved with family carers and working class communities suggested some popular support for the evolving practices that the consensual approach endorsed. Yet the formation of a stronger, but narrower, consensus on the merits of a medical model of care was eventually adopted to bring local practice into conformity with national policy. This introduced additional tension into the statutory–voluntary alliance that was already strained by the inherent contradictions of the funding regime and had far-reaching implications for the delivery of services in the area.

In the community, voluntary social workers deferred to medical opinion but retained a niche in the management of mental deficiency as a social rather than medical problem. Lay professionals working within the criminal justice system tended to work around rather than with the requirements of the MDAs. The Board of Control acquiesced to these arrangements and lay claims to expertise but other lay professionals lost out to the new medical orthodoxy. Teachers tended to lose out to medical control, especially in the management of residential care for sick, disturbed and even delinquent children. The RWCI was not able to maintain its niche market in residential special schooling. Later, the Board of Control came to present the 'moral management' regime at Starcross as increasingly obsolescent and irrelevant. The arrival of a resident medical officer, always viewed by the Board as Mayer's successor, fatally undermined the lay superintendent even before he was finally discredited by a series of events that themselves originated in the medicalization of care.[88]

The transition towards the medicalization of care echoes discussion about other individual institutions and the wider framework of mental deficiency policy. Yet evidence from not just Starcross but its partner local authorities and related voluntary agencies suggests that the trend towards the medicalization of care was not irresistible. The issue remained contentious throughout the inter-war period. Financial and organizational difficulties, well documented in other studies, were compounded by a strong vein of resistance that at different times embraced a variety of lay professionals, and occasionally medical practitioners who also chose to limit the ascendancy of local authority medical officers. For a variety of reasons Devon was slow to adopt the model of local authority-controlled, medically run colonies described by Thomson. This affected the type and number of cases dealt with. Yet the initial failure to develop these services is shown to be a factor behind the later explosion of activity in the 1930s that included issues like criminality, the 'problem family' and mental health services that Thomson and Welshman date to the 1940s and 1950s.[89] Not only was the chronology of mental deficiency work in the Devon area slightly different to that offered by Thomson and also Welshman but the underlying consensus on mental deficiency work is shown to encompass both acceptance of and resistance to the eugenic agenda of mental deficiency campaigners. There were therefore important continuities with the new agenda for mental deficiency work emerging in the late Victorian and Edwardian periods but also an earlier approach focusing on the potential of individual patients and the ability of family carers to provide appropriate levels of care and control.

Notes

1 J. Melling, R. Adair and B. Forsythe, '"A Proper Lunatic For Two Years": Pauper Lunatic Children in Victorian and Edwardian England. Child Admissions to the Devon County Asylum, 1845–1914', *Journal of Social History*, 31, 1997, pp. 371–405.

2 The context for the campaign for and implementation of the Mental Deficiency Act is explored in M. Thomson, *The Problem of Mental Deficiency: Eugenics, Democracy and Social Policy in Britain c. 1870–1959*, Oxford: Clarendon Press, 1998, pp. 10–23.

3 In this volume David Pearce (Chapter 6) and Vicky Long (Chapter 9) demonstrate the importance of the 1930 Mental Treatment Act with regard to all these points. Evidence from Devon suggests that the removal of chronic cases from local mental hospitals was central to attempts to modernize the mental health sector in the 1930s. Devon Record Office (DRO) 153/5/1/2, Devon Mental Deficiency Committee (DMDC), 15 November 1934, minute 39.

4 Thomson, *The Problem of Mental Deficiency*, pp. 1–9.

5 University of Exeter Library, RWCI archive, box 22, casebooks. Adults over the age of 21 accounted for only 14 per cent (346 from a total of 2,503) of RWCI admissions and re-admissions, 1 April 1913 to 31 March 1939.

6 In a written application to the RWCI for the admission of seventeen-year-old Kenneth M. concerns were raised about his alleged delinquencies, but the letter makes it clear that a far more pressing problem was finding suitable accommodation once he was too old for the scattered homes. RWCI archive, box 29, correspondence from Plymouth Voluntary Association (hereafter PVA), Lee to Mayer, 3 June 1938.

7 Files of correspondence sent to the RWCI by PVA give a particularly rich account of the circumstances that led to applications for the admission of individual patients. RWCI archive, box 29, correspondence from PVA.

8 Details of these proposals were outlined by a DMDC sub committee, 23 February 1917. DRO 153/5/1/1, minutes filed after DMDC, 13 February 1917.

9 The admission of Kenneth M., referred to earlier, involved Plymouth City Council Education and Public Assistance Committees as well as the deputy Medical Officer of Health, staff at the scattered homes, Plymouth Voluntary Association and the RWCI. This was treated as a routine application.

10 G. Finlayson, 'A Moving Frontier: Voluntarism and the State in British Social Welfare, 1911–49', *Twentieth Century British History*, 1, 1990, pp. 183–206.

11 Thomson, *The Problem of Mental Deficiency*, p. 155.

12 Occupation centres run by the voluntary associations competed directly with the RWCI for local child cases.

13 D. Wright, 'Getting Out of the Asylum: Understanding the Confinement of the Insane in the Nineteenth Century', *Social History of Medicine*, 10, 1997, pp. 137–155.

14 The RWCI tended to resist the medicalization of care, which lay staff associated with care rather than training.

15 D. Wright, *Mental Disability in Victorian England: The Earlswood Asylum 1847–1901*, Oxford: Clarendon Press, 2001, pp. 21–22 and conclusion.

16 M. Jackson, *The Borderland of Imbecility: Medicine, Society and the Fabrication of the Feeble Mind in Late Victorian and Edwardian England*, Manchester: Manchester University Press, 2000.

17 Jackson, *The Borderland of Imbecility*, pp. 1–20.

18 Thomson, *The Problem of Mental Deficiency*, pp. 10–23.

19 In September 1916 the Devon Mental Deficiency Committee simply received notification of nine ineducable children (minute 75) but discussed WJB who was reported to be a 'deaf mute' and required a place in a state institution following a court appearance (minute 82a). DRO 153/5/1/1, DMDC, 12 September 1916.

20 A list of new admissions, and a brief biography of these patients, was filed with a draft of the RWCI annual report for 1934–35, RWCI archive, box 31. Patients 3094 and 3095 had both been before the courts for theft but were processed under different sections of the MDAs. This reflected their individual circumstances and influenced their future care.

21 In Devon there was particular tension over the future of special education. DRO 153/5/1/2, report of meeting between representatives from DMDC and RWCI, 23 April, 1936, p. 3.

22 See for example RWCI archive, box 36, sub committee to consider final draft of mental deficiency regulations 1935, 9 August 1935, minute 415.

23 This was explicitly communicated to the RWCI at a special meeting with representatives of Devon County Council, 23 April 1936, DRO 153/5/1/2, report of meeting, pp. 1–5.

24 P. Dale, 'Implementing the 1913 Mental Deficiency Act: Competing Priorities and Resource Constraint Evident in the South West of England before 1948', *Social History of Medicine*, 16, 2003, pp. 403–418.

25 When PVA expressed concerns about the farm employment found for Richard C., these centred on the procedures adopted by the town clerk and the undesirable proximity of the farm to Plymouth, and presumably unsuitable friends or family members. RWCI archive, box 29, correspondence from PVA, LJ to Mayer, 17 January 1934.

26 The institution at Starcross changed its name on several occasions as it sought recognition for its changing mission and royal patronage. For the purposes of this chapter it will simply be referred to as the RWCI.

27 Thomson, *The Problem of Mental Deficiency*, pp. 10–16.

28 The transfer of Bertram C. from Stoke Park Colony to the RWCI was encouraged because 'he will be ready for hostel trial fairly soon', but the move was also designed to frustrate his mother's campaign to get him released altogether. RWCI archive, box 29, correspondence from PVA, LJ to Mayer, 21 January 1937, p. 2.

29 The RWCI superintendent outlined the RWCI programme in several speeches to local voluntary organizations. For example, copy of address to Dorset Voluntary Association, 30 March 1936, RWCI archive, box 31.

30 M. Thomson, 'Community Care and the Control of Mental Defectives in Inter-war Britain', in P. Horden and R. Smith (eds), *The Locus of Care: Families, Communities, Institutions and the Provision of Welfare since Antiquity*, London: Routledge, 1998, pp. 198–216.

31 J. Walmsley, D. Atkinson and S. Rolph, 'Community Care and Mental Deficiency 1913 to 1945', in P. Bartlett and D. Wright (eds), *Outside the Walls of the Asylum: The History of Care in the Community 1750–2000*, London: Athlone Press, 1999, pp. 181–203.

32 Thomson, 'Community Care and the Control of Mental Defectives in Inter-war Britain', p. 200. Local services are detailed in DRO, 153/5/1/1, Devon Voluntary Association Ninth Annual Report, 1925–26.

33 This led to an increasing number of applications for re-admission to the RWCI.

34 The early history of the RWCI was frequently recounted in the minutes of the management committee. See also D. Gladstone, 'The Changing Dynamic of Institutional Care: The Western Counties Idiot Asylum, 1864–1914', in D. Wright and A. Digby (eds), *From Idiocy to Mental Deficiency: Historical Perspectives on People with Learning Disabilities*, London: Routledge, 1996, pp. 134–160; and J. P. Radford and A. Tipper, *Starcross: Out of the Mainstream*, Toronto: The G. Allan Roeher Institute, 1988.

35 Gladstone, 'The Changing Dynamic of Institutional Care', p. 149.

36 RWCI archive, box 36, folder marked company members 1915–43. There were seventeen names recorded in 1915, with five additions before the end of 1921. A further fifteen names are recorded for the period 1934 to 1943 although here there is some overlap with committee members.

37 1937 marked the switch to an enlarged joint committee structure. The precise role of the superintendent, the deputy superintendent and the new resident medical officer were subject to heated discussion at a special meeting of the Joint Committee, 18 January 1938, minute 26. RWCI archive, box 36.

38 RWCI archive, box 36, first meeting of the Joint Committee, 30 November 1937. Devon County Council sent five representatives, while Somerset and Dorset County Councils each had one, as did the City of Exeter. Cornwall's single representative sent her apologies and three of the four Plymouth representatives were present. Eleven RWCI members of the former managing committee joined the joint committee. In attendance were the RWCI Superintendent and Secretary as well as the Devon County Medical Officer of Health.

39 Wright, *Mental Disability in Victorian England*, fig. 5.2, p. 87.

40 The position of the RWCI in 1914 is described by Gladstone, 'The Changing Dynamic of Institutional Care', p. 157.

41 In September 1914 the statutory committee heard that a property suitable for a county asylum had already been identified and inspected but the war then prevented its acquisition. DRO 153/5/1/1, DMDC, 1914, minutes 3, 7, 11 and 15. The indefinite postponement of the scheme is outlined in a separate document filed with minute 38, 1915.

42 In May 1919 the Devon Mental Deficiency Committee (DRO 153/5/1/1, 20 May 1919, minute 170) resolved that the Chairman and Clerk should interview the

Board of Control on the matter of accommodation. Significantly plans to take over the RWCI (rejected in April 1919) were successfully amended to a partnership agreement at the next meeting (DRO 153/5/1/1, DMDC, 1 September 1919, minute 182b). The detail of this agreement (DRO 153/5/1/1, DMDC, 11 May 1920, minute 215) notes that the Board of Control had been closely involved.

43 The nomination of Devon County Council representatives to the RWCI managing committee did much to facilitate this. DRO 153/5/1/1, DMDC, 17 February 1920, minute 202, outlined these arrangements and the managing committee minutes (RWCI archive, box 36) show long-serving Devon representatives playing a key role in its deliberations after this date.

44 Devon County Council eventually made the admission of 100 trainable cases to the new Langdon Colony dependent on the RWCI creating 100 additional beds for 'helpless' cases and a further fifty for 'low-grade' cases. RWCI archive, box 25, Devon County Council colony file, Miller to Mayer, 18 June 1936.

45 Dale, 'Implementing the 1913 Mental Deficiency Act' pp. 412–413.

46 This policy was discussed at a fairly acrimonious meeting between the RWCI and representatives of Devon County Council, 10 June 1937. RWCI archive, box 31, draft notes from special meeting.

47 In the report of the superintendent for the year ending 31 March 1931 the disappointing test results for recent admissions were noted alongside a strategy for making the most productive use of all patient labour. RWCI archive, box 31, Annual Report 1931, p. 9 and p. 17.

48 The RWCI Annual Report for the year ending 31 March 1931 drew together ideas about the ability, potential for training and possible discharge of patients. RWCI archive, box 31, Annual Report 1931, pp. 1–25.

49 Dale, 'Implementing the 1913 Mental Deficiency Act', p. 410.

50 P. Dale, 'Training for Work: Domestic Service as a Route out of Long-stay Institutions before 1959', *Women's History Review*, 13, 2004, pp. 387–405.

51 Mathew Thomson attributes these remarks to F. D. Turner, Medical Superintendent of the RECI, but Mayer adopted them as his own and used the theme in many of his speeches and reports.

52 A good example of this approach is Mayer's address to the Dorset Voluntary Association AGM, 30 March 1936. RWCI archive, box 31.

53 Plymouth Voluntary Association used the occasion of a visit to Plymouth Mental Hospital to discuss the future of a former RWCI patient being treated there. The RWCI superintendent ruled out any possibility of her return because of a history of troublesome behaviour and self-harming incidents. RWCI archive, box 29, correspondence from PVA, LJ to Mayer, 8 March 1934; and reply, 24 March 1934.

54 DRO 153/5/1/1, DMDC, special sub committee appointed to make any necessary arrangements in connection with the first meeting of the voluntary association, 23 February 1917.

55 DRO 153/5/1/1, figures included in the minutes for the DMDC meeting 1 June 1915, showed there had been no expenditure on 'guardianship'.

56 A significant resource was the unpaid labour of lady visitors but financial contributions from organizations like the RWCI also helped.

57 The brother of LF was described by PVA as 'a thoroughly good hardworking young man' but his ability to care was compromised by reports that both parents were dead and a sister was suspected of being feeble-minded and having an illegitimate child. LF was admitted in 1934 and was still at the institution in 1958. RWCI archive, box 29, correspondence from PVA, LJ to Mayer, 21 March 1934. In a similar way licence for female patient 2933 was opposed because PVA staff thought 'the home is one of the worst in Plymouth' and her

mother 'alcoholic, addicted to fighting, and I believe immoral'. RWCI archive, box 29, correspondence from PVA, LJ to Mayer, 21 July 1934.

58 The superintendent stressed the benefits of early institutional training and the dangers of leaving people at home until they proved uncontrollable. RWCI archive, box 31, Annual Report 1931, p. 2.

59 The letter accompanying the application for Henry H. mentioned that PVA had been trying to help his mother by providing advice on her housing situation as well as caring for her disabled son and new baby. A type of respite care had been tried but since the mother was a 'complete nervous wreck' a more permanent solution was being sought. RWCI archive, box 29, correspondence from PVA, Lee to Mayer, 24 August 1937.

60 The application for Michael's admission to the RWCI was made 'on behalf of the mother' who was in constant pain and struggling to do the necessary lifting. RWCI archive, box 29, correspondence from PVA, LJ to Mayer, 22 June 1937.

61 Dale, 'Implementing the 1913 Mental Deficiency Act', pp. 409–410.

62 The PVA was instrumental in finding a 'very suitable situation' for Mary (RWCI patient 2839), and promised to report on her progress. RWCI archive, box 29, correspondence from PVA, LJ to Mayer, 4 May 1934.

63 The RWCI hoped to use holidays and other incentives for patients to bolster its own training programmes but needed the DVA and PVA to approve and organize these. Thus Mayer stressed he wanted 'Margaret' to have a holiday because she was 'so well behaved' and it 'would encourage her'. RWCI archive, box 29, correspondence from PVA, Mayer to LJ, 31 May 1934.

64 Dale, 'Implementing the 1913 Mental Deficiency Act', p. 412.

65 A change in format makes it difficult to compare statistics but it appears from the minutes of the statutory committee that Devon County Council had 111 defectives under order in January 1921 and 777 in January 1937. DRO 153/5/1/1 and DRO 153/5/1/2, DMDC.

66 Report of the Interdepartmental Committee on Mental Deficiency, 1925–29 (Wood Report), London, HMSO, 1929.

67 The current location and preferred destination of these patients was discussed at a series of meetings between various statutory and voluntary organizations. The main conclusions were summarized by the chairman in a 1935 report. DRO 153/5/1/2, Devon County Council Joint Sub Committee 13 September 1935, points 4, 5 and 10; and DRO 153/5/1/2, DMDC, 18 November 1935.

68 Reference has already been made to a fairly acrimonious meeting between the RWCI and representatives of Devon County Council, 10 June 1937. It is notice-able that the MOH and his assistant were very vocal on this occasion. RWCI archive, box 31, draft notes from special meeting.

69 DRO 153/5/1/1, DMDC, 7 September 1915. Outlined role of different doctors in document detailing plans for mental deficiency work for year ending 31 March 1916. Appointment of specialist discussed DRO 153/5/1/1, DMDC, 1 September 1919, minute 179.

70 An early example of this was discussion about accommodation for three 'crimi-nal defectives' and a 'morally defective' female identified by the Board of Control. DRO 153/5/1/1, DMDC, 26 May 1914, minute 8.

71 New responsibilities in relation to court work and guardianship are outlined in DRO 153/5/1/2, DMDC, 7 February 1935, minutes 55 and 58. Investigations into chronic cases resident at Devon Mental Hospital and additional cases housed in workhouses discussed at Devon County Council Joint Sub Commit-tee, 13 September 1935, minutes filed with DRO 153/5/1/2, DMDC, 1935.

72 When the Clerk reported that Mrs H. decided not to take up a place for her son at the RWCI in 1914, the statutory committee simply resolved to request

repayment of expenses incurred in connection with the case. DRO 153/5/1/1, DMDC, 16 November 1915, minute 45b.

73 The RD and E had taken more Starcross patients 1938–40, but as soon as the hospital was busy with 'convoy and civilian casualties', the RWCI was instructed not to send any more cases. RWCI archive, box 36, Joint Committee 25 June 1940, minute 237.

74 RWCI archive, box 36, Joint Committee 29 June 1943, minute 652.

75 RWCI archive, box 29, Schneider to Mayer, 27 November 1935, noted a visiting nurse had been very impressed by the school.

76 The likely number of special school pupils moving into long-term care was discussed at a meeting between the RWCI and representatives of Devon County Council, 10 June 1937. RWCI archive, box 31, draft notes from special meeting.

77 RWCI archive, box 25, Davies to Mayer, 10 October 1938, discussed admission of a severely disabled child currently 'attending school in a wheeled chair'.

78 The fact that WHB's headmaster was 'furious' about his incarceration was noted by the PVA but apparently had no influence over his admission to Starcross. RWCI archive, box 29, correspondence from PVA, LJ to Mayer, 12 September 1934.

79 See case of John J., RWCI archive, box 25, correspondence with Devon County Council Medical Department, Dr L. M. Davies to Mayer, 11 November 1938.

80 P. Cox, 'Girls, Deficiency and Delinquency', in Wright and Digby (eds), *From Idiocy to Mental Deficiency*, pp. 184–206.

81 RWCI archive, box 25, Withycombe to Mayer, 25 October 1935.

82 Two important examples of this occurred in 1934. RWCI archive, box 29, correspondence from PVA, LJ to Mayer, 11 September 1934; and LJ to Mayer, 23 November 1934.

83 Charges of arson against Albert H. were withdrawn when Devon County Council agreed to pursue an order under the MDAs, presumably with the consent of relatives. RWCI archive, box 25, Miller to Mayer, 17 June 1933.

84 RWCI archive, box 25, Miller to Mayer, 1 June 1933. When the mother of 'Leslie' repudiated consent for institutional care the statutory committee instructed the clerk to suggest the police charge him with theft.

85 RWCI admission and discharge data suggests that approximately 80 per cent of male criminal cases were discharged to the care of their relatives or employers while only 53 per cent of all 'feeble-minded' male patients left in this way.

86 This policy was explicitly outlined in the RWCI managing committee minutes, 25 February 1933, minute 112. RWCI archive, box 36.

87 Senior staff at the original five voluntary idiot asylums offered mutual support through a regular conference and warm correspondence. RWCI archive, box 29.

88 Mayer was encouraged to take early retirement after a Board of Control investigation revealed unproven allegations of staff brutality and excessive sedation in the care of a group of women patients exhibiting symptoms of mental disturbance.

89 Thomson, *The Problem of Mental Deficiency*; J. Welshman, 'The Social History of Social Work: The Issue of the "Problem Family", 1940–1970', *British Journal of Social Work*, 29, 1999, pp. 457–476.

9 'A satisfactory job is the best psychotherapist'

Employment and mental health, 1939–60

Vicky Long

Introduction

Reflecting in 1956 on the limitations of psychiatric services for people with chronic mental health problems, community care worker Michael Power explained:

> Often there *is* nothing to be done. The person with chronic schizo-phrenia or a psychopathic state whose symptoms frustrate generations of social workers is a constant problem ... it is a bone of contention that hospitals all too easily label a patient as chronic, and then pass the responsibility back to the social agencies serving the area to deal with as best they can. We frequently meet resentment amongst relatives and social workers because the hospital has failed to cure the patient. It is difficult for them to understand intellectually and accept emotion-ally the limitations of psychiatry, because of a natural tendency to regard specialists and hospitals as omnipotent and refuse to accept knowledge as limited and incomplete.

Nevertheless, after painting this bleak picture of provision for such chronic patients, Power continued, 'often there is a great deal to be done, but socially rather than medically'.[1]

This chapter will explore how efforts were made by one group of mental health workers in the growing field of community care to assist the social recovery of such chronic patients by helping them to gain employment. These projects were underpinned by the belief that employment formed a key aspect of an individual's identity. The chapter will also examine the interrelationship between work and health, situating these schemes within the broader context of economic conditions and the inter-est in work and the workplace as a site for the production of health. Employment was often perceived as a major rehabilitative agent, and thus unemployment, which threatened to undermine people's sense of identity, was believed to have a negative impact upon mental health. However, while the beneficial effects of employment upon people's health were often lauded, concern was expressed about the detrimental effects of repetitive work. These anxieties will be explored through projects to help the long-term unemployed gain employment by meeting their emotional needs.

Michael Power was a psychiatric social worker (hereafter PSW), part of a professional group whose roots could be found in the activities of earlier charitable organizations such as the Mental After-Care Association (hereafter the MACA) that worked with the mentally disordered and their families within community settings, often seeking to remedy people's difficulties by providing solutions to their economic problems.[2] One factor which contributed to the emergence of psychiatric social work was the growing acceptance of psychological explanations for people's behaviour and problems, and the emergence of the mental hygiene movement, which sought to prevent mental illness from occurring by tackling the underlying causes.[3] Another factor that influenced the development of psychiatric social work was the growing interest in the 'problem' child, which paved the way for the development of child guidance clinics. PSWs became part of the team in these newly established clinics which aimed to prevent juvenile delinquency.

Professional training for social workers in psychiatric fields was first developed in America in 1914 at the Boston Psychopathic Hospital.[4] When the American Commonwealth Fund agreed to finance the establishment of child guidance in Britain, they stressed the need to train social workers in a university setting.[5] In 1929, the London School of Economics established the Mental Health Course to train social science graduates with some experience in social work in psychiatric social work. The Association of Psychiatric Social Workers (APSW) was also formed in 1929 with seventeen members. By 1944, only 257 people had qualified as PSWs. Approved courses then started in Edinburgh (1945), Manchester (1947) and Liverpool (1954). From 1958, students who had qualified through generic courses were accepted as members of the APSW, provided they undertook an additional psychiatric placement. The profession established its own periodical, the *British Journal of Psychiatric Social Work*, in 1947. In 1970, the Association and its 1,550 members were absorbed into the British Association of Social Work. Initially, more PSWs were employed in the field of mental hospital work than in child guidance, although the disparity became less marked as the child guidance service developed. The field of community care was slow to develop, only really equalling the other two fields by 1969.[6] In 1962, the number of trained PSWs had reached 1,202, of which 136 were men.

The newly emerging profession of psychiatric social work arguably played a pivotal and pioneering role in the development of services for patients outside of hospital, operating in the space between medical establishments and the community and liaising between different organizations, families and communities as they sought to assist people with mental health problems to live and work within the community. The primary aim of these interventions was not so much to cure the medical symptoms of their patients but to assist their social adjustment. The methods and approach adopted by PSWs to their work can be understood in the context of their specialized training, which drew on the methodologies of both psychiatry and social work, orientating the outlook of PSWs towards patients' families and their lives within the community.

This chapter will focus on the initiatives of three PSWs who, working in different settings and in collaboration with different organizations, sought to help the mentally disordered into work in the community. M. L. Ferard, a PSW attached to a mental hospital in the 1940s, attempted to help maintain chronic schizophrenics in the community; she argued that employment was an essential cornerstone in their social readjustment. Her work illustrates how even PSWs nominally based within institutions sought to assist patients to live outside the hospital. Kathleen Laurie was also a qualified PSW who worked as the employment officer of the MACA, a charity established in 1879 to rehabilitate discharged asylum patients.[7] The charity had a long history of helping its cases into work, seeing this as one of the primary factors to measure the successful rehabilitation of former patients and thus the secretary of the charity claimed 'it is so important to enable these saddest of sad cases to once more take their place among the workers of the world'.[8] However, Laurie used her appointment to develop a theory of the psychological significance of work, suggesting that it might both precipitate illness and promote recovery. Finally, the chapter will discuss PSW Eugene Heimler's collaborative project with the National Assistance Board (hereafter the NAB) to help the long-term unemployed into work. Heimler was one of the first PSWs to work in local authority community services. He developed Kathleen Laurie's theories on the psychological significance of work, believing that meaningful employment might alleviate past frustrations.

Nineteenth and early twentieth-century initiatives

The roots of these initiatives to help the mentally disordered into employment stretch back into the nineteenth century. The asylum solution to mental disturbance was based upon a medical ideology which stressed the beneficial effects of occupation as part of a regime of moral therapy.[9] Asylum medical superintendents attacked the idea that pauper lunatics could be treated outside of the asylum, suggesting that the asylum system made the idle mentally disordered economically productive. In an article in the *Journal of Mental Science*, T. L. Rogers refuted claims that the asylum routine could make lunatics of men, citing this case:

> Here is a man who, whilst under the restraint of an asylum, behaves in an entirely rational manner, and, doing a good day's work, may be

regarded as a producer instead of a consumer. The stability of his condition is tested by a month's liberty, which allows for a debauch, the
consequences of which are that all the benefits of seven month's treatment are dissipated, and, for the next two years or more, he becomes a
consumer and destroyer instead of a producer.[10]

This excerpt emphasizes how the medical function of the nineteenth-
century asylum and moral therapy was inexorably linked with its social
disciplinary role. Thus while employment was believed to alleviate the
symptoms of mental illness by distracting the patient from his or her trou-
bles, it was also seen as a way to inculcate responsibility within the patient.
These aspects of the asylum system have been noted by historians and
sociologists such as Andrew Scull, who viewed the nineteenth-century
process of incarceration as an attempt by the ruling classes to instil the
values of labour discipline and bourgeois rationality into unproductive and
inconvenient people in an attempt to restore them to the productive work-
force.[11] Laurence Ray, meanwhile, has argued that asylum authorities constructed the asylum population as impaired, rather than sick, and thus not
justifiably allowed to withdraw from social responsibilities. Whether the
disorder of the patient was ascribed to environmental stresses such as
debt, alcoholism and family disagreements or the patient was viewed as
physically impaired, case notes dwelled favourably upon inmates who
worked within the asylum and after an assessment of the degree of dangerousness posed by a patient, the medical superintendent considering a discharge would ask 'whether the inmate was likely to be a further charge on
the poor rate. Would the discharged patient be able to support him/her
self outside the asylum? Other aspects of recovery were secondary.'[12]
Peter Bartlett has suggested that a 'productive alliance' existed between
the asylum and the Poor Law.[13] He argues that the asylum was viewed primarily as a Poor Law institution, containing members of a social residuum
whose insanity was frequently viewed as instigated by alcoholism or
immorality. The role of the asylum was to fit these people back into their
place in society by making them productive. Similar concerns appear to
have pervaded and shaped the development of such mental deficiency services as working colonies in the early decades of the twentieth century, in
which therapeutic ideals sat uneasily next to the morally reformative
nature of productive work and a desire to reduce expenditure.[14]

Just how much attitudes towards mental illness and productivity had
changed by the first few decades of the twentieth century is questionable.
Caseworkers for the MACA who sought to help the mentally ill gain
employment in the late nineteenth and early twentieth centuries viewed
mental disorder as socially rather than biologically determined. They trod
a line between depicting their clients as respectable victims of a social situation in need of help to re-establish their position and suggesting that deficiencies in character were the precipitating cause of breakdown. The

annual report of the MACA for 1887–88 for example described a 'respectable' case where mental breakdown was ascribed to a social, not hereditary, cause and the girl was placed in a suitable occupation: 'A most respectable girl. Became ill through worry and deprivation in helping her father – a small tradesman who lost his capital. Is now in service in a house of a member of the committee.'[15] However, cases like this appeared alongside others such as this case from 1917, which related 'another striking example of personal influence', describing a young woman who:

> Before she went to the asylum, had been four times in prison with a very bad record. This girl, after weeks of patient endeavour, responded to the better influence brought to bear ... she has voluntarily undertaken the support of her child ... her situation is down in the south, away from her unsuitable friends.[16]

In this instance the caseworker's role was to use their personal influence to help restructure the character of their client and enable them to support themselves through work. It is clear however that this approach was not universal amongst voluntary social workers: indeed, Pamela Dale's chapter (Chapter 8) demonstrates that voluntary social workers in Devon began to medicalize their delivery of mental deficiency services in the same era as a means to enhance their professional status with respect to other lay professionals.

A case study prepared by the APSW for discussion at a conference in 1932 considered the case of R. D., a married man with children who had lost his job after displaying nervous symptoms. The APSW writer considered that by resolving R. D.'s personal difficulties, 'apart from the hope of relieving a distressing personal situation, R. D. seems capable of contributing, as an intelligent and responsible citizen, to the community on which he has so long parasitically depended'.[17] Fifteen years later in the *British Journal of Psychiatric Social Work*, similar ideas were cited: 'We have to help the patient to assume social responsibilities for himself, his family and the community, to bear strains and pressures.'[18]

Following the economic downturn of 1929–32, efforts to help people with mental disorders gain employment were no longer simply focused on a desire to make such people productive. The psychological effects of unemployment upon people's mental health and their families had become a major area of interest and research.[19] Now it appeared that employment was a requirement in order to remain healthy. Studies such as that undertaken by Paul Lazarsfeld, Marie Lazarsfeld-Jahoda and Hans Zeisel in the 1930s suggested that the effects of unemployment on even healthy, mentally sound people led stage by stage to a psychological demoralization or deterioration of the unemployed individual who became incapacitated to seek work effectively.[20] Similarly, *The Memoirs of the Unemployed*, published in 1934, sought to elucidate the psychological trauma and resultant physical and mental illness experienced by the unemployed.[21]

Conversely, other developments began to suggest that work might not only be detrimental to physical health but mental health as well. Beliefs began to be expressed by a range of organizations that the deskilling of labour entailed by new production methods and mechanization led employees to view employment as simply a necessary means to obtain money for satisfactions outside of work. The 1931 Factory Inspectorate, for example, claimed that mechanization had led to an increase in nervous disabilities and mental weariness.[22] Established in 1918 and emerging from war-time concerns to maximize worker productivity, the Industrial Fatigue Research Board and its successor organization, the Industrial Health Research Board, explored the impact that fatigue and environmental conditions within the workplace could have upon workers' health and productivity.[23] The Trades Union Congress, which had traditionally been concerned to secure compensation for workers who had experienced physical injuries or illnesses as a result of their occupation, also began to explore the impact that work could have on mental health and corresponded about the possibility of establishing mental hygiene clinics for workers who had experienced emotional trauma as a result of their work.[24]

Employment as a form of psychiatric social treatment in the 1940s

Drawing on ideas which had emerged in the 1930s, but mostly working in a time when there was a significant demand for labour, a new approach to the employment of the mentally disordered was formulated by PSWs handling cases affected by long-term or recurring forms of mental disorder for which there was no definable mental breakdown and no clear recovery. It was in this climate that PSW M. L. Ferard described her experience of working with four paranoid schizophrenics outside of the hospital in the 1940s.[25] Ferard recognized that her cases all still exhibited the symptoms of their disorder, but instead chose to focus on trying to

> help the patients to the best social adjustment which their symptoms permit. Psychiatric social treatment interpreted in this way is not concerned with 'curing' mental illness, nor even necessarily with trying to reduce symptoms, it is less ambitious, frankly palliative, and more directed to assessing a degree of health rather than a degree of ill health.[26]

One of Ferard's cases was C. D., a single woman aged forty-nine who had been in hospital for twelve years. C. D. managed to retain two long-term jobs, as a canteen assistant and then as a waitress, despite 'the "voices" all telling her to do different things at the same time and threatening her with her "notice".' Ferard's role was to discuss the hostile voices that C. D. still heard and persuade her to disregard them. C. D. was not officially discharged from certificate, but perhaps the main criterion Ferard used to assess whether she should remain living out of the hospital was her capacity to hold down a job, judging that 'the patient's symptoms are probably unabated, but she has learnt to manage them up to a point. She earns her own living and has made a partial social adjustment.'[27] E. F., a single man of forty-two, retained the belief that 'influences' affected his work and caused him to make mistakes. He found work in a bakery and was officially discharged from certificate after six months, although Ferard's assessment again emphasized the importance of successful employment in her decision and the lesser importance of E. F.'s symptoms: 'he has been earning his own living, was less disturbed by his symptoms and assumed a tolerant aloofness towards other people'.[28]

Even individuals who were seen as too disordered to ever support themselves might be assessed according to their capacity to undertake productive tasks. An examination of the MACA permanent care homes for residents believed to be incapable of remunerative employment and self support reveal that from 1948 admission registers for the homes used medical classifications such as schizophrenia and chronic neurosis to describe their cases. However, reports of the caseworker on the home and decisions regarding individual cases were based more on the appearance of residents and their willingness to do domestic chores in the household. Considering the future of A. H. after the closure of a MACA home in 1961, the social worker emphasized her social usefulness, describing her as

> clean, tidy, and dresses nicely. Helps a bit in things like wiping the dishes, and also is reliable in taking messages, keeping an eye on a patient in bed or other socially useful things . . . I think she would be a nice person to have about and worth sticking a point for as she is one of our successes.[29]

Patients in twentieth-century mental hospitals were also encouraged to occupy themselves with work. Diane Gittins, in her study of Severalls Hospital, noted that virtually all patients were persuaded to work, but that the occupations assigned to them remained rigidly divided by gender. Women were trained in housewifery in the Department of Household Management that was established in 1960, or were given small jobs such as sewing bows on Marks and Spencer's lingerie. Men were assigned to carpentry and made doll's houses. By the 1930s, Colney Hatch had also started to substitute employment with occupational therapy. This move was championed by the Board of Control who attacked the assumption 'that unless a patient can be employed in some immediately useful or remunerative way, it is a matter of indifference whether he does anything or nothing'.[30] There does appear to have been a shift in emphasis from late nineteenth-century ideas and practices. In Severalls and Colney Hatch, patients were still believed to benefit from a course of work, which could restore their 'independence and self-respect in an active rehabilitation programme'.[31] However, the results of the patients' economic productivity no longer went to financially support the institution and were given back to them as wages. The activity may have been seen as more useful in giving institutionalized patients an idea of work outside of the hospital rather than a method of measuring which patients were sufficiently recovered to be discharged.[32]

Working for the MACA from 1939–40, another PSW was developing similar ideas to those of M. L. Ferard in her attempts to get the mentally disordered successfully employed during the period of high unemployment in the inter war years. Kathleen Laurie published a report of her work as the employment officer of a department placing recovered mental and nervous breakdown cases and what she termed 'occupational misfits'. Laurie felt she might be dealing in a new way with 'the hard core of unemployment'.[33] Laurie suggested both that her work had other potential applications than the employment problems of the mentally disordered, and that the problem of the 'hard core unemployed' could be explained by more widespread psychological disturbance than hitherto thought. Like her MACA predecessors, Laurie also justified her work on the basis of potential monetary savings for the community: it would 'show a saving of Government money. Its results would be still more important in re-establishing people in normal life.'[34]

Laurie believed that being placed in the wrong job led to dissatisfaction and frustration. Unskilled workers might be wrongly placed into positions that were beyond their capacity while skilled workers placed in a position not demanding enough might lose interest. Either scenario, Laurie argued, could lead to a loss of confidence, emotional or intellectual dissatisfaction and finally maladjustment. In this situation, unsuitable work could precipitate mental disorder. In order to counter the possible harmful effects of unsuitable work, Laurie argued that an 'employment history' of the case should be taken. This should uncover where difficulties in employment arose in the past and whether the patient's home environment was harming their health, and establish the nature of the illness or the 'psychological motive' behind a breakdown. The caseworker also needed to assess any continuing impairment of the personality that had to be allowed for, although like Ferard, Laurie did not believe that continuing symptoms of disorder necessarily debarred an individual from successfully undertaking work in the right environment. Laurie argued that '*recovery and yet a certain impairment are not incompatible*', claiming that a person could be taught to deal with their delusions, thus a case might

> have quite a dangerous or stupid attitude to one person (possibly his wife) and towards no one else. One such man is a good works foreman and is a reliable worker, but at all costs he must be kept away from his

wife. His judgment on everything else in life is utterly sane and sound. To his wife he is still really dangerous.[35]

Having taken an employment diagnosis, Laurie's next stage was to create a social treatment plan. This needed to take account of any remaining symptoms and remove any possible conditions that might cause them, for example by placing people whose home environments were hostile into residential posts. Laurie also stressed the importance of a tolerant and understanding employer and the need to provide after-care for some cases still affected by emotional or personality problems. One of the case studies cited demonstrates Laurie's approach:

> (4) A man once in specialised government work, always on night duty, is now a porter in a hospital, taking his turn as a roof spotter. His illness seemed to be the rebellion of a conscientious person's body and mind against the abnormality of his life conditions. These allowed no social amenities and very few human contacts even with his family ... his new employment had to remove these wrong conditions and provide company for him so that he could strike roots. He had an excellent character, both generally and in the army, and we used this to get him a well-paid job, allowing of contacts.[36]

In this narrative, the illness was ascribed to a social cause, the man's previous employment, and was remedied by a more suitable position.

Laurie's work was interrupted by the war, but a glance at the kind of positions that her clients were placed in is informative. Of the 285 women, 220 were placed in domestic work, most of these positions being residential. Although this might be partly explained by Laurie's desire to place her clients in residential positions away from unsuitable home environments, this trend reflected a more general move of women into domestic service in the 1930s as other fields of work for women were hit by the depression. In 1931, 1,142,655 women were working in private service. However, service remained an unpopular and low-status occupation among female workers and by 1951 only 350,000 women were employed in domestic service.[37] Laurie's reliance upon a disappearing sphere of work for the accomplishment of her project ties its success specifically to the economic conditions of the 1930s. Laurie perhaps failed to address the lack of training and experience required for industrial work that handicapped many former asylum residents and may have encountered further difficulties with her project had she undertaken it in 1960, not 1940.

Work, satisfaction and functioning in the 1950s

While Laurie developed her plans to assist people with mental health problems gain employment, future PSW Eugene Heimler observed at first hand the impact that enforced unemployment and purposeless activity could have on people. Writing over forty years later, Heimler described how his father had been forced out of practising law, commenting 'my concern in unemployment started when I impotently had to witness my father's totally useless existence which had been imposed on him by the National Socialists'.[38] In 1944 Heimler was forced to take part in an experiment in the Concentration Camp at Troglitz. He was among a group of prisoners assigned to move sand from one end of a factory to the other, and then back again, week after week, as an 'experiment in mental health'. Those forced to participate in the experiment experienced a substantial increase in mental disturbance, and the growth in suicide rates amongst the group of prisoners led the camp commandant to joke ' "now there is no more need to use the crematoria". 'It was clear,' wrote Heimler, 'that meaningless tasks and pointless work destroyed people'.[39] The corollary, Heimler deduced, could be that being given some purpose in life might help the mentally ill and they might be 'encouraged to find some new satisfaction in a meaningful task'. This view was based on the belief that man was a product of both the past and the present.

> The PSW tries to enable his patient to function better in his present life and uses the present as a therapeutic tool. If the patient can be induced to adopt a new pattern of functioning, this assists him to *feel* different about his past ... Frustration reinforces past patterns of frustration. Satisfaction can alleviate past frustrations.[40]

To this end, Heimler argued, 'a satisfactory job is the best psychotherapist'.[41]

In 1954, Eugene Heimler led a project in Hendon, Middlesex, to tackle the employment problems of unemployed people exhibiting emotional difficulties. The Hendon NAB referred forty-one people who had been unemployed for a long period to Heimler, all of whom exhibited serious emotional problems. Heimler divided the difficulties of his cases into four groups. First, those whose deep-rooted emotional problems blocked their ability to work; second, people employed in unsuitable work which failed to satisfy them, leading to frequent job changes and spells of unemployment, often causing family relationship difficulties; third, people unable to get work due to the modernization of industries and automation: this situation could aggravate anxiety and lead to emotional problems within the family. Heimler's recognition of the changing employment market and the difficulties this might pose to the mentally disordered marked a break from Kathleen Laurie's approach. Finally, Heimler isolated a group he defined as 'work shy' in the traditional sense – having no desire to work and being more satisfied when not employed. Within six months, twenty of the forty-one cases – Heimler referred to them as 'patients' – had returned to work, and were still employed by 1961. The work expanded so that by the end of 1956, 301 people had been referred. Another initiative of the Hendon project was the establishment in 1958 of a Human Relations Course for NAB officers. This course aimed to make officers aware of their applicants' emotional needs and to help them recognize applicants with mental or emotional problems who might require specialized services.

Heimler developed his observations on the emotional significance of work by creating a Social Function Scale. This test measured the client's levels of satisfaction in the areas of financial security, sexual satisfaction, satisfaction through family relationship, satisfaction through friendship, satisfaction through work and through hobbies. Heimler's approach embraced the ability of the present to change the way a person may feel about negative events in the past. 'Satisfactions, properly used and expressed, are "sending back messages" to a somewhat frustrated childhood', Heimler argued. 'The damage is in fact being "repaired".'[42] For Heimler, a certain level of frustration in people's lives was helpful, acting as a spur to achieve more satisfaction. The Social Function Scale could be used to facilitate communication, enabling the client to think about his problems and formulate a plan of action, and thus it was not simply a diagnostic tool. Created initially to measure the levels of frustration and satisfaction amongst the long-term unemployed referred to him by the NAB, Heimler subsequently enhanced the sophistication of the scale by testing it on different groups such as people who had experienced mental or emotional illness, churchgoers, people who had spent their childhood in Barnardo's homes, students and attendees at jazz clubs.[43] Scored out of 100, Heimler concluded that scores below sixty on the scale indicated significant frustration which might inhibit a person's ability to experience satisfaction and function in the community without assistance. Crucially, Heimler's work severed the link between mental illness and the ability of an individual to function adequately in society, by distinguishing between the clinical illness and social illness. As Heimler explained to journalist Christopher Driver, 'people who were revealed to be hopelessly neurotic when scored by Doctor Eysenck's Maudsley personality inventory could score correspondingly high on "social functioning". Their satisfactions, it seemed, could counterbalance their sickness.'[44] Heimler argued that given the appropriate environmental conditions even people diagnosed with paranoid schizophrenia could successfully hold down work: 'Given the conditions which suit them, people with apparently crippling delusions can live normal lives. For instance, a man may have a fixed idea, immune to psychotherapy, that he is being persecuted by the police. An employer who has himself been a refugee, with experience of persecution, may be able to accept him.'[45]

The motivations underlying the project were by no means clear-cut. Heimler often portrayed the primary aim of the NAB project as an attempt to reduce emotional distress and to assist people to find meaningful work that would satisfy them. 'Money is an inadequate way of expressing human happiness or unhappiness', Heimler argued in 1961, and by 1980 he was expressing similar qualms: 'we have agencies like Job Centres but they lack the human element of saying to people "who are you, what do you want in life?"'[46] However, at other times the financial benefits of the project were accentuated: 'in this experiment £1,600 was saved, and had it been carried out on a national scale ... the total saving would have been £600,000 per annum.'[47] Studying the actual clientele addressed by Heimler's project raises another interesting issue. Of the 301 cases dealt with by the project, eighty-two were referred by the NAB, ninety-four by general practitioners and medical specialists, and the rest from sources such as mental hospitals, out-patient clinics, voluntary agencies or self-referred. Around half of the cases had never seen a psychiatrist or received treatment in a mental hospital. Indeed, it is questionable whether Heimler's primary aim was to develop a psychological approach to the emotional problems of the unemployed or to tackle the employment problems of the mentally disordered. Yet again, tension arose between the objective of helping people to find meaningful work which would resolve their emotional problems and the objective to get people off benefits. Under Section 51 of the 1948 National Assistance Act the NAB could prosecute people they felt had failed to try and get work yet still claimed benefits, a measure derived from concerns to save public money rather than to assist people to find satisfying work. Moreover, it is difficult to assess whether Heimler did indeed assist people to find work that gave meaning to their lives, as his analysis of the cases detailed only the length of time that each case had been out of work, their cost to the NAB in benefits, whether they had successfully found long-term employment and the savings thus achieved to date. Indeed, Heimler's summary of the aims of the project for an article in 1955 hinted that his own aims diverged from those of the NAB: 'the aim of psychiatric social work in relation to the NAB was to adjust the patient to work, which meant the easing of some emotional difficulty in the patient.'[48]

To properly evaluate the Hendon project it needs to be contextualized within the economic climate of the early 1950s, mostly a time of full employment when there was a significant demand for labour. According to Richard Warner's research on the relationship between schizophrenia and the economy, efforts to rehabilitate people with schizophrenia are most extensive during times of a labour shortage when the perceived value of the mentally ill increases. Thus, Warner links the move to deinstitutionalize psychiatric patients in the 1950s and 1960s to the demand for labour.[49] It is however unclear how many of the cases assisted through the Hendon project fell into the category of patients who experienced chronic mental health problems.

Heimler's focus on the emotional satisfaction to be gained from employment was challenged in an APSW conference of 1963, where the real financial problems of the mentally disordered, resulting from unemployment, were addressed:

Social workers are being asked to help people adjust to society in cases where society should be doing a better job for the individual … When the welfare services fail, social workers are expected to make life bearable, but it is housing, National Assistance and other national needs which are unfulfilled … Why should people on national assistance, when they are given less than their previous subsistence-level wage, be adjusted to living within scales that would tax the ingenuity and health of the best managers? It can be said that adjustment is necessary because reality has to be accepted, but the social workers would like to do a little adjustment of reality for a change.[50]

As levels of unemployment began to climb in the 1970s, even Heimler began to reevaluate his approach to unemployment. Concerned at the dramatic shifts in the nature and availability of work, Heimler began to consider the fates of young people who might not be able to find their true vocation and of older workers who found themselves made redundant and unable to compete in the changing workplace. 'The modern crisis of Man is that of an existential vacuum, which needs to be filled if we are to prevent the collapse of our society', Heimler wrote in 1980. 'Modern industrial life with its strains and stresses is creating a similar "mental health experiment" that the Nazis did with us during the summer of 1941.'[51] Heimler proposed that people unable to find meaningful work should be encouraged to undertake 'lifetasks', producing goods and services for people unable to afford those offered through the standard economy.

Discussion

PSWs, like the nineteenth-century MACA workers before them, stressed the importance of getting their cases into employment, often citing the financial savings that could be made to society. Yet it is clear that employment had a far greater significance. Despite the transition of mental health services from under the auspices of the Poor Law to an integral part of the National Health Service, the ability of a mentally disordered individual to hold down full employment has been and possibly remains a key signifier of an individual's recovery and reintegration into society: conversely, unemployment might indicate the continuing disorder – and isolation – of an individual.

The approaches to unemployment examined in this chapter largely relied on a social definition of disorder. Mental illness was viewed in the late nineteenth century as the result of a bad environment or economic pressures. By the 1930s PSWs were depicting mental disorder as the outcome of damaged family relationships and unsuitable work. Those workers engaged with clients affected by long-term disorders started to focus on a social approach to maximize health as opposed to a medical approach focusing on illness. These views were typified by Margaret Eden, a PSW from the 1940s to the 1960s, who wrote: 'treatment needs have increasingly come to be seen in terms of the restoration of the patient's social function and work capacity'.[52] Thus Eugene Heimler differentiated between clinical and social illness, arguing: 'psychiatric community care is less concerned with removing the symptoms of mental illness than with creating conditions, in the family and its wider environment, to enable the patient to live a more or less normal life with or without his symptoms'.[53] Employment was seen as one means to help restore the patient's social balance and facilitate his or her recovery. As the asylum population peaked in the 1950s and government responses to mental illness became more orientated around community-based services and measures, work was again viewed as an active therapeutic agent. Inside psychiatric hospitals, industrial therapy became more widespread, supplementing the existing occupational therapy. Research suggested that paid industrial work was more likely to assist the rehabilitation and resettlement in employment of patients. Day hospitals also focused on restoring patients' work capacity.[54] The Uffculme Day Hospital in Birmingham, which opened in 1957, operated under a criterion of occupational adaptation. Patients were not removed from work to enter the day hospital, while absence from work was viewed as a positive reason for admission. Of thirty patients persistently unemployed before treatment, fifteen were returned to 'gainful employment'. The writers of the paper concluded that 'the change of attitude to employment taking place while day patients seemed of far greater importance for return to work than the degree of psychiatric disability'.[55]

The extent to which these projects sought to alleviate the difficulties experienced by people diagnosed with chronic and severe mental health problems is hard to quantify. Ferard's paper clearly indicated that her work was undertaken amongst patients diagnosed with paranoid schizophrenia and discussed both the limitations of working with such patients and how psychiatric social treatment such as she proposed could potentially assist their social reintegration. As the excerpt from Michael Power's 1956 article at the start of this chapter indicates, such patients often benefited little from the interventions offered by mainstream psychiatric practice in this era and PSWs may have seen work with such patients as a way to make a distinctive contribution in the field of community care and mental health services.[56] Laurie's work however was largely undertaken with cases who had nominally recovered, although many continued to experience personality disorders and difficulties gaining employment unassisted. Although her report did not indicate the diagnostic categories under which her cases fell, she did note that 60 per cent had been referred by hospitals and clinics. Heimler's figures meanwhile indicate that half the cases assisted through the Hendon project had not been in contact with a psychiatrist or the mental health services.

The successes of the projects undertaken by PSWs should be evaluated in relation to the levels of unemployment and the types of work available to the mentally ill. Unemployment rose in the 1930s making the task of finding work for those already stigmatized by mental disorder more difficult. However, research suggesting that unemployment led to mental deterioration was also published in this period. This may have made the employment of individuals already affected by mental disorder seem more crucial if further attacks of illness were to be avoided. Another interesting feature in this period was the temporary resurgence of domestic service amongst women as other positions became more difficult to obtain. The fall in unemployment levels from the 1940s made the task of starting the mentally disordered into employment much easier, while the growth of mechanization in this period may have fuelled concerns that factory work could lead to emotional disorder and stress.

Richard Warner has linked the recovery rates for schizophrenia in industrialized societies to economic cycles and the requirements of the labour market, arguing: 'efforts to rehabilitate and reintegrate the chronically mentally ill will only be seen at times of extreme shortages of labour'. During a period of depression, Warner suggests that the recovery rate for schizophrenia drops as 'the reduced demand for labour results in a deterioration of rehabilitation and reintegration efforts'.[57] Thus, in the 1960s when the economy was still buoyant and unemployment remained below 2.5 per cent of the labour force, state investment in an institutional approach to the care of the mentally ill was displaced by the policy of care in the community. The mentally disordered were to be reintegrated into society as valued members; however, the success of this project has been questioned. In *Closing the Asylum*, Peter Barham noted that the institution of community care policies had failed to properly integrate the mentally disordered into the community:

> The legacy of the Victorian Asylum is, in an important sense, the abolition of the *person* who suffers from mental illness. In place of the person we have been given mental patients, their identities permanently spoiled, exiled in the space of their illness on the margins of society.[58]

Barham's interviewees suggested there remained an expectation amongst mental health professionals and the employment services that people with mental disorders should not work. Simon, a mental health service user, described the attitude of the Job Centre to his predicament:

> (I) went to the job centre and said, 'Look I want a part-time job at the very least, can you help us?' and they said, 'Well, why aren't you signing on?' of course, 'Are you signing on?', and I said not, and they said 'Well, what's the problem?' and I told them and they said, 'Oh, we usually find people from "that place",' as they put it – the hospital – 'can't cope with a job'.

Vaughan related a confrontation with his doctor: 'I said I was going to look for a job and he said, "I wouldn't bother looking for a job, just get an hour or two's rest every day." I said, "That's no good, I want to get out and get a job." He said, "Oh no, I should take it easy." '[59]

The exclusion of an individual from participation in employment does not simply mark their social exclusion. It is important to recognize the financial difficulties caused by low benefit payments that can also act to stigmatize the mentally disordered. Barham, commenting on the failure of psychiatrists to establish a framework whereby the long-term mentally ill can participate in society, refers to 'the belief that individual worth is determined by the market-place and only those who show themselves to be economically capable are to be valued as integral to society', and suggested that for mental health service users in the 1980s and 1990s, 'release from the stigmatizing discourse of psychiatry may not entail much more than the freedom to be picked up in the stigmatizing discourse of poverty'.[60]

Barham's work on the economic and social exclusion of former mental hospital patients was undertaken in another period of depression when the mentally disordered were once more liable to be excluded from the employment market. According to Warner's analysis, efforts to rehabilitate psychiatric patients depend upon three interrelated factors: government mental health policy, the psychiatric paradigm of mental disorder and public opinion towards people who experience mental illness. An economic boom will orientate these factors towards the consensus that mental distress can be alleviated by social integration.[61] Data gathered by MIND on levels of unemployment in 2001 suggested that 'only 13 per cent of people with serious mental health problems are working'.[62] The absence of a social approach in the 1980s and 1990s seems to be illustrated by the people interviewed by Peter Barham. Speculatively, their continuing unemployment and isolation may have rested upon the biological paradigm operating within psychiatric practice. Illnesses such as schizophrenia are now less likely to be seen as the result of social tensions and faulty family relationships. Instead, they are more likely to be viewed as the result of faulty biology or genes, internalizing the disorder within the physiology of the sufferer and making a social diagnosis and cure more difficult.

However, since Barham's research was undertaken, levels of unemployment have fallen. The recent Social Exclusion Unit Report commissioned by the Government, *Mental Health and Social Exclusion*, asserted that difficulties experienced gaining employment was a key factor in the social exclusion of people with mental health problems, devoting two chapters to the role that work played in the lives of mental health service users and ways in which barriers to employment might be overcome.[63] The report identified public prejudice, the low expectations of mental health professionals regarding the capabilities of their clients and a lack of support and services to enable people to work as major factors which reinforce the social exclusion of people with mental health problems. Acknowledging that only 24 per cent of adults with long-term mental health problems were employed, one of the two main questions that the report sought to address was 'what more can be done to enable adults with mental health problems to enter and retain work?'[64] It appears that with the upturn in the labour market, efforts to socially rehabilitate people with mental health problems and assist them to work have yet again become a priority, although it is not certain that these efforts extend to people with severe and chronic mental health problems.

Acknowledgements

The research for this chapter was funded by an Arts and Humanities Research Board Postgraduate Doctoral Award and was undertaken in the Modern Records Centre at Warwick University, the Wellcome Library at London and the archives at the University of Southampton. I wish to thank all the archivists for their kind assistance. I would like to thank my thesis supervisors Hilary Marland and Mathew Thomson for their helpful comments and advice on drafts of this chapter, and the editors of this volume for their thoughtful suggestions. Earlier versions of this chapter were presented at the 'Fresh Perspectives on Inclusion and Exclusion' Conference (Sussex University, 2002) and at the 'Themes in Twentieth-Century Psychiatry' Workshop (Exeter University, 2002): I would like to thank the participants at these events for their helpful comments.

Notes

1 M. Power, 'Community Care: A New Service', *British Journal of Psychiatric Social Work*, 3, 1956, pp. 4–10. Quoted on p. 7. Italics in original text.
2 The MACA deployed lady volunteers to visit its charity cases in their homes or places of work to check on the progress of their recipients and resolve any difficulties with their employers. The primary aim of the charity was for many years to enable its cases to gain employment. See V. Long, 'Chapter Three: Psychiatric Social Workers', in 'Changing Public Representations of Mental Illness in Britain 1870–1970' (unpublished PhD thesis, University of Warwick, 2004), pp. 178–232. The Central Association for Mental Welfare (founded in 1913 as the Central Association for the Care of Mental Deficiency) was also engaged in work with the mentally disordered within the community. Their work is discussed in L. Westwood, 'Avoiding the Asylum: Pioneering Work in Mental Health Care 1890–1939' (unpublished DPhil thesis, Sussex University, 1999).
3 The role of the mental hygiene movement in the emergence of psychiatric work is discussed in K. Woodroofe, *From Charity to Social Work in the United States and England*, London: Routledge & Kegan Paul, 1962, pp. 124–139.
4 For more information on the development of psychiatric social work training in America see E. Lunbeck, *The Psychiatric Persuasion: Knowledge, Gender and Power in Modern America*, Princeton: Princeton University Press, 1994, pp. 35–45.
5 The origins and development of psychiatric social work and child guidance in

Britain, and in particular the role that American influences played, is discussed in J. Stewart, 'US Influences on the Development of Child Guidance and Psychiatric Social Work in Scotland and Great Britain during the Inter-War Period', in A. Andresen, K. Tove Elvbakken and W. E. Hubbard (eds), *Public Health and Preventive Medicine 1800–2000: Knowledge, Co-operation and Conflict*, Bergen: Rokkan Centre, 2004, pp. 85–95. See also D. Thom, 'Wishes, Anxieties, Play and Gestures: Child Guidance in Inter-War England', in R. Cooter (ed.), *In the Name of the Child: Health and Welfare, 1880–1940*, London: Routledge, 1992, pp. 200–219. For a history of psychiatric social work in Britain, see N. Timms, *Psychiatric Social Work in Great Britain, 1939–1962*, London: Routledge & Kegan Paul, 1963. The role that psychiatric social workers played in shaping public ideas about mental illness is considered in Long, 'Chapter Three: Psychiatric Social Workers', in 'Changing Public Representations of Mental Illness', pp. 131–177.

6 A thorough examination of the numbers of PSWs entering different fields of work and their geographical location can be found in Timms, *Psychiatric Social Work in Britain*, pp. 66–89. The chart illustrates only the main trends in the employment of PSWs: not all qualified PSWs went in to these three fields of work and Timms should be consulted for more details of other sectors of employment for PSWs.

7 See Long, 'Chapter Four: The Mental After-Care Association', in 'Changing Public Representations of Mental Illness', pp. 178–232.

8 H. Thornhill Roxby, 'The After Care Association for Poor Female Convalescents on Leaving Asylums for the Insane', unpublished paper SA/MAC/A.1/2, Archives and Manuscripts, Wellcome Library, London.

9 See for example A. Digby, *Madness, Morality and Medicine: A Study of the York Retreat, 1796–1914*, Cambridge: Cambridge University Press, 1985, pp. 57–87.

10 T. L. Rogers, 'A Chapter on Broken Bones', *Journal of Mental Science*, 20, 1874–75, pp. 81–89. Quoted on p. 85.

11 A. T. Scull, *Museums of Madness: The Social Organisation of Insanity in Nineteenth-Century England*, London: Allen Lane, 1979.

12 L. J. Ray, 'Models of Madness in Victorian Asylum Practice', *Archives of European Sociology*, 22, 1981, pp. 229–264. Quoted on p. 256.

13 P. Bartlett, 'The Asylum and the Poor Law: The Productive Alliance', in J. Melling and B. Forsythe (eds), *Insanity, Institutions and Society, 1800–1914: A Social History of Madness in Comparative Perspective*, London: Routledge, 1999, pp. 48–67.

14 See for example M. Thomson, *The Problem of Mental Deficiency: Eugenics, Democracy, and Social Policy in Britain c.1870–1959*, Oxford: Clarendon Press, 1998, pp. 110–148.

15 *The After Care Association for Poor and Friendless Female Convalescents Upon Leaving Asylums for the Insane: Report of the Council 1887–1888*, London, 1888, p. 7.

16 *The Mental After-Care Association for Poor Persons Convalescent or Recovered from Institutions for the Insane: Report of the Council 1917*, London, 1918, p. 7.

17 The APSW, *Psychiatric Social Work and the Family Part II Illustrative Material: A Study in Preparation for the Second International Conference on Social Work*, London: APSW, 1932, p. 7.

18 G. Hamilton, *Theory and Practice of Social Casework*, New York: Columbia University Press, 1940. Cited in P. Armstrong, 'Aspects of Psychiatric Social Work in a Mental Hospital', *British Journal of Psychiatric Social Work*, 1, 1947, pp. 36–44. Quoted on p. 44. Armstrong gives no page reference for Hamilton's quotation.

19 These developments are discussed in P. Miller, 'Psychotherapy of Work and Unemployment', in P. Miller and N. Rose (eds), *The Power of Psychiatry*, Cambridge: Polity Press, 1986, pp. 143–176.

20 P. Lazarsfeld, M. Lazarsfeld-Jahoda and H. Zeisel, *Die Arbeitslosen von Marienthal. Ein soziographischer Versuch uber die Wirkungen langdauernder Arbeitslosigkeit. Mit einem Anhang zur Geschichte der Soziographie*, Leipzig: Osterrichischen Wirtschaftspsychologischen Forschungsstelle, 1933. This is discussed in R. McKibbin, *The Ideologies of Class: Social Relations in Britain 1880–1950*, Oxford: Oxford University Press, 1991, in Chapter 8 'The Social Psychology of Unemployment in Inter-War Britain', pp. 228–258.

21 H. L. Beales and R. S. Lambert (eds), *Memoirs of the Unemployed*, London: Gollancz, 1934.

22 J. Stevenson, *British Society, 1914–45*, Harmondsworth: Penguin, 1984, pp. 187–191.

23 The Industrial Fatigue Research Board was renamed the Industrial Health Research Board in 1929 when it came under the control of the Medical Research Council.

24 Papers of the Trades Union Congress: Mental Health 1935–39, MSS.292/140.1/2, Modern Records Centre, University of Warwick.

25 M. L. Ferard, 'Notes on the Psychiatric Social Treatment of Mental Hospital Patients: Four Paranoid Schizophrenics', *British Journal of Psychiatric Social Work*, 1, 1947, pp. 45–56.

26 Ferard, 'Notes', p. 54.

27 Ferard, 'Notes', p. 52.

28 Ferard, 'Notes', p. 53.

29 Mrs M., 'Everley' 1948–62, MACA Home Files, SA/MAC/F/1/9, Archives and Manuscripts, Wellcome Library, London.

30 Board of Control Report 1932. Cited in R. Hunter and I. Macalpine, *Psychiatry for the Poor: 1851 Colney Hatch Asylum – Friern Hospital 1973; a Medical and Social History*, Folkestone: Dawsons, 1974, p. 152.

31 Ibid., p. 154.

32 D. Gittins, *Madness in its Place: Narratives of Severalls Hospital, 1913–1997*, London: Routledge, 1998, pp. 107–111.

33 K. Laurie, *Employable or Unemployable? Report on Pioneer Experimental Work Covering the Period February 6 1939–August 1 1940*, London: the Mental After-Care Association, 1941, p. 2.

34 Laurie, *Employable or Unemployable?* p. 2.

35 Laurie, *Employable or Unemployable?* p. 20. Italics in original text.

36 Laurie, *Employable or Unemployable?* p. 30.

37 P. Horn, *The Rise and Fall of the Victorian Servant*, Dublin: Gill and Macmillan, 1975, pp. 170 and 179.

38 Papers of Eugene (John) Heimler: Publications by Heimler: University of Southampton Libraries Special Collection, MS 220 A859/3/6/7 'The Gift of Unemployment' 1983–87 Folder 1 of 3.

39 E. Heimler, *Mental Illness and Social Work*, Harmondsworth: Penguin, 1967, pp. 107–108.

40 Heimler, *Mental Illness*, pp. 118–119.

41 A. Driver, 'Concentration Camp Graduate', *Guardian*, 8 April 1961.

42 E. Heimler, 'The Emotional Significance of Work', *Concilium*, 1982–83, pp. 17–23. Quoted on p. 22.

43 E. Heimler and N. Davies, 'An Experiment in the Assessment of Social Functioning', *Medical Officer*, 20 January 1967, p. 32.

44 Driver, 'Concentration Camp Graduate'.

45 Driver, 'Concentration Camp Graduate'.

46 E. Heimler, 'Psychology and Common Sense', Typescript submitted to the Guildhall Gazette 22 November 1961, Papers of Eugene (John) Heimler: University of Southampton Libraries Special Collection, Publications, Lectures by Heimler: General Sequence MS 220 A859/3/5/4 1956–80. E. Heimler, 'The Human Meaning of Work and the Impact of Redundancy', Typescript of talk delivered by Heimler at Edinburgh University on 24 September 1980, MS 220 A859/3/5/4.

47 Heimler, *Mental Illness and Social Work*, p. 117.

48 E. Heimler, 'Psychiatric Social Work with NAB Cases', *Medical Officer*, 16 December 1955, pp. 351–353. Quoted on p. 351.

49 R. Warner, *Recovery from Schizophrenia: Psychiatry and Political Economy*, 3rd edn, Hove: Brunner-Routledge, 2004.

50 From unnamed, undated paper, 'Social Work – Who's Out of Step?' APSW Press Cuttings, MSS.378/APSW/14/4/120, Modern Records Centre, University of Warwick.

51 E. Heimler, 'Possibilities of Treatment out of the Psychiatric Hospital', in *Alternatives to Mental Hospitals: European Workshop Papers*, Ghent: Nationale Vereniging voor Geestelijke Gezondheidszorg, 1980, pp. 27–33. Quoted on p. 31.

52 M. Eden, 'A Short Stay Psychiatric Treatment Unit', in APSW, *New Developments in Psychiatry and the Implications for the Social Worker*, London: APSW, 1971, pp. 6–11. Quoted on p. 9.

53 Heimler, *Mental Illness and Social Work*, pp. 9–10.

54 For an overview of developments in occupational and industrial therapy, especially in the post Second World War era, See D. Bennett, 'Work and Occupation for the Mentally Ill', in H. Freeman and G. E. Berrios, *150 Years of British Psychiatry Volume II: The Aftermath*, London: Athlone Press, 1996, pp. 193–208.

55 J. A. Harrington and W. Mayer-Gross, 'A Day Hospital for Neurotics in an Industrial Community', *Journal of Mental Science*, 105, 1959, pp. 224–234. Quoted on p. 233.

56 The proportion of patients within the mental health services who might be diagnosed with a chronic mental illness is hard to quantify on a national level. Curiously, this information was not included in the Annual Reports of the Board of Control. Statistics on the prevalence of chronic conditions such as schizophrenia vary greatly, although Warner in his summary of existing statistical studies suggested that the incidence of schizophrenia increased during the nineteenth century, peaked, and has been on the decline since the early 1960s: the current incidence rate of schizophrenia in the West has been averaged at around one in 200 of the general population (Warner, *Recovery from Schizophrenia*, pp. 206–230). If mental health problems such as schizophrenia were particularly prominent during the 1940s and 1950s, this may help explain the development of programmes to help assist people diagnosed with these conditions.

57 Warner, *Recovery from Schizophrenia*, pp. 145 and 151.

58 P. Barham, *Closing the Asylum: The Mental Patient in Modern Society*, 2nd edn, London: Penguin, 1997, p. xiii.

59 Barham, *Closing the Asylum*, pp. 45 and 47.

60 Barham, *Closing the Asylum*, p. 105.

61 Warner, *Recovery from Schizophrenia*, pp. 145–148.

62 MIND 'Creating Accepting Communities: Executive Statement' was available at http://www.mind.org.uk/information/about_government_policy/creating_accepting_communities.asp (accessed 3 December 2001). This page has since been taken down from the MIND website.

63 The Social Exclusion Unit, *Mental Health and Social Exclusion*, London: Office of the Deputy Prime Minister, 2004. See Chapter 5 'Mental Health and Employment', pp. 51–58 and Chapter 6 'Overcoming Barriers to Employment', pp. 59–71.
64 The Social Exclusion Unit, *Mental Health and Social Exclusion*. Statistic given on p. 52, research question quoted from the inside cover of the report.

10 Inside the walls of the hostel, 1940–74

John Welshman

Introduction

This chapter is an attempt to move from the question of what went on outside the walls of the asylum, to that of what went on inside the walls of the hostel. There has been much research in the history of learning disability and mental health in recent years. Work has for instance explored the history of mental deficiency, both in terms of institutional care, and with regard to care in the community. Similarly the history of mental health has both continued its fascination with institutions, notably the Victorian asylum, but has also begun to look at the care that was provided outside its walls.[1] In both cases, but notably with regard to learning disability, there has been an attempt to place the 'official history' alongside the experience of service users, mainly through oral history interviewing. Nevertheless it is fair to say that the role of smaller institutions in the community has been more neglected by historians, and this chapter is a preliminary attempt to try to remedy that neglect. By 'smaller institutions', I mean the Occupation Centres that were later called Adult and Junior Training Centres, Special Schools, and hostels that together formed a notional network of care in the community in the postwar period.

The role played by the hostel in the emergence of care in the community has been considered by some writers. Kathleen Jones points out that in 1939 there were nine hostels in operation, and more recently Charles Webster mentions hostels as part of the range of services provided in the community.[2] In terms of local studies, Hugh Freeman notes the opening of a hostel in his study of mental health services in Salford in the period up to 1974, arguing that it was more geared towards rehabilitation, and better integrated into the psychiatric service, than may have been the case elsewhere.[3] But local authority hostels were not included in Pauline Morris's famous survey of institutions for the 'mentally retarded', published as *Put Away* (1969). Indeed in the foreword to that study, Peter Townsend recommended that detailed studies were required of numerous aspects of mental health, including 'the social structure of both the hospital and the hostel'.[4] Similarly Mathew Thomson says little about hostels in his otherwise masterly survey of mental deficiency, or about the processes within hostels that made them possible stepping stones to the community.[5]

The role of the small institution, typically the residential home, has been well covered by writers working on contemporary social care. The 1989 White Paper drew attention to the role of 'homely settings in the community'.[6] Craig Gurney and Robin Means have written about the meaning of home in later life for older people, arguing there is a hierarchy based on the cultural, intermediate and personal meanings attached to home.[7] Joan Higgins has examined the concept of 'home' in residential care, and questions the extent to which the domestic ideal has been realized in institutions. She suggests that in homes, gender and class inequalities persist and reflect those in domestic settings in the outside world.[8] Dorothy Atkinson, too, has shown how 'institutional' can refer to a style of care that denies individual choice, as much as to the type or size of a building. She also includes hostels in a useful, if brief, history of residential care.[9] This work has drawn attention to the importance of defining the word 'hostel'. Since the medieval period, hostels have usually been seen as a place of lodging for students or travellers, especially those not run for commercial gain.[10] What has been most important, arguably, is the temporary nature of the period of residence, and it is this that has been one of the points of contention in the use of the hostel for mental disorder. Moreover by the end of this period there were suggestions that the term 'hostel' should be replaced by that of 'home'.

The subject of this chapter, then, is that of the role of the hostel in the implementation of policy for mental health and learning disability, between roughly 1940 and 1974. The chapter explores how hostels fit in with the rest of policy relating to the care and treatment of mental disorder. It is not concerned with residential homes for older people, nor with hostels for other types of service user, such as drug users and homeless people. The research was inspired by a photograph of the interior of a hostel in an annual Medical Officer of Health report – a room with a few armchairs, and a television set. This led me to wonder how much might be discovered about hostels and their residents. The chapter is concerned not just with the way that the hostel was perceived by policy makers and social policy analysts, but also with the question of what actually went on within these small institutions. How were they seen by service users, and did they actually function as halfway houses between the institution and the community? How did their role change over time? And what differences were there in the role of the hostel for mental illness compared to learning disability? At the start of this period, there were very few hostels; at the end there was a network. This chapter is an account of what shaped the way the network developed, and accounts for its form at the end of the period.

Hostels in policy and practice before 1948

Although the main theme of this chapter is the role of the hostel after the Second World War, it is important to locate these later changes in the context of the hostel system before 1939. The influence that eugenics had in the field of mental deficiency is one that has attracted much research.[11] Furthermore developments in institutional care provide some models for the later hostel ideal. Mathew Thomson has shown how the colony was considered as a solution to the 'problem' of mental deficiency, though he has been pessimistic about its influence before the Second World War. In the nineteenth century, the institution had been revived by the addition of 'wings', 'pavilions' and 'villas', and Thomson argues the 'colony' was the last of these. In the second half of the nineteenth century, the term 'colony' was used to describe mental hospitals that were built in the style of smaller 'cottages' or 'villas', with shared central administrative facilities. The villas were aimed to be small enough to maintain an intimate atmosphere, while the community would also socialize the patients. The colony seemed to offer a new form of institutional care which would be more humane and efficient than the closed asylum.[12] The colony had a much broader appeal, however, being drawn on in relation to labour colonies for the 'social residuum', and being incorporated into tuberculosis sanatoria.[13] As Thomson has demonstrated, colonies were associated with the 1913 Mental Deficiency Act, making the legislation appear more progressive than it might otherwise have done.

The colony provided a new design and ethos for the housing of groups already provided with institutional care, but it appeared particularly suitable for the feeble-minded. It seemed to offer a sheltered environment in which defectives could be protected from the community and also contribute to their own support. Other models were offered by the Gheel colony in Belgium; the practice of 'boarding out' in Scotland; and the colony model in the United States. The Royal Commission on the Care and Control of the Feeble-Minded (1908) also considered systems of small voluntary-run hostels and refuges for feeble-minded girls. Nevertheless Thomson argues the Royal Commission came down in favour of a closed industrial villa colony – one that took on some of the features of the colony, but did not open its walls to the outside world. This model was chosen because it was the only one that could guarantee medical control over care and secure segregation of the residents. In this it reflected the influence of the psychiatric profession, which opposed small homes run by lay organizations, but which also wanted to align itself with progressive social policy.[14] Thomson argues in the interwar period there was no wholesale adoption of the colony model. In 1937, for example, only eighteen institutions had adopted the title of 'colony', and most institutions remained under non-medical management.[15]

In the 1930s however there was a move towards the more open colonies that had been considered but rejected by the Royal Commission. Mathew Thomson has written of the interwar period that 'the division between the colony and the community was ... broken down through the development of hostels, outside the walls of institutions'.[16] The Superintendent of the Royal Eastern Counties Colony called in 1928 for institutions to become 'flowing lakes' rather than 'stagnant water', stressing a more open system. The Wood Report on Mental Deficiency (1929) was enthusiastic about colonies, and it argued that 'the hostel affords valuable training and an opportunity of testing the defectives' fitness for more responsibility and increased liberty'.[17] Winifred Gibson wrote in 1930 of Eagle House, opened as a hostel for feeble-minded girls by the Surrey Voluntary Association for Mental and Physical Welfare in May 1924. She wrote of potential residents that 'such cases should be of stable temperament, without serious physical disabilities, and sufficiently intelligent to be able to perform ordinary household duties without a very great amount of supervision'. Most 'girls' worked in domestic service, but the work for 'boys' was more varied – farm labourers, gardeners and carpenters. Given the emphasis attached to saving the money earned through work, Gibson concluded that the hostel system 'while making for happiness and self-respect, should also prove an economical method of dealing with the highest-grade of mental defectives in the community'.[18]

Evidence from the Board of Control indicates a complex picture in terms of the number of mental defectives and forms of provision. In 1938, for example, there were 1,475 defectives in state institutions for the violent or criminal; 34,290 in certified institutions (local authority); 9,445 in approved (Poor Law) institutions; 173 in certified (private) houses; and 671 in approved (charitable and religious) houses. There had been a shift towards local authority provision. Most of the approved (Poor Law) institutions held under fifty patients, and the approved houses were also small, none with more than fifty residents. Thomson concludes that if institutions are assessed in terms of who controlled and managed them, their scale and their design, they failed to live up to the colony ideal of 1908–13. He suggests this is also true in a qualitative sense – the sixty-bed villas that were built were really barrack blocks on a smaller scale. Moreover nursing and medical care were poor, and occupational therapy degenerated into work. Medical Superintendents remained cautious about a shift to the community. Thomson suggests that despite some changes in the 1930s, the British colony system continued to be a primarily segregative regime divorced from the outside community.[19]

Nevertheless the certified and approved institutions created opportunities that have been emphasized by other writers. Sheena Rolph has argued that Thomson does not pay much attention to the hostels, nor to the processes within hostels that made them stepping stones to the community. She notes that the 'certified institutions' were generally small, with some being run by voluntary organizations, and others by local authorities. Rolph points out that in 1923 and in 1930 Evelyn Fox, Honorary Secretary of the Central Association for Mental Welfare, turned to the idea, popular in America, of 'working hostels'. These working hostels for boys and girls were seen as providing an organized and supervised way back into the community from institutions, and were regarded as a form of short-term provision.[20] Rolph therefore locates the origins of the hostels of the 1950s in the smaller institutions of the interwar years, and is generally more optimistic about their rehabilitation functions.

Local case studies provide support to both the Thomson and Rolph interpretations, showing that there were small voluntary hostels and refuges for feeble-minded girls, but that these were incorporated into larger local authority colonies in the 1920s. In the Midlands city of Leicester, for example, the After-Care sub-committee of the Education Committee in 1907 established 'Sunnyholme', a small residential unit for twelve feeble-minded girls, based on similar institutions in Ipswich and Clapton. The aim was to provide 'a safe shelter from the dangers of the outside world, in a permanent home, to girls whose mental infirmity prevents them from taking responsible care of their own lives'.[21] The girls were taught domestic work and gardening, and parents and relatives paid monthly visits. Apart from local authority provision for mental defectives, voluntary organizations were also active in the provision of after-care for the mentally ill. The Mental After-Care Association (MACA) provided an after-care service, mainly in London and the South East of England. These homes tended to be owned by ex-matrons or ex-nurses, and they were paid by the MACA on a per capita basis. In general, these homes were very small, taking only an average of four patients at a time, but in the 1920s the MACA began to accept residents directly from the community, and place them in the hostels. Nevertheless voluntary organizations such as the MACA were also influential, through the evidence they provided to the Royal Commission (1957).

Finally, it is important to note that the Second World War, and the evacuation of schoolchildren and other vulnerable groups, provided an opportunity for experiment and innovation in the use of hostels. The term 'hostel' had become more generally known from the late 1920s through the work of the Youth Hostels Association (YHA). By 1939, there were some 397 hostels in Britain, and the YHA had some 106,524 members.[22] Moreover the potential uses of hostels were further highlighted during the Second World War, when evacuation drew attention to the psychological needs of children. Child Guidance Clinics had been established in cities in the 1920s, but during the war, children deemed to be 'maladjusted' or 'difficult' who could not be placed with private families were billeted in hostels. The Board of Education claimed that by July 1943 there were 3,400 children in 325 hostels. In February 1945, there were 235 hostels, forty-five of which provided psychiatric treatment; 109 where psychiatric advice was available; and eighty-two other hostels for 'difficult' children.[23]

Although most children remained unprovided-for, the war in this respect did provide an experiment in the potential use of hostels. For adults, too, voluntary organizations such as the Central Association for Mental Welfare developed agricultural hostels for patients from the mental deficiency institutions who worked on the land to assist home food production.[24]

The hostel as a component of policy on mental disorder, 1948–74

In the period before the Second World War, the colony, the certified and approved institutions and the small homes that were opened for feeble-minded girls all provided models for the hostel. At the same time, the numbers of hostels and their functions remain unclear, and before the 1959 Mental Health Act no single agency was active in providing hostels.[25] It has been suggested that the postwar period saw the development of a 'modern domestic ideal', so that by the 1980s, being 'at home' meant something quite different from what was understood by that phrase in the 1940s.[26] Similarly, the discourse of the family after the Second World War was reflected in familial models, and hostels were constructed as 'homely' or 'home-like'. With the revived postwar interest in rehabilitation, the hostel was seen as ideal for resocialization and training.[27] This came in the context of an increasing emphasis on care in the community, underpinned by a pharmacological revolution, and a critique of institutional care. All of the major policy documents of the period stressed the potential role that hostels might play.

The Piercy Committee, for instance, had been appointed in March 1953 to review the existing provision for the rehabilitation, training and reset-tlement of disabled persons, and to make recommendations.[28] The need for hostels for the disabled was stressed in much of the evidence the Com-mittee received. These were seen to be needed as, first, short-stay hostels for people leaving hospital and second, permanent hostels for the 'depend-ent' disabled. The short-stay hostel could be for hospital patients who were ready for discharge, but had no homes to go to – it would provide accommodation and board – and a 'breathing space'. This would be of value to hospitals. But it was essential to include a mechanism to transfer into permanent hostel accommodation those disabled people who were unable to move on into normal housing.[29] The Piercy Committee discussed hostels for other types of service user, such as patients with tuberculosis and paraplegics, but its main focus was on physical disabilities, and it was cautious about hostels for the mentally ill and defective, pointing out that the level of need was not known, and they would only be justified in the larger local authority areas.[30] Given this uncertainty about demand, a policy of experimentation was perceived as being the most sensible one to adopt.[31]

In addition to the emphasis on rehabilitation, new forms of treatment meant that the management of patients was made easier, and patients with family ties were able to leave hospital. Electro-convulsive therapy had been used from the 1930s. But deep insulin therapy and brain operations, which had been used regularly in the 1950s, were rarely used by the 1960s, mainly because better results could be achieved through the use of drugs. Several drugs established themselves as effective in the treatment of mental illnesses such as schizophrenia and severe depression, but also of neurotic disorders such as anxiety and tension states. Although some of these developments were not to occur until the 1960s, this 'pharmacological revolution' provided part of the context in which the Royal Commission on Mental Health (1957) argued that whatever form care in the community might take, the aim should be to reorient away from institutions, towards residential homes in the community.

The Royal Commission listed hostels as among the services that local authorities should be providing, along with training centres, occupation centres and residential accommodation.[32] Many witnesses to the Royal Commission said that local authorities should be providing residential hostels for people who needed a home and advice, but not psychiatric intervention or nursing care. Potential users might include young people leaving schools for the educationally subnormal, feeble-minded adults, older people who were mentally ill and patients recovering from mental illness. Residence in a hostel was seen as useful for patients who could not benefit from further hospital treatment, but for whom living in the community was possible, if they had a home and some support. And the Royal Commission saw this as a local authority responsibility, given their role in after-care.[33] Some organizations agreed, such as the Association of Municipal Corporations and London County Council, but others, notably the County Councils Association, disagreed, arguing this should be the responsibility of hospitals, not local authorities.[34] Assessing potential need was seen as a further difficulty.

An important influence on the development of hostels was the emerging critique of institutionalization. In *Institutional Neurosis* (1959), Russell Barton had documented the symptoms of a syndrome he regarded as being characterized by apathy, loss of interest in the future, submissiveness, loss of individuality and an acceptance of things as they were.[35] Goffman was later to write (1968) that entry into institutional care entailed what he called 'curtailment of the self' – the individual cast off one set of roles (mother, daughter, husband, wife) and took on others (resident, patient, inmate).[36] Attempts were being made, by the early 1960s, to break down some of the mental hospital hierarchies by creating 'therapeutic communities', in which patients took more responsibility for the running of the ward.[37]

This critique of institutional care was supported by empirical evidence, including, in Britain, Peter Townsend's study *The Last Refuge* (1963), an important ethnographic study of residential homes for older people. Townsend was concerned with the relationship between the size of the institution and the quality of care that was provided. He suggested the smaller homes were of higher quality than the larger. They were better staffed, and had a more liberal regime, with fewer restrictions on what residents might do, and better opportunities for social living. Townsend wrote that homes with twenty or thirty beds had advantages that were often overlooked – relationships between staff members and between the staff and the residents were often closer and more informal. It was easier to simulate the customs and practices of home and community life.[38] Pauline Morris's study *Put Away* (1969) was based on institutions for the mentally retarded. This showed that the larger institutions continued to cater for large numbers of residents. Of patients, 61 per cent were in hospital complexes of more than 1,000 beds each, and only 1 per cent were in single rooms – 38 per cent were in wards with sixty beds or more.[39] Morris also provided a devastating picture of conditions in the larger institutions. To take one example, she found that in many institutions, the stock of clothing was communal, meaning that after laundry it was not returned to individuals. Hospitals did not provide many items of clothing, and most was 'dull, unimaginative and often ill-fitting'. Often the clothes that were worn were poorly matched – in one large hospital, clothing was described as 'nondescript and baggy'.[40] At the same time, Morris showed that although the smaller homes seemed more comfortable and less regimented, the psychological implications of 'subnormality' were neglected, and in this respect the smaller homes were more isolated from theories of rehabilitation than the larger institutions.[41] Nonetheless, Morris recommended that the larger institutions should provide accommodation and treatment for those who required constant medical and nursing care. In most cases however, they should provide out-patient treatment for the majority of patients who would live in hostels.[42]

Commentators on care in the community noted that Peter Townsend had argued for the advantages of small institutions, which need not be more expensive. They tended to advocate hostels as small and inexpensive, alongside sheltered workshops. In 1961, Jack Tizard, then based at the Medical Research Council's Social Psychiatry Research Unit, at the Maudsley Hospital in London, wrote that in an ideal hospital service for the mentally handicapped the units would be small, and situated close to the community they served. Admission and discharge would be easy and visiting would be informal. The adults too might work in industry or in sheltered workshops right outside the hostels they lived in.[43] In 1964, Tizard argued that large institutions tended to be remote from the centres of population; they easily became isolated from developments in medicine, psychiatry and education; they wasted specialist services; it was difficult to attract and keep good staff; and visiting was also difficult. Tizard made the important point that the costs of small units need not be greater than that of larger establishments, if specialist services were pooled.[44] He recommended hostels for 'high grade defectives who are working out', and for 'lower grade dependent defectives'. But he recognized hostels should cater for both men and women since their function would be 'to prepare school-leavers and young adults for independent living in ordinary lodgings or their own homes'.[45] The residents of these hostels would normally go out to work in the daytime. But the main need was for long-stay homes for adults who were mentally subnormal. Again, this provision should be in small family-type units, close to sheltered workshops. Part of the argument was that day and residential services should be integrated, so that services might be used by both patients living in their own homes and those in residential care. If schools and workshops catered for larger numbers, it might be possible to keep hostels small.[46]

The role of hostels was again emphasized in the major policy documents issued in the early 1960s, including the *Hospital Plan*, and the *Health and Welfare* White Paper. The *Hospital Plan*, for example, noted that the number of hospital beds for the mentally ill was expected to decline markedly over the following ten years, but that there were relatively few residential hostels for them.[47] Similarly the *Health and Welfare* White Paper (1963) included hostels as a vital part of the network of care in the community. In the case of the mentally ill, accommodation was seen as valuable where the patient needed supervision and help before returning to ordinary life. Similarly the White Paper argued that for the 'mentally disordered', alternative homes would always be needed, though it was important these should be 'real' homes.[48] One consultant in 1965 distinguished between 'custodial' and 'rehabilitatory' hostels, the former providing life-long care for 'welfare' cases, the latter acting as a halfway house between the hospital and the outside world. He recommended that wardens need not be mental nurses, but should have some experience in hostel management, while food should not be of high quality, since this made discharge difficult.[49] The main organizational change in this period was the creation of Social Services Departments, and the reduction in the scope of local authority Health Departments, reflecting the recommendations of the Seebohm Committee.[50] The Seebohm Committee observed that most patients were able to live with their families or in hostels if medical supervision was provided by hospital out-patients departments or by general practitioners, but it also noted that the functions of hostels needed to be reviewed.[51]

The emphasis on hostels was again reiterated in the White Papers on the Mentally Handicapped (1971) and the Mentally Ill (1975), where more attention was given than previously to their internal dynamics and vocabulary. The White Paper on the Mentally Handicapped recommended they should be small, with a maximum of twenty-five adults and twenty children, and contain residents of both sexes. Most adults should have single rooms, and no rooms should have more than four beds. There should also be plenty of space for recreation, both inside and outside. The White Paper noted that 'in such surroundings a family atmosphere can be created, where individuals can develop within a small group and with their own interests and possessions'.[52] More importantly, the White Paper advocated the word 'home' in place of 'hostel'. It argued that the word 'hostel' had the ring of 'impermanence and a certain austerity'. It usually described a place where people stayed while working or studying, away from their home. But residential homes were a permanent substitute family home for most of the residents, even though they kept in touch with their own families and visited them as often as possible. The White Paper argued that the staff and residents became a 'substitute family group', so that the 'the home should be homely'.[53] Nevertheless it conceded that most local authority hostels lacked this family atmosphere. One minor improvement would be to know them by their individual name or street number. In this, the White Paper reflected moves towards a policy that would later come to be known as 'normalization'. Writing in 1972, the social worker Howard Lovejoy argued that the standing of the hostel in the community would be enhanced if it could gain a reputation for 'quality and value'.[54] The White Paper on the Mentally Ill again emphasized that hostels had to be small if an institutional atmosphere was to be avoided. Hostels needed to be outward looking, and residents should spend most of the day elsewhere, at day centres, day hospitals and so on. There should be a maximum of one to fifteen residents. In order to facilitate this, hostels should be located in residential areas where they would fit in with other houses. Residents should participate in the running of the hostel, they should have their own rooms and reasonable expectations of privacy.[55]

There was, therefore, much support for the concept of the hostel in this period, both for people with mental health needs, and for those with learning difficulties. Successive policy documents and White Papers included the hostel as part of the network of smaller institutions that, along with services in the home, made up care in the community. The potential of the hostel was underlined by moves towards care in the community, notably through the Royal Commission on Mental Health and the 1959 Mental Health Act. In attempting to explain the popularity of the hostel as a policy option in the postwar period, four reasons can be put forward. First, the hostel fitted in with the postwar emphasis on the family, with hostels being constructed as being 'homely' or 'home-like'. Second, the hostel seemed an ideal vehicle through which to provide rehabilitation and socialization. Third, the attractiveness of small hostels was strengthened by the increasing critique of institutions, not least since commentators such as Jack Tizard argued that smaller institutions were not necessarily more expensive. Fourth, the development of new types of drugs, including tranquillizers, made care in hostels rather than hospitals possible, in some cases for the first time. What is perhaps surprising, with hindsight, is that there was not a more rigorous evaluation of the functions of the hostel. As

Richard Titmuss remarked of the idea of care in the community, the hostel seemed attractive and comforting, but also remained a vague and ambiguous concept.[56]

The implementation of hostel policy, 1948–74

But while the hostel became part of community care rhetoric, it is important to explore how far this policy was implemented. With the creation of the National Health Service in 1948, many of the institutions previously run by local authorities passed into the control of the new Regional Hospital Boards (RHBs). Nevertheless, Section 29 of the 1946 National Health Service Act confirmed the responsibilities of local authorities under the Mental Treatment Acts, 1890–1930, and under the Mental Deficiency Acts, 1913–38. Under Section 28 of the 1946 Act, local authorities also had permissive powers for the prevention, care and after-care of mental illness and mental deficiency. Local authorities established Mental Health Committees and appointed Mental Welfare Officers, and slowly began to assume responsibility for care in the community.[57] The other main legislative change in this period was the 1959 Mental Health Act which reflected many of the aims of the Royal Commission, in moving from institutions to care in the community. However the legal precedents set by the 1959 Mental Health Act were not matched by rapid changes to services at the local level. In particular, the provision of services remained permissive, and local authorities were not provided with major grants with which to improve mental health services.[58]

The provision of hostels thus represents a case study in the wider development of care in the community in the postwar period. A circular issued by the Ministry of Health in January 1952 authorized local authorities to remove mental defectives from families, and it claimed that some had shown interest in the potential of hostels.[59] Over the next twenty years both the Ministry and its successor, the Department of Health and Social Security, were to repeat this exhortation periodically, generally listing hostels as part of a potential network of community care services that embraced training and occupation centres, social centres, clubs, home visiting services and also residential homes. Nevertheless, as others have pointed out, the Ministry provided local authorities with very little guidance on what the functions of hostels should be, including the extent to which they would be long-stay institutions, or engage in rehabilitation.

Correspondence between the Ministry and individual local authorities and RHBs about hostels was revealing. In the mid-1950s, the Ministry viewed the building of hostels as largely experimental – while it would not discourage local authorities, it was not likely to put pressure on those that were reluctant. It remained unclear whether hostels should best be run by local authorities or by the RHBs, and the Ministry used the impending publication of the Report of the Royal Commission to play for time.[60] As ever, the policy of the Ministry was one of gentle exhortation, rather than coercion to conform to a more uniform policy. In many respects, the main pressure came from the RHBs which were running the large institutions, rather than the local authorities who were potentially responsible for the community services.[61] But some local authorities were also seeking support for proposals.[62] At a meeting in August 1959, the Ministry agreed on some points of principle on the provision of hostels for various categories of service user.[63] Comments in the rather thin 'hostels' file held in the Ministry of Health records at the Public Record Office indicate it was frequently mislaid, providing further evidence that the Ministry did not view hostels as being of major policy importance in this period, its exhortations in the published reports notwithstanding.

The result was that the pace of change at the local level was extremely slow. Between July 1959 and April 1962, for example, eight hostels for the mentally ill were opened, in places such as Birmingham, Bradford, Sheffield, York and Leeds.[64] The *Health and Welfare* White Paper (1963) indicated that at 31 March 1962, there were only forty-seven hostels for the mentally 'subnormal' in England and Wales, providing 947 places, and only eighteen hostels for the mentally ill, providing 340 places.[65] The plan was that over the next ten years the number of hostels for the mentally 'subnormal' would increase to 464 by 31 March 1972, providing 9,907 places, and hostels for the mentally ill to 211, with 4,812 places. The cost of this capital building programme was estimated as £7.6m in the period 1962–63 to 1971–72.[66] However the approach taken in *Health and Welfare* was actually very tentative, since no attempt was made to establish a general ratio of places in homes or hostels to either population, or to places in training centres for children and adults. Peter Mittler, then a lecturer in psychology at Birkbeck College, London, later commented that *Health and Welfare* was 'one of the most disappointing publications in the mental health field for many years'.[67] In England and Wales as a whole, there were only thirty-one local authority hostels for the mentally ill by the end of 1964, eight of which had been purpose-built, and twenty-three in adapted premises. The inevitable result was dramatic geographical variations in the level of provision. Wales, for example, had only eleven homes or hostels for the mentally disordered in 1964, which together provided only 190 places.[68]

A report by the Ministry in 1965, based on a questionnaire and visits to some local authorities, provided some more information on how the Ministry viewed hostels. Nearly all local authorities had co-operated with hospital psychiatrists, but effective co-operation between hospital and local authorities was only evident in a few cases. In four-fifths of the admissions, the cases had been referred from mental hospitals. The hostels were viewed by the Ministry in the same way as they had been by the Royal Commission – as catering for patients discharged from hospital who could not live independently in the community. The Ministry argued that the hostel should be an integral part of mental health services; there should be good co-operation between the local authority and the hospitals; and a 'team' approach was needed to the selection of residents, and their care and rehabilitation. Selection should not be confined to hospital in-patients, but should be widened to include any mentally ill person living in the community. Finally, the approach should be a flexible one, with alternative forms of residential accommodation, since some might require long periods of hostel care.[69]

The White Paper on the Mentally Handicapped (1971) for the first time produced more definite planning targets, based on the number of places required per 100,000 total population. These estimated that ten places were required for children (birth to fifteen), and sixty places for adults (sixteen and over), per 100,000 population. Nevertheless as with *Health and Welfare*, what was more interesting was the way these calculations gave some sense of the deficits in provision that remained at the end of the 1960s. Using the figure of ten places per 100,000 population, 1,800 places were provided for children in England and Wales in 1969, against an estimated 4,900 required. Using the figure of sixty places per 100,000 population, 4,300 places for adults had been provided in 1969, against an estimated 29,400 that were required.[70] Nevertheless even this provision was recognized as failing to meet need. As Barbara Castle, Secretary of State for Social Services, noted in the foreword to the White Paper on the Mentally Ill (1975) there were many problems in shifting the emphasis to community care, and social services facilities – hostels, day centres, group homes – had to be built up from minimal levels.[71]

The earlier restrictions on capital expenditure that had been a serious obstacle to the building of hostels did loosen in the early 1970s, to an extent. In 1973–74, for instance, the Department of Health and Social Security devoted £3.9m to homes and hostels for mentally handicapped adults; £1m to homes and hostels for mentally handicapped children; and £1.4m to homes and hostels for mentally ill adults, as part of a package of expenditure of £48.3m.[72] DHSS statistics for 1975 (for England) indicated there were 167 homes and hostels for the mentally ill, with some 2,091 places, and 302 homes and hostels for the mentally handicapped, with some 5,960 places.[73] Even so, independent reviews of hostels continued to paint a pessimistic picture. A review published in 1978, on behalf of the Campaign for the Mentally Handicapped, was based on visits to hospitals, hostels, homes and other units in 1975–76. It concluded that the range and extent of provision was 'patchy and inconsistent', and that the response of local authorities had been 'characteristically opportunistic'. In particular it attempted to measure the quality of life of residents, with a checklist that included personal identity, privacy, relationships and activities.[74]

Local studies indicate that in many areas, hostels were not opened until the mid-1960s. In the Midlands city of Leicester, for instance, which had established a home for feeble-minded girls in 1907, hostels for the mentally ill and mentally subnormal were opened only in November 1965 and June 1970 respectively.[75] The main question therefore, in reviewing policy from the Second World War to the early 1970s, is why so little progress was made in the building of hostels. Local authorities were generally overwhelmed by the increase in their responsibilities for mental health, particularly as they received so little guidance from central government for their emerging responsibilities for care in the community.[76] But there were three particular problems that together explain the slow development of hostels in this period. First, there were the difficulties in starting a new capital programme, getting permission for building, recruiting staff and getting local support for plans. In the case of hospitals, restrictions on capital expenditure limited the provision of new institutions, meaning that provision continued to reflect the legacy that RHBs had inherited from the pre-NHS era.[77] Other writers have made the same point about health centres, which were not built on a widespread scale until the late 1960s, even though they were included as a local authority provision in the 1946 NHS Act.[78] While hostels were much cheaper to build, or indeed could arguably have been provided in converted buildings, similar factors are likely to have been evident in the failure of the hostel building programme. Second, there was the resistance of local authorities to enter the field of institutional care, not least because it was claimed many hostels failed to fill their beds. Third, there were the organizational difficulties that the tripartite structure of the NHS created for joint planning of services between the local authorities and the RHBs. Most local authorities generally had poor links with the RHBs, including the Hospital Management Committees. Together these factors meant that relatively few hostels were built before the late 1960s.

The hostel as a halfway house: mental health

The policy documents thus contain only fleeting references to hostels, and in order to provide a more sustained investigation of what actually went on inside their walls, it is necessary to turn to other sources. In the space available here, it is possible to look only at two of these – social surveys and secondary work based in part on oral interviews. In the case of the first, we look at the survey *Halfway Houses*, published in 1968 by Robert Apte, later Lecturer in Community Mental Health at the University of California, Berkeley. With the second, we use the recent thesis by Sheena Rolph, exploring the functions of hostels in Norfolk. While the Apte survey was based on hostels for the mentally ill, the work by Rolph has been concerned with hostels for people with learning difficulties.

Richard Titmuss, Professor of Social Administration at the London School of Economics, was one of the most perceptive commentators on the development of care in the community in the postwar period. One of the most useful studies of hostels, or halfway houses, was completed by his

American graduate student, Robert Apte. The Apte survey was based on twenty-four local authorities, and on twenty-five halfway houses that were in operation at the end of 1963. Apte pointed out that at that time, no major research had been carried out on the way that they operated. He regarded halfway houses or transitional hostels as temporary residences, that provided ex-hospital patients with sheltered accommodation, that helped them to meet the community and thus become more independent. They had a rehabilitative function, based on the reintegration of the individual into society. But they were also places that mentally ill individuals living in their own homes could go to, during a period of crisis, rather than into hospital. The word 'hostel' could thus refer to halfway houses, that were transitional hostels, or long-stay hostels that were non-transitional.[79]

Apte located hostels as part of a group of transitional institutions that included day hospitals, night hospitals, foster care homes, sheltered rehabilitation workshops, therapeutic social clubs, and out-patient psychiatric clinics.[80] Apte only focused on hostels that served as halfway houses or transitional facilities, and he pointed out that neither the Piercy Report, the Royal Commission nor the Mental Health Act had defined what was meant by 'short-stay' or 'long-stay' hostels. Defining what was meant by a transitional hostel was particularly difficult – some hostels had started with the aim of providing a time-limited service, but their experience with chronic patients had required a change in their aims.[81] In the end, Apte used the time definition based on one year. The twenty-five transitional hostels had 851 individuals living in them.[82]

Although it might be thought that hostels with an average of three staff and eighteen residents were simply organized, Apte found that their location between the hospital and the community, and the way they had been shaped by social and economic factors, meant they were complex.[83] The Apte survey was particularly interesting on the question of the role of the staff, including how qualified they were for this type of work. The wardens were seen alternatively as parental figures as people who could help the residents find employment, as a source of education in citizenship and as people who had psychotherapeutic roles. Most had some previous experience in nursing, but eleven had no relevant training after secondary school. Of the twenty-five, only one had some previous experience in psychiatric rehabilitation. Apte claimed that there was little level of agreement, between the different levels of staff, on what the objectives for the hostel should be. Although most hostels had established social clubs, the wardens seemed to take little active part in these. Three-quarters of the wardens had previously been employed in medical or nonmedical institutions, and they brought into the hostels values and modes of behaviour towards the mentally ill typical of institutional environments.[84]

In terms of variety of psychiatric disorders of the residents, most of the hostels were replicas of the mental hospitals. Employment for residents was generally unskilled, including gardening, factory work and domestic service for women – in only a few cases were the residents learning trades.[85] Apte pointed out that residents needed help from social workers and psychiatrists to make the decision about moving on. Otherwise, hostels could actually reinforce dependency, 'in this situation the halfway house can become for the patient a *custodial ward*'.[86] Apte was also concerned to study the restrictive practices evident in the hostels, and the responsibility that the staff expected from residents. He attempted to compare the twenty-five hostels with seventeen hospital wards, to see if they had become a logical bridge into the community. This exposed practices in some hostels, for example over dress, where in one case it was clear residents were expected to wear slippers, both during the day and in the evening.[87] From this, Apte created a typology of halfway houses, what he called 'restrictive' and 'permissive' halfway houses. Fifteen (60 per cent) seemed broadly restrictive, and ten (40 per cent) more permissive. He wrote that the 'permissive' halfway houses had humanitarian attitudes and high expectations of responsibility from their residents, whereas the 'restrictive' halfway houses had more custodial attitudes and expected considerably less responsibility.[88]

Arguably the main question that underlay the Apte survey was that of what happened to the residents, and whether the hostels actually functioned as halfway houses. In terms of outcome, Apte thought there were three – a return to the hospital, a return to the community and remaining in the hostel after one year. More women returned to the hospital or community, whereas a higher proportion of male residents remained in the hostel as long-stay residents. Employment played a crucial role in the idea of the hostel as a stepping stone. However 46 per cent of the residents were totally unemployed while living in the hostels – 'there was little opportunity to fit the job to the resident; the emphasis was rather on expecting him to take what could be found'.[89] Moreover, 40 per cent of men, and 42 per cent of women, had no jobs at the point of moving to the community, indicating that rehabilitation was incomplete.[90] There certainly were important differences between hostels in the proportion of residents returned to the community, and one problem highlighted was that of low occupancy rates. Apte found that the more restrictive environments were associated with blocking of places with long-stay residents, while a more permissive environment was associated with the movement of residents into the community. But it was the 'change inducing' aspects of the hostel that influenced the resident to return to the community, rather than just institutional controls.[91]

Apte concluded that it was necessary to clarify the role of the halfway house and also of the mental hospital. Local authorities and hospitals needed to plan halfway houses together and with specific types of patients and services in mind. Otherwise there seemed to be a danger of building too many halfway houses. Apte concluded that 'without a clarification of purpose, the halfway house could turn into a diffuse and aimless institution, similar to the *workhouse* of former years'.[92] Similarly Titmuss himself asked in the foreword if halfway houses represented a new component of community care policy, or whether the rejection of a chronic role by the mental hospitals, aware of the need for a rapid turnover, was leading to the development of new 'chronic wards' in the community.[93]

Experiences in hostels: learning disability

A rather different, but equally interesting, question is that of what actually went on in hostels, and how they were perceived by service users. Here local case studies, drawing on oral history interviews, are particularly valuable. In her work on the history of care in the community in Norfolk, Sheena Rolph throws valuable light on care, control and community through the internal history of hostels for people with learning disabilities. These were Eaton Grange, opened as a local authority hostel for women in 1930, and Blofield Hall, opened as a hostel for men in 1951. Rolph has noted, for example, that little is known about the meaning of work in hostels for people with learning disabilities, or about the gendering of work. One of Rolph's main aims was to see both the rehabilitative and the controlling nature of hostel work, and its role in community care.[94]

Rolph suggests that at different times, and perhaps at the same time, Eaton Grange was seen as a hostel, an institution, a home, a family, an asylum, a place of control, a halfway house and a rehabilitative home. When opened in September 1930, the local Mental Deficiency Committee wrote that its policy was to develop Eaton Grange as a hostel, not as an institution, so that in Eaton Grange the girls felt that they had a real home.[95] The twin aims of care and control appeared to be one of the main themes in life at Eaton Grange. Even if the Matrons were liberal, they had to abide by the Mental Deficiency Acts that ensured that women's lives were monitored and freedoms curtailed. For example, no relationships with men were permitted. Similarly, women could have experience of work and opportunities for outings, but again these were strictly supervised. In the case of Eaton Grange, it appears that in some respects the Matrons tried to create a home rather than an institution, but that for others the hostel remained a restrictive and controlling arm of community care, and the familial discourse led to infantilism and control. The hostel filled a gap in provision between the institution and family care, but while it was a home it was also a segregated and compulsory placement. Women were able to have a role in the community, and in this respect, it is claimed that the hostel prefigured the normalization ideas that would become much more influential in the 1970s. At the same time, the tensions between care and control increased as the role of the hostel changed from a long-term home to that of a halfway house.

Rolph's work on Eaton Grange is particularly interesting in relation to employment, suggesting it always had a symbolic value for people with learning difficulties. Work provided a means to cross boundaries, a progression route through care settings, access to wider social networks, a means to gain independence, and a source of friendship, care and family life. At the same time, work could also have a darker side as an instrument of punishment, imposed redemption and atonement, exploitation and a means of control.[96] Rolph claims that from its earliest days, the staff at Eaton Grange encouraged as many women as possible to go out to work on licence, although while the women had a degree of independence, they were also supervised closely, through the licence arrangements, visits and supervision. This emphasis on training also continued after 1948, including domestic training in the 1970s. Some women had work as carers that offered a kind of passport to a normal life, but more typically, women worked in local factories as the domestic jobs tended to be phased out. Rolph suggests that work could act as a kind of progression route, where women earned their way out of the hostel through successfully negotiating work placements. In the 1970s, this was accelerated with the increasing availability of group homes, Adult Training Centres and lodgings that together offered supported accommodation. Some women were able to move out of the hostel into flats. Work could function as a form of atonement for their disability, and earn their way to a more independent life. At the same time, work was a means by which the women formed important friendships outside the hostel.[97]

It is interesting to contrast provision for women with that for men. The other hostel that Rolph examined, Blofield Hall, was opened in 1951, and was run by a Hospital Management Committee of the East Anglican RHB until 1974. Unlike Eaton Grange, it was located in the countryside, but in many other respects it seems very similar. The hostel was both a home for men going out to daily work and a stepping stone for those on their way out through long-term licence. However the theme of the hostel as offering a 'homely atmosphere' was less of a feature of Blofield Hall, perhaps because of gender differences. For similar reasons, sport seems to have had an important socializing function, providing opportunities for interaction with the community. Camping and holidays, for example, were an important aspect of life at Blofield Hall, and by the 1970s the activities included holidays abroad. This attempt to give the men greater choice and independence in their leisure activities was reflected in other changes made to the use of leisure time in the hostel. Efforts were made to transform the hostel into a more normal living environment, through the provision of sofas, television sets and radios, and the creation of a social club that included a bar.[98] This was seen as useful as it provided training in the handling of money; and in fact leisure forms tended to be seen as training mechanisms. Nevertheless, as at Eaton Grange, some of the tensions between care and control remained unresolved. Surveillance in the hostel and at work, and monitoring when men were out on licence, aimed to prevent opportunities for interaction with women. The men still tended to be treated like children, so that one of the main punishments continued to be loss of parole.

Again, as at Eaton Grange, work placements provided one of the main means for the men to build links with the community.[99] Like Eaton Grange, it was a residential home with residents that went out to daily work, or who were prepared for long-term work placements. The types of work included domestic training and gardening, and factory work was included from the 1960s. There certainly seemed to be strong demand for workers prepared to do jobs that were menial and poorly paid. Travelling to work by bicycle was an important source of independence for the men, some of whom were boarded out with local families. Overall, the work for men seemed more varied than that for the women. Here too, work seemed to offer them a kind of progression route, so that well before the 1959 Mental Health Act, men were encouraged to move out of the hostel on licence. This was further accelerated after 1971, with the Psychiatric Social Worker playing a key role. Oral interviews indicated that work was valued by residents as providing a sense of identity, pride and a wage. Nevertheless Rolph also points out that work could also function as a form of atonement, since the men did not receive full pay, and much of the work was hard and menial. While she claims that employment at Blofield Hall seemed to prefigure ideas on normalization, the economic value of labour to the local community also served to delay progress to independence. Despite campaigns against the economic exploitation of people with learning disabilities, the idea that residents owed society a debt for their disability thus remained influential.

Thus the experience of the two hostels, Eaton Grange and Blofield Hall, had many similarities in the postwar period. Rolph argues that in both cases, the hostels had the dual function of providing long-term care and a stepping stone to further independence. Community care was an adjunct to institutional care, with Rolph writing that 'hostels were a distinctive part of provision with their own ideology and role, not just small replicas of hospitals'.[100] Her claim that ideas that might be deemed 'normalization' occurred earlier than might have been expected at the two hostels seems more difficult to substantiate, given the twin aims of care and control.[101] Perhaps most importantly, the study of the Norfolk hostels shows how oral interviews with service users, and other documents including photographs from family albums, can be most usefully integrated with the 'official' history.

Conclusion

This chapter has explored the role of the hostel in the implementation of policy for mental health and learning disability, between roughly 1940 and 1974, and considered how hostels fit in with the rest of policy relating to the care and treatment of mental disorder. At the start of the period there were very few hostels; at the end there was a network. Before the Second World War, the emphasis on the colony, the opening of homes for feeble-minded girls, the certified and approved institutions and the move towards more open hostels in the 1930s all provided models for the hostel. At the same time, the influence of the colony was limited, and it is unclear how far hostels were genuine halfway houses. This chapter has considered why the hostel emerged as important in policy for care in the community, suggesting that this reflected the postwar emphasis on the family and 'homely' environments; a new concern with rehabilitation and socialization; the critique of institutionalization; and new drugs that made the management of patients possible in the hostel environment. Nevertheless there were delays in actually achieving this at the local level. Local authorities were overwhelmed by their responsibilities for mental health; they were reluctant to go into the institutional field; building hostels required getting support for new proposals and a financial commitment; and their relationships with Hospital Management Committees and RHBs were poor.

It is important to explore how the hostels actually functioned in practice. Here the evidence of both the Apte survey and the Rolph thesis show some of the problems and contradictions evident in the hostels in practice. The Apte survey illustrates how hostels for the mentally ill worked imperfectly as vehicles for rehabilitation. Wardens had little training and there was little agreement on what the aims for the hostel should be. Apte regarded fifteen of his twenty-five hostels as being broadly restrictive, and evidence on employment suggested that rehabilitation was incomplete. Rolph, on the other hand, has been more optimistic about hostels for people with learning difficulties, being keen to stress their role as stepping stones to life in the community, and regarding them as predating the normalization theories of the 1970s. While Rolph acknowledged that work could have a redemptive function, she is keen to stress its potential as a kind of progression route, both for men and women. She also shows the impact that living in a hostel actually had on service users, and this is an important corrective to the official history, with its over-reliance on documentary sources. This suggests that exploring similarities and contrasts between hostels for the mentally ill and for people with learning difficulties is one important area for further research.

But the chapter has also been concerned with the study of hostels as providing a new direction for the study of the history of mental illness and mental disability in Britain. While preliminary in scope, the approach of this chapter, and its suggestions, might usefully be extended to the other small components – Occupation Centres, Junior and Adult Training Centres, social clubs and homes – that together formed the network for care in the community. Very little is known, for example, about the role of Occupation Centres, and about the way that they were repackaged as Special Schools. Nor does recent work acknowledge the important role of the Junior and Adult Training Centres, and the way these fitted around family life. We need to know more about the relationship between the hospital and the hostel; between service users and their families; about the extent to which work functioned as a means of rehabilitation; and about how far the concept of the hostel changed from that of a longstay institution to a stepping stone to the community. Local studies are important in this respect, in illustrating the way that local factors impinged on the construction and function of these small institutions, and in exploring the experiences of service users. The volume *Outside the Walls of the Asylum*, edited by Peter Bartlett and David Wright, marks an important attempt to focus attention on the history of care in the community, and away from the history of the asylum. However in the process, the contributors tend to juxtapose the asylum against the family. Switching the focus from outside the walls of the asylum to inside the walls of the hostel thus usefully problematizes the meaning of both 'institution' and 'community'.

Acknowledgements

An earlier period of research was funded by the Wellcome Trust. I would also like to thank Sheena Rolph, Jan Walmsley and Dorothy Atkinson for their encouragement.

Notes

1 P. Bartlett and D. Wright (eds), *Outside the Walls of the Asylum: The History of Care in the Community 1750–2000*, London: Athlone Press, 1999.
2 K. Jones, *Mental Health and Social Policy, 1845–1959*, London: Routledge and Kegan Paul, 1960, p. 86; C. Webster, *The Health Services Since the War: Volume 1: Problems of Health Care: The National Health Service Before 1957*, London: HMSO, 1988, p. 340.
3 H. Freeman, 'Mental Health Services in an English County Borough Before 1974', *Medical History*, 28, 1984, pp. 111–128, p. 124.
4 P. Townsend, 'Foreword', in P. Morris, *Put Away: A Sociological Study of Institutions for the Mentally Retarded*, London: Routledge and Kegan Paul, 1969, p. xii.
5 M. Thomson, *The Problem of Mental Deficiency: Eugenics, Democracy, and Social Policy in Britain, c.1870–1959*, Oxford: Clarendon Press, 1998, pp. 144, 273.
6 Department of Health, *Caring for People: Community Care in the Next Decade and Beyond* (Cmd. 849) London: HMSO, 1989, p. 3, para. 1.1.
7 C. Gurney and R. Means, 'The Meaning of Home in Later Life', in S. Arber and M. Evandrou (eds), *Ageing, Independence and the Life Course*, London: Jessica Kingsley, 1993, pp. 119–131.
8 J. Higgins, 'Homes and Institutions', in G. Allan and G. Crow (eds), *Home and Family: Creating the Domestic Sphere*, Basingstoke: Macmillan, 1989, pp. 159–173.
9 D. Atkinson, 'Living in Residential Care', in A. Brechin, J. Walmsley, J. Katz and S. Peace (eds), *Care Matters: Concepts, Practice and Research in Health and Social Care*, London: Sage, 1998, pp. 13–26.
10 *Oxford English Dictionary*, Oxford: Oxford University Press, 1989, volume

VII, pp. 418–419; *Chambers English Dictionary*, Edinburgh: W. & R. Chambers, 1990, p. 688.

11 See for example, G. Jones, *Social Hygiene in Twentieth Century Britain*, London: Croom Helm, 1986.

12 Thomson, *The Problem of Mental Deficiency*, pp. 110–125.

13 See for example, J. Brown, 'Charles Booth and Labour Colonies', *Economic History Review*, Second Series, XXI(2), 1968, pp. 349–361; L. Bryder, *Below the Magic Mountain: A Social History of Tuberculosis in Twentieth-Century Britain*, Oxford: Clarendon Press, 1988.

14 Thomson, *The Problem of Mental Deficiency*, pp. 113–125.

15 Thomson, *The Problem of Mental Deficiency*, p. 130.

16 Thomson, *The Problem of Mental Deficiency*, p. 144.

17 Board of Education and Board of Control, *Report of the Mental Deficiency Committee*, London: HMSO, 1929, Part III, p. 26, para. 25.

18 W. Gibson, 'The Hostel Method for Feeble-Minded Young Men and Women', *Mental Welfare*, II, 1930, pp. 75–77.

19 Thomson, *The Problem of Mental Deficiency*, pp. 128–147.

20 S. Rolph, 'The History of Community Care for People with Learning Difficulties in Norfolk 1930–1980: The Role of Two Hostels' (PhD thesis, the Open University, 2000), pp. 9–10.

21 Leicestershire Record Office, Wigston, Leicester (hereafter LRO): DE 3107/168, '1908 Report', pp. 2–4.

22 O. Coburn, *Youth Hostel Story*, London: National Council of Social Service, 1950, p. 13; J. Stevenson, *British Society 1914–45*, Harmondsworth: Allen Lane, 1984, p. 393.

23 Evelyn Fox, ' Emergency Hostels for Difficult Children', *Mental Health*, 1(4), 1940, pp. 97–102; I. M. Leslie, 'Some Problems of a Hostel in a Reception Area', *Social Work*, 1(5), 1939–41, pp. 307–312; Board of Education, *Health of the School Child, 1939–45*, London: HMSO, 1947, pp. 64–70. See also R. Titmuss, *Problems of Social Policy*, London: HMSO and Longmans, 1950, pp. 378–387.

24 H. Lovejoy, 'Community Hostels', in M. Adams and H. Lovejoy (eds), *The Mentally Subnormal: Social Work Approaches*, London: Heinemann, 1960, second edn, 1972, p. 220; Thomson, *The Problem of Mental Deficiency*, p. 273.

25 R. Z. Apte, *Halfway Houses: A New Dilemma in Institutional Care*, London: G. Bell & Sons, 1968, pp. 12–13.

26 G. Crow, 'The Post-War Development of the Modern Domestic Ideal', in Allan and Crow (eds), *Home and Family: Creating the Domestic Sphere*, 1989, pp. 14–32.

27 Rolph, 'The History of Community Care', pp. 44–45, 234–235.

28 Ministry of Labour and National Service, *Report of the Committee of Inquiry on the Rehabilitation, Training, and Resettlement of Disabled Persons* (Cmd. 9883) London: HMSO, 1956, pp. ii, 1.

29 *Report of the Committee of Inquiry on the Rehabilitation, Training, and Resettlement of Disabled Persons*, pp. 29–30, paras 119–120.

30 *Report of the Committee of Inquiry on the Rehabilitation, Training, and Resettlement of Disabled Persons*, pp. 69–70, 72, paras 282, 286, 295–296.

31 *Report of the Committee of Inquiry on the Rehabilitation, Training, and Resettlement of Disabled Persons*, pp. 211–212, paras 613, 618.

32 *Royal Commission on the Law Relating to Mental Illness and Mental Deficiency 1954–1957* (Cmnd. 169) London: HMSO, 1957, pp. 17–18, paras 47–48.

33 *Royal Commission on the Law Relating to Mental Illness and Mental Deficiency 1954–1957*, pp. 217–218, paras 632–636.

34 *Royal Commission on the Law Relating to Mental Illness and Mental Deficiency 1954–1957*, pp. 212–214, paras 619–625.

35   Apte, *Halfway Houses*, p. 19.
36   Higgins, 'Homes and Institutions', p. 171.
37   P. Mittler, *The Mental Health Services*, London: Fabian Society, 1966, p. 4.
38   J. Tizard, *Community Services for the Mentally Handicapped*, London: Oxford University Press, 1964, p. 157.
39   Morris, *Put Away*, p. xxiv.
40   Morris, *Put Away*, pp. 95–97.
41   Morris, *Put Away*, p. 276.
42   Morris, *Put Away*, pp. 314–315.
43   J. Tizard and J. C. Grad, *The Mentally Handicapped and Their Families: A Social Survey*, London: Oxford University Press, 1961, p. 131. See also N. O'Connor and J. Tizard, *The Social Problem of Mental Deficiency*, London: Pergamon Press, 1956, pp. 147–161.
44   Tizard, *Community Services for the Mentally Handicapped*, p. 161.
45   Tizard, *Community Services for the Mentally Handicapped*, p. 174.
46   Tizard, *Community Services for the Mentally Handicapped*, pp. 175–176.
47   Parliamentary Papers (hereafter PP) 1961–62, XXXI, *A Hospital Plan for England and Wales* (Cmnd. 1604) London: HMSO, 1962, p. 11, para. 41.
48   PP 1962–63, XXXI, *Health and Welfare: The Development of Community Care: Plans for the Health and Welfare Services of the Local Authorities in England and Wales* (Cmnd. 1973), pp. 25–26, paras 87, 91.
49   F. J. S. Esher, 'Subnormality Hostels – Two different Functions', *Mental Health*, 24(3), 1964, pp. 124–125.
50   PP 1967–68, XXXII, *Report of the Committee on Local Authority and Allied Personal Social Services* (Cmnd. 3703), pp. 116–117.
51   *Report of the Committee on Local Authority and Allied Personal Social Services*, para. 337.
52   Department of Health and Social Services, *Better Services for the Mentally Handicapped* (Cmnd. 4683) London: HMSO, 1971, p. 35, para. 163.
53   *Better Services for the Mentally Handicapped*, p. 35, paras 161–163.
54   Lovejoy, 'Community Hostels', p. 227.
55   DHSS, *Better Services for the Mentally Ill*, pp. 37–39, paras 4.36–4.47.
56   R. M. Titmuss, 'Community Care – Fact or Fiction?' in H. Freeman and J. Farndale (eds), *Trends in the Mental Health Services: A Symposium of Original and Reprinted Papers*, Oxford: Pergamon Press, 1963, pp. 221–225.
57   See for example, S. Rolph, D. Atkinson and J. Walmsley, '"A Pair of Stout Shoes and an Umbrella": The Role of the Mental Welfare Officer in Delivering Community Care in East Anglia: 1946–1970', *British Journal of Social Work*, 33, 2003, pp. 339–359.
58   C. Unsworth, *The Politics of Mental Health Legislation*, Oxford: Clarendon Press, 1987, p. 316; Webster, *Problems of Health Care*, p. 340; C. Webster, *The Health Services Since the War: Volume II: Government and Health Care 1956–79*, London: HMSO, 1996, p. 120.
59   Ministry of Health, *Annual Report of the Ministry of Health, Part 1, 1952*, London: HMSO, 1953, pp. 92–95.
60   National Archives, Kew, London (hereafter NA) MH 134/18: W. S. Maclay to H. R. D. Porter, Deputy SAMO, Oxford RHB, 28 June 1955.
61   NA MH 134/18: J. E. Gibbon to Secretary, Ministry of Health, 17 May 1957.
62   NA MH 134/19: minute by M. M. Mason, 15 March 1962.
63   NA MH 134/19: 'Note of Meeting on 27th August, 1959 to Discuss the Provision by Local Health Authorities of Residential Accommodation for the Mentally Disordered'.
64   NA MH 134/19: 'Local Authority Hostels (Mentally Ill)', 11/4/62.
65   PP 1962–63, XXXI, *Health and Welfare*, pp. 366–367.

66 *Health and Welfare*, pp. 366–367.
67 Mittler, *The Mental Health Services*, p. 12.
68 Ministry of Health, *Annual Report of Ministry of Health, 1964* (Cmnd. 2688) London: HMSO, 1965, pp. 67–68.
69 Ministry of Health, *On the State of the Public Health, 1965*, London: HMSO, 1966, pp. 164–169.
70 DHSS, *Better Services for the Mentally Handicapped*, p. 42, table 5.
71 DHSS, *Better Services for the Mentally Ill*, p. iii.
72 DHSS, *DHSS Report for 1973*, London: HMSO, 1974, p. 56.
73 DHSS, *Health and Personal Social Services Statistics, 1975*, London: HMSO, 1976, p. 122, table 7.6.
74 A. Tyne, *'Looking at Life': In Hospitals, Hostels, Homes and 'Units' for Adults who are Mentally Handicapped*, London: Campaign for the Mentally Handicapped, 1978, pp. 6–7.
75 Leicester Health Committee, *Annual Report of the Medical Officer of Health, 1965*, Leicester: Leicester Corporation, 1966, p. 19; LRO: Health Committee minutes, 19 June 1970, p. 58.
76 E. Durkin, *Hostels for the Mentally Disordered*, London: Fabian Society, 1971, p. 3.
77 J. Mohan, *Planning, Markets and Hospitals*, London: Routledge, 2002, pp. 132–157.
78 See for example, P. Hall, 'The Development of Health Centres', in P. Hall, H. Land, R. Parker and A. Webb, *Change, Choice and Conflict in Social Policy*, London: Heinemann, 1975, pp. 277–310.
79 Apte, *Halfway Houses*, pp. 9–10.
80 Apte, *Halfway Houses*, pp. 26–27.
81 Apte, *Halfway Houses*, pp. 28–29.
82 Apte, *Halfway Houses*, p. 36.
83 Apte, *Halfway Houses*, p. 41.
84 Apte, *Halfway Houses*, pp. 42–46, 113.
85 Apte, *Halfway Houses*, p. 56.
86 Apte, *Halfway Houses*, p. 57.
87 Apte, *Halfway Houses*, pp. 65 and 69.
88 Apte, *Halfway Houses*, p. 100.
89 Apte, *Halfway Houses*, p. 118.
90 Apte, *Halfway Houses*, p. 85.
91 Apte, *Halfway Houses*, pp. 102 and 110.
92 Apte, *Halfway Houses*, p. 119.
93 R. M. Titmuss, 'Foreword', in Apte, *Halfway House*, p. 4.
94 Rolph, 'The History of Community Care', p. 47.
95 Rolph, 'The History of Community Care', p. 152, from the *Eastern Daily Press*, 22 June 1037.
96 Rolph, 'The History of Community Care', p. 184.
97 Rolph, 'The History of Community Care', p. 231.
98 Rolph, 'The History of Community Care', pp. 250–254.
99 Rolph, 'The History of Community Care', pp. 267–268.
100 Rolph, 'The History of Community Care', pp. 315–319.
101 Rolph, 'The History of Community Care',

Landmarks in the care of the mentally disordered

Selected legislation in chronological order

Lunatics Act, 1845 (8 & 9 Vic., c. 100) (An Act for the regulation of the care and treatment of lunatics)

Lunatic Asylums Act, 1845 (8 & 9 Vic., c. 126) (An Act to amend the laws for the provision and regulation of lunatic asylums for counties and boroughs and for the maintenance and care of pauper lunatics in England)

Lunacy Regulation Act, 1853 (16 & 17 Vic., c. 70)

Lunatics Care and Treatment Amendment Act, 1853 (16 & 17 Vic., c. 96)

Lunatic Asylums Amendment Act, 1853 (16 & 17 Vic., c. 97)

Lunacy Regulation Act, 1862 (25 & 26 Vic., c. 86)

Idiots Act, 1886 (49 & 50 Vic., c. 25)

Local Government Act, 1888 (51 & 52 Vic., c. 41)

Lunacy Act, 1890 (53 & 54 Vic., c. 5)

Lunacy Act, 1891 (54 & 55 Vic., c. 65) (Together the Lunacy Acts, 1890 and 1891)

Elementary Education (Defective and Epileptic Children) Act, 1899 (62 & 63 Vic., c. 32)

Mental Deficiency Act, 1913 (3 & 4 Geo. V, c. 28)

Mental Deficiency and Lunacy (Scotland) Act, 1913 (3 & 4 Geo. V, c. 38)

Elementary Education (Defective and Epileptic Children) Act, 1914 (4 & 5 Geo. V, c. 45)

Mental Deficiency (Amendment) Act, 1927 (17 & 18 Geo. V, c. 33)

Local Government Act, 1929 (19 Geo. V, c. 17)

Mental Treatment Act, 1930 (20 & 21 Geo. V, c. 23)

National Health Service Act, 1946 (9 & 10 Geo. VI, c. 81)

National Assistance Act, 1948 (11 & 12 Geo. VI, c. 29)

Mental Health Act, 1959 (7 & 8 Eliz. II, c. 72)

Mental Health Act, 1983 (31 & 32 Eliz. II, c. 20)

National Health Service and Community Care Act, 1990 (38 & 39 Eliz. II, c. 19)

Health and Social Care (Community Health and Standards) Act, 2003 (51 & 52 Eliz. II, c. 43)

Select bibliography and further reading

Adair, R., J. Melling and B. Forsythe, 'Migration, Family Structure and Pauper Lunacy in Victorian England: Admissions to Devon County Pauper Lunatic Asylum, 1845–1900', *Continuity and Change*, 12, 1997, pp. 373–401.

Andrews, J., A. Briggs, R. Porter, P. Tucker and K. Waddington, *The History of Bethlem*, London: Routledge, 1997.

Andrews, J. and A. Digby (eds), *Sex and Seclusion, Class and Custody: Perspectives on Gender and Class in the History of British and Irish Psychiatry*, Amsterdam: Rodopi, 2004.

Barham, P., *Closing the Asylum: The Mental Patient in Modern Society*, 2nd edition, London: Penguin, 1997

Bartlett, P., 'The Asylum, the Workhouse and the Voice of the Insane Poor', *International Journal of Law and Psychiatry*, 21, 1998, pp. 421–432.

Bartlett, P., 'The Asylum and the Poor Law: The Productive Alliance', in J. Melling and B. Forsythe (eds), *Insanity, Institutions and Society: A Social History of Madness in Comparative Perspective, 1800–1914*, London: Routledge, 1999, pp. 48–67.

Bartlett, P., *The Poor Law of Lunacy: the Administration of Pauper Lunatics in mid-Nineteenth Century England*, London: Leicester University Press, 1999.

Bartlett, P. and D. Wright (eds), *Outside the Walls of the Asylum: The History of Care in the Community 1750–2000*, London: Athlone Press, 1999.

Bartlett, P. and D. Wright, 'Community care and its antecedents', in P. Bartlett and D. Wright (eds), *Outside the Walls of the Asylum: The History of Care in the Community 1750–2000*, London: Athlone Press, 1999, pp. 1–18.

Berrios, G. and H. Freeman (eds), *150 Years of British Psychiatry, 1841–1991*, London: Gaskell, 1991.

Busfield, J., *Men, Women and Madness: Understanding Gender and Mental Disorder*, Basingstoke: Macmillan, 1996.

Bynum, W. F., R. Porter and M. Shepherd (eds), *The Anatomy of Madness: Essays in the History of Psychiatry*, vol. I and vol. II, London: Tavistock, 1985 and vol. III, London: Routledge, 1988.

Cherry, S., *Mental Health Care in Modern England: The Norfolk Lunatic Asylum/St Andrew's Hospital c.1810–1998*, Woodbridge: Boydell Press, 2003.

Cox, P., 'Girls, Deficiency and Delinquency', in D. Wright and A. Digby (eds), *From Idiocy to Mental Deficiency: Historical Perspectives on People with Learning Disabilities*, London: Routledge, 1996, pp. 184–206.

Digby, A., *Madness, Morality and Medicine: A Study of the York Retreat, 1796–1914*, Cambridge: Cambridge University Press, 1985.

Finlayson, G., *Citizen, State, and Social Welfare in Britain, 1830–1990*, Oxford: Clarendon Press, 1994.

Forsythe, B., J. Melling and R. Adair, 'Politics of Lunacy: Central State Regulation and the Devon Pauper Lunatic Asylum, 1845–1914', in J. Melling and B. Forsythe (eds), *Insanity, Institutions and Society, 1800–1914: A Social History of Madness in Comparative Perspective*, London: Routledge, 1999, pp. 68–92.

Freeman, H. and G. E. Berrios (eds), *150 Years of British Psychiatry. Vol. II: The Aftermath*, London: Athlone Press, 1996.

Freeman, H., 'Mental Health Services in an English County Borough Before 1974', *Medical History*, 28, 1984, pp. 111–128.

Gittins, D., *Madness in its Place: Narratives of Severalls Hospital, 1913–1997*, London: Routledge, 1998.

Gladstone, D., 'The Changing Dynamic of Institutional Care: The Western Counties Idiot Asylum, 1864–1914', in D. Wright and A. Digby (eds), *From Idiocy to Mental Deficiency: Historical perspectives on People with Learning Disabilities*, London: Routledge, 1996, pp. 134–160.

Goffman, E., *Asylums: Essays on the Social Situation of Mental Patients and other Inmates*, New York: Anchor Books, 1961.

Horden, P. and R. Smith (eds), *The Locus of Care: Families, Communities, Institutions and the Provision of Welfare since Antiquity*, London: Routledge, 1998.

Ignatieff, M., 'Total Institutions and the Working Classes', *History Workshop Journal*, 15, 1983, pp. 167–173.

Jackson, M., *The Borderland of Imbecility: Medicine, Society and the Fabrication of the Feeble Mind in Late Victorian and Edwardian England*, Manchester: Manchester University Press, 2000.

Jones, K., *Mental Health and Social Policy, 1845–1959*, London: Routledge and Kegan Paul, 1960.

Jones, K., *A History of the Mental Health Services*, London: Routledge and Kegan Paul, 1972.

Jones, K. and A. J. Fowles, *Ideas on Institutions: Analysing the Literature on Long-term Care and Custody*, London: Routledge and Kegan Paul, 1984.

Jones, K., *Asylums and after: A Revised History of the Mental Health Services from the Early 18th Century to the 1990s*, London: Athlone Press, 1993.

Lees, L. H., *The Solidarities of Strangers: The English Poor Laws and the People, 1700–1948*, Cambridge: Cambridge University Press, 1998.

MacKenzie, C., *Psychiatry for the Rich: A History of Ticehurst Private Asylum, 1792–1917*, London: Routledge, 1992.

Melling, J., 'Accommodating Madness: New Research in the Social History of Insanity and Institutions', in J. Melling and B. Forsythe (eds), *Insanity, Institutions and Society, 1800–1914: A Social History of Madness in Comparative Perspective*, London, Routledge, 1999, pp. 1–30.

Melling, J. and B. Forsythe (eds), *Insanity, Institutions and Society, 1800–1914: A Social History of Madness in Comparative Perspective*, London: Routledge, 1999.

Melling, J., B. Forsythe and R. Adair, 'Families, Communities and the Legal Regulation of Lunacy in Victorian England: Assessments of Crime, Violence and Welfare in Admissions to the Devon Asylum, 1845–1914', in P. Bartlett and D.

Wright (eds), *Outside the Walls of the Asylum: The History of Care in the Community 1750–2000*, London: Athlone Press, 1999, pp. 153–180.

Morris, P., *Put Away: A Sociological Study of Institutions for the Mentally Retarded*, London: Routledge and Kegan Paul, 1969.

Murphy, E., 'The Lunacy Commissioners and the East London Guardians, 1845–1867', *Medical History*, 46, 2002, pp. 495–524.

Porter, R., 'The patient's View: Doing Medical History from Below', *Theory and Society*, XIV, 1985, pp. 175–198.

Porter, R., *Mind-forg'd Manacles, a History of Madness in England from the Restoration to the Regency*, London: Athlone Press, 1987.

Porter, R., *A Social History of Madness: Stories of the Insane*, London: Weidenfeld and Nicolson, 1987.

Porter, R., *Madness: A Brief History*, Oxford: Oxford University Press, 2002.

Porter, R., (ed.), *Patients and Practitioners: Lay Perceptions of Medicine in Pre-industrial Society*, Cambridge: Cambridge University Press, 1985.

Porter, R. and D. Wright, *The Confinement of the Insane: International Perspectives, 1800–1965*, Cambridge: Cambridge University Press, 2003.

Scull, A. T., *Museums of Madness: The Social Organization of Insanity in Nineteenth-Century England*, London: Allen Lane, 1979.

Scull, A., *The Most Solitary of Afflictions: Madness and Society in Britain, 1700–1900*, New Haven, CT: Yale University Press, 1993.

Showalter, E., *The Female Malady: Women, Madness and English Culture, 1830–1980*, London: Virago, 1987.

Smith, L. D., *Cure, Comfort and Safe Custody: Public Lunatic Asylums in Early Nineteenth-Century England*, London: Leicester University Press, 1999.

Sturdy, H. and W. Parry-Jones, 'Boarding-out Insane Patients: the Significance of the Scottish System 1857–1913', in P. Bartlett and D. Wright (eds), *Outside the Walls of the Asylum: The History of Care in the Community 1750–2000*, London: Athlone Press, 1999, pp. 86–114.

Suzuki, A., 'The Household and the Care of Lunatics in Eighteenth-century London', in P. Horden and R. Smith (eds), *The Locus of Care: Families, Communities, Institutions and the Provision of Welfare since Antiquity*, London: Routledge, 1998, pp. 153–175.

Suzuki, A., 'Enclosing and Disclosing Lunatics within the Family Walls: Domestic Psychiatric Regime and the Public Sphere in Early Nineteenth-century England', in P. Bartlett and D. Wright (eds), *Outside the Walls of the Asylum: The History of Care in the Community 1750–2000*, London: Athlone Press, 1999, pp. 115–131.

Thomson, M., 'Community Care and the Control of Mental Defectives in Inter-war Britain', in P. Horden and R. Smith (eds), *The Locus of Care: Families, Communities, Institutions and the Provision of Welfare since Antiquity*, London: Routledge, 1998, pp. 198–216.

Thomson, M., *The Problem of Mental Deficiency: Eugenics, Democracy, and Social Policy in Britain, c. 1870–1959*, Oxford: Clarendon Press, 1998.

Ussher, J. M., *Women's Madness: Misogyny or Mental Illness?*, London: Harvester Wheatsheaf, 1991.

Walton, J., 'Casting Out and Bringing Back in Victorian England: Pauper Lunatics 1840–70', in W. F. Bynum, R. Porter and M. Shepherd (eds), *The Anatomy of Madness: Essays in the History of Psychiatry*, vol. II, London: Tavistock, 1985, pp. 132–146.

Webster, C., *The Health Services Since the War: Volume 1: Problems of Health Care: The National Health Service Before 1957*, London: HMSO, 1988.

Wright, D., 'Getting Out of the Asylum: Understanding the Confinement of the Insane in the Nineteenth Century', *Social History of Medicine*, 10, 1997, pp. 137–155.

Wright, D., 'The Discharge of Pauper Lunatics from County Asylums in mid-Victorian England: the Case of Buckinghamshire, 1853–1872', in J. Melling and B. Forsythe (eds), *Insanity, Institutions and Society, 1800–1914: A Social History of Madness in Comparative Perspective*, London: Routledge, 1999, pp. 93–112.

Wright, D., *Mental Disability in Victorian England: The Earlswood Asylum 1847–1901*, Oxford: Clarendon Press, 2001.

Wright, D. and A. Digby (eds), *From Idiocy to Mental Deficiency: Historical Perspectives on People with Learning Disabilities*, London: Routledge, 1996.

Index

Printed in Australia
Ingram Content Group Australia Pty Ltd
AUHW011933201124
403088AU00004B/94